Rehabilitation of the Severely Brain-Injured Adult

A practical approach

Second Edition

Edited by
Gordon Muir Giles and Jo Clark-Wilson

Consultant Editor
Jo Campling

Stanley Thornes (Publishers) Ltd

First edition published in 1988 by Croom Helm

Second edition published in 1999 by:
Stanley Thornes (Publishers) Ltd
Ellenborough House
Wellington Street
Cheltenham
Glos.
GL50 1YW
United Kingdom

99 00 01 02 03 / 10 9 8 7 6 5 4 3 2 1

A catalogue record for this book is available from the British Library

ISBN 0 7487 3352 3

Typeset by Gray Publishing, Tunbridge Wells, Kent
Printed and bound in Great Britain by T.J. International Ltd, Padstow, Cornwall

Rehabilitation of the Severely Brain-Injured Adult

CONTENTS

Contributors   xi

Preface   *Gordon Muir Giles, Jo Clark-Wilson*   xiii

Acknowledgements   xvii

1   Brain-injury rehabilitation: from theory to practice   1
Gordon Muir Giles
Severity of brain injury   2
Family and social consequences of brain injury   7
Theories of recovery after brain injury   8
Restitution   9
Substitution   10
Is rehabilitation effective?   12
Cognitive rehabilitation models   16
Models of therapy   18
A functional behavioural-learning approach to brain-injury
    rehabilitation   21
Conclusion   25
Summary   26

2   Medical considerations in brain-injury rehabilitation   27
Martyn J. Rose
Introduction   27
Mechanisms of injury   29
What goes wrong?   30
Natural history of recovery   31
Mechanisms of recovery   33
Organization of services   33
General principles of management   34
Medical assessment   35
Conclusion   38

3 **The pharmacotherapeutic management of behavioural and emotional disturbances following brain injury** *Tom W. Freeman* **39**
Behavioural syndromes 41
Strategies for intervention 46

4 **The practice of behavioural treatment in the acute rehabilitation setting** *James C. Wilson, William Dailey* **54**
Acute rehabilitation 55
Initial assessment and philosophy 55
Specialized management of behaviours related to medical
  complications 57
Cognitive impairments 59
Types of problem 61
Behaviour-management approaches 67
Interventions 69
Conclusion 79

5 **Management of behavioural disregulation and non-compliance in the post-acute severely brain-injured adult** *Gordon Muir Giles* **81**
Types of behaviour disorder 81
Basic principles of learning theory 84
Behavioural interventions 85
Applications of learning principles to behavioural change 88
Summary 96

6 **Functional skills training following severe brain injury** *Gordon Muir Giles, Jo Clark-Wilson* **97**
Assessment 99
Retraining methods 100
Antecedent control 101
Engaging the patient in therapeutic activities 102
Elimination of unwanted behaviours 104
Skill building 106
Assessment and training in specific areas 110
Outcome studies 134

7 **Motor learning following brain injury**   135
   Mary Beth Badke, Gordon Muir Giles, Jill Kerry
   Motor control   135
   Components of a motor control model and related dysfunctions   136
   Assessment   141
   Motor learning principles   145
   Factors affecting performance and learning   146

8 **Rehabilitation of physical deficits in the post-acute brain-injured adult: four case studies** *Jennifer Hooper-Roe* 153
   Introduction   153
   Case studies   155
   Conclusion   163

9 **Treating cognitive/language and oral motor dysfunction in the brain-injured adult** *Ann L. Dill, Gordon Muir Giles* 164
   Evaluation of the minimally responsive patient   165
   Coma   166
   Formal rating and assessment systems   167
   Acute evaluation and treatment   170
   Treatment principles and methods   178
   Conclusion   183

10 **Lack of insight following severe brain injury**   184
   Gordon Muir Giles
   Definition of terms   186
   The nature of self-awareness   188
   Dynamic theories of denial   190
   Metacognition   191
   Cognitive behavioural models of self-awareness   191
   Stress and coping   192
   Denial in neurological illness   193
   The neuropsychological account of lack of insight   198
   The psychological account of lack of insight   202
   Assessment   206
   Treatment   207
   Summary and conclusions   209

11 **Vocation and occupation** *Jo Clark-Wilson* **211**
Factors influencing work entry or re-entry after brain injury 211
Approaches to facilitate work entry 216
Occupational activities and leisure time 227
Conclusion 228

12 **Problems in implementing an integrated programme
for brain-injury rehabilitation** *Gordon Muir Giles, Ian Fussey* **229**
The rehabilitation team 229
The problem of role definition 230
Functional behaviour management: a user's guide 232
Functional assessment 233
Specific techniques in functional behaviour management 234
Why behavioural management may fail 238
A note on working with the families of brain-injured people 239
Conclusion 240

13 **The social and emotional consequences of
severe brain injury: a social work perspective** **241**
Mary Roberts Lees
Introduction 241
Family needs in the acute stage of recovery 241
The social work role 246
Counselling 248
The experience of readjustment – some family profiles 251
The family and the rehabilitation team 257
The social worker and the rehabilitation team 258
Planning for future needs 259
Conclusion 261

14 **Community reintegration after brain injury** **263**
Catherine Johnson
Background 263
What is community reintegration? 264
Community reintegration – how to do it? 265
Conclusions 271

15 **Future directions in brain-injury rehabilitation**   272

  Gordon Muir Giles

  Introduction   272
  Developments in rehabilitation   274
  The structure of service provision   277

References   280

Index   310

Contributors

Mary Beth Badke
Director of Outpatient Rehabilitation Services, UW Health, University of Wisconsin Hospital and Clinics, 600 Highland Avenue, Madison, Wisconsin 53792, USA.

Jo Clark-Wilson
Occupational Therapist and Brain Injury Case Manager, Director of Head First, Northgrove Road, Hawkhurst, Cranbrook, Kent TN18 4AN, UK.

William Dailey
Behavior Specialist, Garfield Neurobehavioral Center, 1451 28th Avenue, Oakland, California 94601, USA.

Ann L. Dill
Regional Therapy Director, Guardian Health Group, 5725 Paradise Drive Suite 900, Corta Madera, California 94925, USA.

Tom W. Freeman
University of Arkansas for Medical Sciences, John L McClellan Memorial Veterans Hospital, 2200 Fort Roots Dr, North Little Rock, Arkansas 72114-1706, USA.

Ian Fussey
Consultant Psychologist, BUPA Hospital, Gartree Road, Leicester LE2 2FF, UK.

Gordon Muir Giles
Director of Neurobehavioral Programs, Guardian Health Group, 5725 Paradise Drive Suite 900, Corta Madera, California 94925, USA, and Assistant Professor of Occupational Therapy, Samuel Merritt College, 370 Hawthorne Avenue, Oakland, California 94609, USA.

Jennifer Hooper-Roe
Senior Physiotherapist, St Andrew's Hospital, Northampton NN1 5DG, UK.

Catherine Johnson
Brain Injury Case Manager and Director of Rehab Without Walls, 27 Presley Way, Crownhill, Milton Keynes, Bucks MK8 0ES, UK.

Jill Kerry
Physical Therapist, Guardian Health Group, 5725 Paradise Drive Suite 900, Corta Madera, California 94925, USA.

Mary Roberts Lees
Social Work Team Manager, St Andrew's Hospital, Northampton NN1 5DG, UK.

Martyn J. Rose
Consultant in Neuropsychiatric Rehabilitation, Formerly Clinical Director of the Brain Injury Rehabilitation Division of St Andrew's Hospital, Northampton, UK. Northampton General Hospital, Cliftonville, Northampton NN1 5BD, UK.

James C. Wilson
Neuropsychologist and Clinical Director, Garfield Neurobehavioral Center, 1451 28th Avenue, Oakland, California 94601, USA.

PREFACE

Since the publication of the first edition of *Rehabilitation of the Severely Brain-Injured Adult: A practical approach* the field of brain-injury treatment has seen rapid change. There has been a growing research interest in traumatic brain injury with a concomitant increase in knowledge. The study of risk factors has demonstrated that there are groups of individuals who are at special risk for brain trauma and that some individuals (such as those with a history of alcohol or drug abuse) may be especially susceptible to its effects. Researchers concerned with the acutely traumatized patient have explained in detail the types of neuronal damage which may occur following various types of trauma (mechanical, anoxic), and there has been considerable interest in attempts to interrupt or reverse the neurochemical events which follow the original trauma. It has been recognized that even very severely injured individuals can achieve remarkably good outcomes (Whitlock, 1992).

New psychological models of brain functioning are influencing how we think about the problems of brain-injured people. For example parallel distributed processing theories, used to model learning systems, are leading to re-evaluations of much of cognitive psychology.

The first edition of this book was the earliest attempt to present a functionally oriented interdisciplinary model of brain-injury rehabilitation based on learning theory. Since that time behaviourism has gone from being a pariah amongst intervention models to a recognized subspecialty in brain-injury rehabilitation. There has been progress in our understanding of how to apply behavioural methodology to the brain-injured population. Our early behaviourism was not very sophisticated, there was little consideration given to the constraints imposed by the brain-injury itself and operant conditioning was the predominant intervention (Wood, 1987; Giles and Fussey, 1988). There is increasing sophistication in the application of behavioural theory to patient treatment. Interventions developed for other client populations have been adapted for use with the brain injured and cognitive behavioural approaches have been developed to help patients use their retained cognitive abilities to develop more adaptive behaviours. The first edition of this book also represented the first serious attempt to advocate for a functional skills retraining model after brain injury. At the time there was considerable excitement about computer-based cognitive retraining and the use of memory retraining and other cognitive rehabilitation models (Gianutsos, 1980; Wilson and Moffat, 1984). Advocates of behavioural and functional skills retraining approaches were regarded as on the margins of accepted rehabilitation practice. Over the last 10 years the array of techniques used in functional skills training has increased as has the research supporting the effectiveness of the approach (Mills *et al.*, 1992; Giles and Clark-Wilson, 1993; Giles, 1998).

There has been increasing recognition of the importance of an informed pharmacological approach in the rehabilitation and management of the severely brain-injured adult (see Chapter 3). Unfortunately our understanding of the neuro-chemical changes which may follow brain damage remains meagre. The uniqueness of each patient's difficulties means that only an empirical approach (informed by a knowledge of the relationships between neurotransmitter systems and behavioural and affective syndromes) is likely to be fully effective with these patients. This is an area likely to enjoy much further development.

Currently the pattern of service provision to the brain-injured population is changing. It is important to keep in mind what we have learned during this period of rapid development (Giles, 1994a, b). Acute medical management has advanced and there are more brain-injured individuals surviving. Most rehabilitation workers are convinced of the importance of energetic management in the acute recovery period. In the USA the status of acute rehabilitation has suffered in part from economic factors but also due to an inability to carry out randomized controlled trials. Despite the lack of strong evidence of a positive treatment effect we do know that the effects of not intervening are disastrous both for the patient and the family.

As pointed out by Tom Freeman an educated pharmacological intervention can prepare the patient for retraining but it cannot teach a patient to perform functional tasks (Chapter 3). There has been some increased interest in how to train specific functional skills. Both our own work (Giles and Clark Wilson, 1988a, b; Giles and Shore, 1989a, b; Giles et al., 1997) and that of others (Katzman and Mix, 1994; Pulaski and Emmett, 1994) have demonstrated that patients can be trained to perform specific functional skills of real practical importance to themselves and their caregivers. At the time of the first edition of this book functional behavioural rehabilitation was regarded as something that you did when your other rehabilitative interventions had failed. The predominant model was one of cognitive retraining. Outcome studies were few and far between. Current evidence shows that functional behavioural retraining may produce a significant change in patient's functional behaviours. Piecemeal behavioural engineering may not return the patient to their previous level of functioning but it can make the difference between living in an institution and living in the community. Interestingly even when cognitive change is the target of intervention it is functional behaviours that improve (Giles, 1998). In the post-acute phase of treatment we know that services should be functionally, behaviourally and socially oriented. Specific task training, behaviourally oriented social skills retraining and behavioural control retraining, when carefully selected and obsessively applied, can affect meaningful aspects of real world functioning.

Despite the increased number of books on the treatment of individuals with traumatic brain injury many of these remain descriptive and focus on evaluation rather than treatment. From reading most books on brain-injury rehabilitation one would get the impression that everybody gets better and goes home to resume productive and meaningful lives. Sadly the reality for many patients is quite different. Again in this second edition we focus on practical treatment approaches for the severely injured.

Many brain-injured individuals are underserved (Giles, 1994a, b, 1998). In the USA treatment is often grossly inadequate for the uninsured or under-insured. The long-term situation of the brain-injured patient is often far worse than it is acutely. The problems of the severely impaired brain-injured adult do not go away and in some cases become worse through time. This constitutes an immense human cost for the patient and their carers – often the patient's family. For those living in the community the situation is often bleak. Pre-established social networks often disintegrate as friends distance themselves from an individual whom they no longer fully recognize. In addition the brain-injured person is often unable to gain or maintain access to community service organizations because of problems in initiation, interpersonal skills, insight, or psychiatric or behavioural impairment. Patients often become increasingly socially isolated and desperate. New models of care and greater resources are required for long-term care services.

A NOTE ON TERMINOLOGY AND PURPOSE

In research it is important to limit variables so that inferences can be made with certainty. This has lead some authors to limit their writings to specific populations such as closed brain injury and to eliminate from their studies patients who have associated problems (such as multiple brain injury or a pre-morbid psychiatric history) that could complicate treatment. In this book, since we are more interested in the effects of brain injury and its treatment than its cause, a wider definition is adopted. This has the disadvantage of imprecision but the advantage of being more like the real world as experienced by most therapists. For example in a substantial minority of patients traumatic brain injury occurs against a background of other factors which affect neurological status (in a series of patients treated in a community-based transitional living programme 40% had factors which complicated the injury (Giles and Clark-Wilson, 1993)). These factors included depriving and abusive childhood environments, learning deficits, previous brain injury, alcohol and drug abuse, psychiatric disturbance and mental retardation. Here the discussion includes patients whose history is positive for significant or repeated brain injury where brain injury includes:

1 trauma – open or closed, focal or diffuse
2 anoxia, ischaemia or hypoglycaemia
3 infections such as herpes simplex encephalitis
4 vascular damage such as aneurysms, AV malformation surgery
5 other space occupying lesions such as non-progressive tumours.

All of which may occur against a background of multiple risk factors. Different symptom complexes are associated with different pathologies (for example patients with marked anoxia tend to have very severe memory disorders due to the susceptibility of the hippocampus to anoxia). The central principles of intervention remain similar but are applied differently due to the different symptom complexes and natural histories of the disorders. Evidence from post-acute rehabilitation suggests that there is remarkable uniformity in response to learning-based approaches across diagnostic category (Cope *et al.*, 1991a, b). The central focus of this book is traumatic brain injury. Discussion in this book is limited to adults due to the complexity of the issues involved in the interaction of development and damage. Work conducted with a mature nervous system is easier to evaluate.

Once again both the editorship of this book and its chapters represents a transatlantic collaboration. We believe that the chapters travel well but some of them are influenced by local practice. The editors hope that the reader will be stimulated by seeing how problems are approached on the other side of the Atlantic. Although not intended to be a training text this book does attempt to present a coherent, interdisciplinary and practical approach to the rehabilitation of the severely injured. From this book the reader should gain the understanding that:

1 a balanced functional behavioural/cognitive behavioural approach should include; a medical/pharmacological element and a culture/environment which maximizes the patient's chances for learning
2 a consistent functional behavioural/cognitive behavioural approach can help patients maximize their functional ability despite relatively fixed cognitive deficits
3 behavioural disorders need not stand in the way of functional skills training
4 a functional behavioural/cognitive behavioural approach can provide a model for interdisciplinary practice.

A note of caution: any intervention powerful enough to produce change in a patient is powerful enough to do harm. We strongly recommend that the interventions described in this book be used only by clinicians experienced in rehabilitation of persons with traumatic brain injury or under the supervision of such a person.

Gordon Muir Giles
San Francisco, California, USA

Jo Clark-Wilson
Hawkhurst, Kent, UK

Acknowledgements

We wish to thank those who have guided our thinking and helped us in the preparation of this book. Special acknowledgement is due to Peter Eames and Rodger Wood who led the Kemsley unit in the early days of developing a new approach to brain-injury rehabilitation. Ian Fussey, co-editor of the first edition contributed a chapter to this edition and his common-sense approach to patient treatment remains influential. As editors we of course wish to thank our contributors, particularly Jim Wilson and Bill Dailey, who read chapters not their own. Thanks to David Manchester for many helpful discussions particularly regarding the content of Chapter 10 and to J.D. Mohr who assisted with Chapter 12. Thanks are also due to Keith Hart for preparation of the graphics, to Austin Thompson for research assistance and to the Library staff at Samuel Merritt College and to all the staff at Head First. Any errors of fact or interpretation remain the responsibility of the authors.

Gordon Muir Giles
San Francisco, California, USA

Jo Clark-Wilson
Hawkhurst, Kent, UK

1 BRAIN-INJURY REHABILITATION: FROM THEORY TO PRACTICE

Gordon Muir Giles

Cognitive, physical, and psychiatric disorder are common consequences of brain injury affecting functional abilities and restricting role participation. Although there has been considerable progress in the past 10 years the services available to persons with brain injury are frequently inadequate. Only a minority of individuals receive specialized services (Dombovy and Olek, 1996). For those patients with continuing needs, specialized long-term settings exist but are often difficult to access with the limited financial resources available. The type of services a patient actually receives is often determined more by financial resources than need.

In addition to limited financial resources the field of brain-injury rehabilitation is hampered by a number of practical and theoretical problems. Many fundamental questions central to the practices of this new rehabilitation subspecialty remain unresolved (Chestnut *et al.*, 1999). Despite major improvements in neurosurgical management, the mechanisms which underlie recovery following brain injury are largely unknown. Truly adequate demonstrations of the efficacy of acute rehabilitation are lacking. No prospective randomized control trials have been performed and because of ethical concerns these are unlikely to be carried out. As a result evaluative surveys of the field typically conclude that the case for brain-injury rehabilitation is unproved (Chestnut *et al.*, 1999; Giles and McMillan, in press). As a result of this lack of knowledge there is no shared philosophy for rehabilitation. Therapists must choose between a number of competing models, all with different implications for therapy. Controversy continues as to what constitutes adequate and appropriate treatment: Should treatment be applied early or late? Can prognosis be determined and how? Is therapy effective and how long should it be continued? Advocacy efforts are hampered by the limited nature of the scientific evidence supporting rehabilitative intervention. As a result patients usually undergo fragmented approaches to rehabilitation.

Having acknowledged the early stage in the development of the field and the limited state of knowledge the authors are unabashed advocates of a particular approach to rehabilitation. The model presented in this book is that of functionally oriented learning-based treatment. Emphasis is placed on cognitive behavioural interventions and on the importance of contextual factors in assessment and the development of treatment programmes. This model has a number of advantages. It is a well-established and widely used methodology fostering research and a problem-solving approach to maladaptive behaviours. Case methodologies in behaviour therapy offer paradigms for evaluation and treatment, as well as a model for rehabilitation and a uniform approach between staff. Although overall the evidence is limited, the best evidence for the effectiveness of treatment comes from those practising in a behavioural tradition. Single case and small series designs have yielded robust evidence for the effectiveness of learning-based approaches.

Interventions have demonstrated positive effects on the targeted behaviours or skills of even profoundly impaired individuals. The literature regarding functional and behavioural interventions with brain-injured individuals is extensive and expanding rapidly.

The first edition of this book (Fussey and Giles, 1988) was the earliest attempt to provide an integrated multidisciplinary model of rehabilitation for brain-injured people based on learning theory. Interventions based on learning theory have since been recognized as central to rehabilitative efforts with this population. Functional and behavioural methods have multiplied and become far more sophisticated. Intervention strategies have been influenced by theories in cognitive neuroscience and cognitive behaviour therapy. Environmental factors are recognized as being crucial in both understanding and influencing behaviour. A functional behavioural perspective offers a coherent, scientific, multidisciplinary approach to evaluation and treatment of the brain-injured adult.

SEVERITY OF BRAIN INJURY

Severity of brain injury refers to the amount of damage the brain has incurred through trauma. Severity is usually inferred from the extent and duration of altera-tions in responsiveness. It should be recognized, however, that this type of assess-ment does not take into account focal injury where a small area of damage can have significant effects on function. Diffuse and focal damage can occur together obscuring the importance of the focal damage. Severity of injury must also be distinguished from severity of outcome (Giles and Fussey, 1988). For example, cumulative minor trauma, or minor trauma in susceptible individuals, can have severe consequences (Williams et al., 1990). A number of scales have been devel-oped to assess the status of the acutely brain-injured patient which can be useful in charting recovery and in the early detection of complications (Teasdale and Jennett, 1974; Ansell et al., 1989). Other scales look at outcome (Livingston and Livingstone, 1985; Levin et al., 1987) and there have been frequent attempts made to relate the two (Jennett et al., 1981; Rappaport et al., 1982; Hall et al., 1985). Outcome assessment is however fraught with difficulties (Giles, 1994a; Giles and McMillan, in press). A number of groups (Clifton et al., 1992; Hannay et al., 1996) have made recommendations about measures to use in assessing outcome after brain injury. The principle functional measures are reviewed below.

Methods used to assess the severity of brain injury in the acute stages have devel-oped rapidly over the past 20 years. A number of scales have been used extensively; the best-known of which is the Glasgow Coma Scale (Teasdale and Jennett, 1974). In the very acute stages where the issues involved are essentially binary – on one hand death or a persisting vegetative state, and on the other hand, survival – there are some fairly robust indicators such as impaired pupillary reaction, impaired eye movements (oculocephalic reflex), abnormal motor responses, increased intra-cranial pressure and paradoxical arousal (Becker et al., 1977). The type of intracranial lesion also has implications for outcome (Seelig et al., 1981; Gennarelli et al., 1982).

Even here, however, where predictive power is strongest there are individual exceptions. Even prolonged persistent vegetative state (PVS) may in some cases resolve with considerable recovery of function (Jennett and Teasdale, 1981; Arts *et al.*, 1985; Berrol, 1986). There remains no absolute measure of severity of brain injury, and views vary as to how it should be defined. Glasgow Coma Scale (GCS) score, duration of coma and length of post-traumatic amnesia (PTA) are the most accepted criteria (Jennett and Teasdale, 1981). Severe brain injury has been defined as leading to a GCS score of 3–8, coma in excess of 1 h or of 6 h, or to PTA in excess of 24 h (Russell and Smith, 1961; Jennett and Teasdale, 1981). Mild and moderate head injury are variously defined. Duration of coma and length of PTA are correlated, and are both good indicators of severity of brain trauma. However, the two criteria may produce different indicators of severity with PTA being more sensitive (but for obvious reasons not available until later in the recovery process). Children and adolescents have long been thought to have better outcomes than adults with similar injuries (Jennett *et al.*, 1977; Berger *et al.*, 1985). However, this view has been increasingly challenged. Although mortality rates are lower in children than in adults (Luerssen *et al.*, 1988) an increasing amount of evidence from long-term follow-up has shown that significant deficits continue to be evident in individuals injured in childhood. It has been suggested that injury during crucial developmental periods may be more harmful than injury when maturation is complete (Webb *et al.*, 1996). Recent long-term follow-up studies of severely brain-injured children suggest that they do make significant functional improvement but have continuing problems in social and occupational functioning that are comparable to the long-term difficulties that are now recognized as the most debilitating in the adult brain-injured population (Andrews *et al.*, 1988; Cattelani *et al.*, 1998). Similarly it has long been thought that the earlier the injury in adulthood the better the outcome (Teuber, 1975). Individuals injured later in life have been found to have worse outcomes than younger individuals despite apparent comparability of injury (Vollmer *et al.*, 1991). It has however been unclear whether comparable injuries cause more damage in an older brain or whether the poorer outcome is a result of interaction of ageing-related complications (dementia, alcoholism, cerebrovascular disease) and age-related cognitive changes. Johnson *et al.* (1998) evaluated the effects of normal ageing on individuals with traumatic brain injury using age-based normative data to calculate indices of relative decline from pre-morbid levels (expressed as z-deficit scores). The results suggested that the greater neuropsychological impairment noted in older individuals is related to normal ageing, although the data did suggest that increasing age is associated with relatively less impairment in intelligence. The findings were however limited to a comparison of 20–39- and 40–59-year-olds and were not controlled for severity, therefore further more adequately controlled work is necessary before firm conclusions can be drawn (Johnson *et al.*, 1998). However, current findings do suggest that rehabilitation protocols may need to be adjusted to meet the special needs of older people by, for example, extending the duration of treatment and increasing expectations for long-term support. Recently it has been suggested that females may have better outcomes than males with comparable injuries, possibly due to the protective effects of progesterone (Groswasser et al., 1998). Genetic factors may also play a role in differential responses to brain injury. Specifically, presence of apolipoprotein E4, known to be associated with Alzheimer's disease, poor outcome following cardiac surgery (Newman et al., 1995) and dementia pugilistica (Jordan et al., 1997), is associated with poor outcome from traumatic brain injury (Teasdale et al., 1997).

Jennett and Teasdale (1981) have related PTA to outcome at 6 months using the Glasgow Outcome Scale (GOS) (Jennett and Bond, 1975). Although there is a clear trend in the group data, indicating that the longer the PTA the worse the likely outcome, the trend is far too weak to make firm predictions in any *individual* case. Only by using few (and therefore gross) outcome categories can a reasonable level of predictive power be maintained. Although one of the aims of producing an outcome measure such as the GOS is to assess comparative effectiveness of treatment methods (Evans et al., 1981; Hall et al., 1985), it is difficult to accept that a measure as imprecise as the GOS could be used for prediction. Recognition of the limitations of the GOS have led to the attempt to produce more sensitive measures (Hall et al., 1985).

The Glasgow Assessment Schedule (GAS) presents a comprehensive rating which includes the assessment of physical, psychological, social, personality and activities of daily living (ADL) deficits (Livingston and Livingston, 1985) and could be used to note trends in recovery and responses to interventions.

The Disability Rating Scale (DRS) of Rappaport and co-workers (1982) charts the recovery of the severely brain-injured person from coma to the redevelopment of community-living skills. The DRS consists of four categories. The first category measures arousal and responsivity and is adapted from the GCS. The second category rates cognitive ability for self-care (feeding, toileting and grooming) and relates to the patient's knowledge of how and when to perform self-care tasks. Ability is rated as complete, partial or minimal. The third category is level of functioning and is modified from the scale developed by Scranton et al. (1970). The patient is rated as completely independent, independent in a special (modified) environment and mildly, moderately, markedly and totally dependent. The fourth category is degree of independent employability the individual is likely to have on the job market. Major advantages of the DRS are brevity (5–15 min to administer) and the ability to track an individual's entire course of recovery. Reliability and validity of the DRS are excellent (Rappaport et al., 1982; Hall et al., 1993). The principle disadvantages of the DRS is that it is relatively insensitive and fails to capture the types of meaningful changes which can occur in post-acute rehabilitation.

The Functional Independence Measure (FIM), provides a standardized method of documenting patient disability and a measurement tool for programme outcome assessment (Uniform Data Set for Medical Rehabilitation, 1993). The FIM measures six specific functional categories; (1) self-care, (2) sphincter control, (3) mobility, (4) locomotion, (5) communication and (6) social cognition. The six categories are then divided into 18 subcategories. The level of assistance needed for the patient to perform the activities outlined in the subcategories is measured on a seven-point scale ranging from 1 to 7 (1 = total assistance and 7 = complete independence, no helper or device). The FIM is both reliable and valid (Dodds et al., 1993; Heinemann et al., 1994). The FIM has been evaluated as a measure of recovery from traumatic brain injury and has been found to be reliable and valid with greater precision than the DRS (Hall et al., 1993). The failure of the FIM to capture meaningful changes at the higher levels of functioning led to the development of the Functional Assessment Measure (FAM). The FAM was developed to use in conjunction with the FIM with individuals who are post-brain injury. The FAM consists of 12 items which address community skills and cognitive functioning. Reliability of the FIM+FAM is adequate (Hall et al., 1993) with higher agreement for ratings of physical activities than for cognitive, communication and behavioural items (McPherson et al., 1996).

The Community Integration Questionnaire (CIQ) attempts to measure outcome from the injured individual's perspective on the fulfilment of social roles. Using the nomenclature of the World Health Organization the CIQ attempts to measure participation (handicap). Community integration is defined as occurring in three domains: integration into a home-like setting, integration into a social network, and integration into productive activities such as competitive or volunteer employment or schooling (Willer et al., 1993). The CIQ has good test–retest reliability and internal consistency (Willer et al., 1993). However, the CIQ is a pure measure of outcome in terms of community integration and does not measure integration skills such as social skills.

An issue related to the measurement of outcome is the duration of the recovery processes. Until recently it was widely believed that significant recovery of function occurs exclusively in the first 6–12 months following injury. This view has been supported by a series of studies by Jennett's group in Glasgow (Jennett and Teasdale, 1981) but can now be contrasted with a number of studies demonstrating continued improvement beyond this period (Mackworth et al., 1982; Cope, 1995). Long-term improvement has been shown to occur irrespective of treatment methods (Levin et al., 1979; Hall et al., 1985). In treatment, effects have been demonstrated well beyond the period of spontaneous recovery (Prigatano et al., 1984; Eames and Wood, 1985a; Harrick et al., 1994; Eames et al., 1995). To some extent these differences in findings may reflect the insensitivity of the assessment instruments (Hall et al., 1985) and the choice of assessment domain. Results of neuropsychological testing may stabilize earlier than measures of community-living skills. Considerable evidence suggests that following the period of rapid spontaneous improvement, energetic therapeutic intervention can play a vital role in helping patients achieve better social adjustment and in developing appropriate adaptation to disability despite relatively fixed neuropsychological deficits. Much of the improvement seems to be occurring in learning-based functional behaviours which are not the focus of the instruments being used to assess recovery.

The course and extent of recovery from brain injury is variable. Someone with a severe brain injury may achieve an apparently full recovery, while an individual with a 'mild' brain injury may show continuing problems for years following the injury. Mild brain injuries are usually defined as injuries with loss of consciousness for less than 20 min or a GCS score of 13–15 (Rimel et al., 1981; Binder, 1986). Most authorities now accept that the long-term problems found in patients who have sustained apparently minor injury can be organic in nature. Significant neuro-psychological deficits are identifiable in some patients following whiplash injury (Yarnell and Rossie, 1988). The symptoms most frequently associated with mild brain injury or post-concussion syndrome (PCS) are problems with attention and memory, increased fatigue, irritability, anxiety, dizziness and headaches. Rimel *et al.* (1981) examined 424 patients 3 months after minor brain injury (unconsciousness of 20 min or less). Of these 424 patients 79% complained of persistent headaches, and 59% described memory problems. Of those patients employed before the incident, 34% were unemployed 3 months later. Most patients had no impairment on neurological examination but showed persisting deficits in attention, concentration and memory. Litigation and compensation were described as having a minimal role in determining outcome (i.e. patients with pending litigation seemed to do marginally worse). Minor injuries are likely to be more significant when they are repeated (a cumulative effect) and when they occur in already neurologically compromised individuals (Williams *et al.*, 1990). In Rimel's study 31% of patients had a previous brain injury. The mildly brain injured may feel under considerable stress in having to cope with reduced memory, attention and information-processing capacities while having to continue to function in their normal life roles; stresses which do not apply to the more severely brain injured (Fordyce *et al.*, 1985; Giles, 1996). A number of workers have used radiological techniques such as computeriz-ed tomography (CT) scans to look for evidence of brain damage after mild brain injury. Findings indicate that even where patients remain asymptomatic, brain damage may have occurred (see Binder, 1986, for a review). Although the issue of financial compensation should not be discounted, the organic consequences of mild brain trauma have been underestimated in the past (Jennett and Teasdale, 1981).

The effects of repeated brain injury may be explicated by reference to the concept of reserve capacity. An uninjured individual may be considered to have capacity that is over and above the minimum required for daily functioning. An initial brain injury may significantly reduce or eliminate reserve capacity but nonetheless fail to produce functional impairment because the individual retains the minimum capacity to meet their daily needs. Later, even mild, brain injury can have catastrophic effects because of limited or absent reserve capacity. Gronwall and Wrightson (1981) found that patients with a history of previous head trauma recovered more slowly than patients without such a history. Similarly the severity of cerebral atrophy found in professional boxers increased in relation to their number of fights (Casson *et al.*, 1984). Mild injuries may also have significant effects when they coexist with other types of trauma such as spinal cord injuries or alcohol abuse (Davidoff *et al.*, 1985; Giles, 1994a).

Drawing attention to the limitations and complications of attempting to predict outcome should not be taken to suggest that such attempts are of doubtful value. It should serve to underline the limitations of prognostication in any individual case, and should emphasize the fact that assessment of outcome must depend on measures which clearly relate to the disabilities of the individual patient (Brooks *et al.*, 1986b; Spettell *et al.*, 1991). Truly functionally oriented measures that may be used to measure recovery into the post-acute period are needed.

FAMILY AND SOCIAL CONSEQUENCES OF BRAIN INJURY

A significant proportion of individuals with severe brain injury have impairments serious enough to prevent them from living fully independent lives. Impairments resulting from other types of trauma leave an individual cognitively intact and more able to adjust to reduced ability. In the person with brain injury, the ability to compensate for and adjust to their injury is often limited as a result of the brain damage itself. This is particularly tragic as brain injury occurs most frequent among adolescents and young adults whose hopes and expectations may suddenly become unrealistic and go unfulfilled. The fact that the individual may have no memory for the injury and for a considerable amount of the recovery process, complicates adjustment to their new situation. Unlike individuals with stroke, who are frequently older and already possess established social networks to provide care and support, the young brain-injured patient often becomes socially isolated. Studies examining the effect of a brain injury on the patient's family have been consistent in finding that cognitive impairments and personality changes are more difficult for families to cope with than physical impairments (Thomsen, 1974; Bond, 1975; Weddell *et al.*, 1980). Parents may be better able than spouses to tolerate change in the patient (Thomsen, 1974) but will nonetheless experience a period of grieving for the injured family member. It may be much easier for parents to adjust to the increased level of dependence of the severely brain-injured person because they cared for the individual during the period of childhood dependency. Weddell *et al.* (1980) found that only a small proportion of severely brain-injured adults were able to return to their former employment. Nearly 50% were unable to work at all, and in half of these cases care was provided by parents. One or both of the parents gave up work to look after heavily dependent children (Weddell *et al.*, 1980).

Oddy *et al.* (1978) examined stress in relatives of brain-injured patients. Expressed stress level was influenced by the relative's perception of personality change and subjective deficits but not by the severity of brain injury, nor by whether patients had resumed work. Relatives' complaints highlighted poor communication from professionals. Relatives often felt that they were given insufficient information about the extent and nature of injury, a finding which is consistent with the results of earlier studies (Panting and Merry, 1972; Thomsen, 1974). Personality change in the brain injured has been found to be far more significant than other factors in causing families stress (Lezak, 1978; Brooks and McKinlay, 1983). Problems may relate to the person's reduced capacity for social perceptiveness resulting in self-centred behaviour and lack of insight. Lack of self-control and impulsivity, as well as memory problems, can lead to a greatly reduced ability to plan and carry out actions. The injured person may be disinhibited, leading to behaviour which the family find disturbing and embarrassing. Sexual behaviours may be either greatly increased or absent (Miller *et al.*, 1986). Altered emotional responsiveness is frequently a problem, with apathy, silliness and increased touching being reported as common problems (Giles, 1996).

Families may feel trapped and isolated, and are sometimes in physical danger from the brain-injured person (Brooks and McKinlay, 1983). Young children find the presence of a 'changed' father or mother particularly difficult. Spouses may have particular problems because of ambivalent feelings towards a markedly changed individual. Spouses often feel guilty about resenting the demands placed upon them by the need to take care of their partner, further isolating them from family and friends. Unfortunately it is often automatically assumed that the injured person will go home after he or she has 'ceased to make progress' at the rehabilitation setting. Family members should be involved in decisions concerning discharge and placement and supported in their decisions. Ultimately the level of involvement must be a matter for the family to decide but rehabilitation workers can play an important role in helping family members resolve some of the issues involved. When the family members are clear that they wish to care for the relative, training and support should be provided, with the staff having a continuing involvement on an 'as needed' basis.

Social isolation is a major problem for individuals with brain injury. A number of models for the provision of supported living services are now available for those who require continuing residential care (Jackson, 1994). Employment in some form plays a central role in facilitating psychosocial integration but despite improved vocational rehabilitation models many brain-injured persons cannot gain or maintain lasting vocational placement. As a result there are large number of people with brain injury who live in the community, either independently or cared for by family, who do not have ongoing sources of support outside the home. Even persons otherwise classified as having good outcome may require ongoing emotional support to maintain functional independence (Tate *et al.*, 1989). A number of community support delivery models have been proposed (Cole *et al.*, 1985) but the most widely used is the support group. Recommendations as to how to start and run a support group for persons with brain injury are available (Blanchard, 1984). A study by Willer and co-workers found that attending support groups was rated by brain-injured women and wives of brain-injured men as an important coping strategy but this was not true of men who placed greater priority on individualistic coping strategies (Willer *et al.*, 1991). Socialization, support and legitimization of members' experiences are important factors in the group process (Schulz, 1994; Schwartzberg, 1994).

THEORIES OF RECOVERY AFTER BRAIN INJURY

The mechanisms underlying recovery of function after brain injury remain little understood. Immediately following brain trauma (primary brain damage) there is a period of alteration of consciousness (coma). The depth and duration of the coma is indicative of the extent of white matter destruction (Jennett and Teasdale, 1981). The brain's reaction to trauma can initiate secondary processes (such as cerebral oedema) that lead to further damage (secondary brain damage). Pharmacological intervention at this stage may in the future be able to protect partially damaged neurons by making their biochemical environment more favourable. Resolution of these problems with appropriate medical management leads to the beginning of recovery which is marked by a return to consciousness. Following the medical stabilization and emergence from coma there is a period of spontaneous recovery. During this period PTA comes to an end and, in most instances, the individual again starts to remember day-to-day events. There are a number of studies that indicate that most recovery occurs in the first 6 months following injury after which the rate of spontaneous recovery slows (Bond, 1979; Jennett and Teasdale, 1981). The process of recovery, however, is neither uniform nor linear; faculties recover at differing rates and recovery in an area can stop unexpectedly. In some areas recovery may be total and rapid; in other areas recovery may take longer and leave functions impaired. In the case of memory some patients never recover the ability to remember day-to-day events so that there is no trend towards recovery. The mechanisms which underlie the recovery are almost totally unknown, but continue to be the subject of speculation under the general heading of 'plasticity'. It is hoped that increased knowledge of the processes involved will lead to more effective rehabilitation (Bach-y-Rita, 1980, 1983). A vast number of mechanisms have been proposed, but can be grouped into two kinds of explanations of recovery of function: restitution and substitution.

RESTITUTION

Diaschisis

Diaschisis is the hypothesized suspension of function as a reaction of surviving neurons to destruction of remote but functionally related neurons (Von Monakow, 1914). After an unspecified period the 'depressed' neurons recover their responsiveness. Evidence for the existence of diaschisis (although not for its involvement in recovery of function) has come from studies of cerebellar blood flow in relation to space-occupying supratentorial lesions on the contralateral side. This 'crossed cerebellar diaschisis' has been reported by Baron et al. (1980) and others (Pantano et al., 1968; Fukuyama et al., 1986) and is thought to be the result of damage to descending fibres from the cerebral cortex to the cerebellum. This kind of research has only become possible with the introduction of CT, nuclear magnetic resonance (NMR) and positron emission tomography (PET), which allow the possibility of much greater insight into the dynamic processes operating in a living brain. More rigorous evidence for the place of diaschisis in recovery of function after brain injury may await the application of these new techniques. Nevertheless the role of diaschisis in recovery of function after brain injury remains debatable (Schoenfeld and Hamilton, 1977; Finger and Stein, 1982). The notion of diaschisis will probably become redundant as its component processes become known.

Denervation supersensitivity

This theory suggests that when the number of dendrites impinging on an intact neuron is reduced it becomes more sensitive to the ones which remain (Cannon and Rosenblueth, 1949). Denervation supersensitivity has received some support (Glick and Greenstein, 1973), but the duration of the process is unclear. Denervation supersensitivity cannot on its own account for recovery of function since it presupposes sparing of some capacity in a given system and is therefore probably best considered in conjunction with redundancy theories discussed below (Finger and Stein, 1982).

Regeneration

Functional regeneration of severed axons only occurs spontaneously in the peripheral nervous system (Schoenfeld and Hamilton, 1977). To be effective a viable axon would have to reconnect to its previous target cells or to cells serving a similar function. There is little evidence for this type of connection reforming in the human brain. This area of research is currently focused toward the treatment of spinal cord injuries.

Collateral sprouting

Collateral sprouting (or reactive synaptogenesis) concerns non-lesioned neurons which take over the site of a synaptic junction no longer occupied by the lesioned cells. Unlike regeneration there is good evidence that this process does take place. Collateral sprouting may underlie some recovery of function in the central nervous system (CNS), but its effect is probably limited and may not always be beneficial. It has been implicated in spasticity (Liu and Chambers, 1958), and could produce 'noise' in the system by making inappropriate non-functional connections.

SUBSTITUTION

Redundancy–equipotentiality–parallel distributed processing

Redundancy is a theory of sparing rather than of recovery. Redundancy suggests that there was in the brain, prior to injury, functional capacity which was surplus to requirements. The strongest statement of this view is the theory of equipotentiality (Tizard, 1959). According to this theory brain tissue has the capacity to subserve any function. Since functions are distributed across the entire cortex, impairment is a function of the amount of brain damage (Lashley, 1938). It is clear from the sometimes devastating deficits that can be produced by circumscribed lesions that the theory of equipotentiality (when considered on a macrolevel) does not accord with our current knowledge (Powell, 1981). A weaker version of the theory (Pribram, 1968; Powell, 1981) views brain systems in terms of their level of redundancy. A system with high redundancy is one where the importance of any individual neuron is low as many others carry out the same function. A system with low redundancy is one where neurons subserve different functions so that the loss of even a small number results in loss of function. Contemporary theories of brain function are influenced by computer network models (Churchland, 1995). Computer networks have properties which appear similar to properties associated with human brain functioning, including the ability to continue to function despite damage to a portion of a network with only gradual debasement in the quality of the discriminations.

Although the human brain is highly connected it does not function as a single network but as multiple interconnected networks. Network theory is therefore easily reconciled with the evidence for localization of function. On a micro level functions are diffuse, subserved by often large neuronal networks, however on a macro level damage to a discrete area of the brain may result in very specific impairments (Giles, 1996).

Neurological substitution

The theory of neurological substitution suggests that brain systems can change function and that the brain can relearn a lost function in an undamaged area of the brain. New imaging techniques allow an analysis to be made of the brain areas which are most active during tasks involving cognitive processing. One interesting strategy using this technique is to examine patients whose lesions suggest that they should have certain cognitive or behavioural deficits but who are able to perform the task without difficulty (see Raichle, 1997 for a discussion of the strengths and weaknesses of these techniques). Miller (1985) has highlighted some of the difficulties involved in determining the possible role of neurological substitution in recovery of function. For neurological substitution to be clearly responsible for recovery of function it would be necessary to demonstrate that (1) a part of the brain not previously involved in a function becomes involved, (2) that the part of the brain subserving the new role never had the role in the past, and (3) that the function is not simply being performed by use of substitute strategies. These factors have not been adequately taken into account in most work claiming to demonstrate neurological substitution (Miller, 1985).

Neural Darwinism

Neural Darwinism, associated with the work of Edelmen (1987) and others (Calvin, 1996), is a neural developmental and selectionist theory of brain function. It suggests that optimal neural response patterns develop in the human cortex as a result of a process of selection analogous to Darwinian natural selection. The development of neuronal interconnections occurs via a process of 'boot-strapping' similar to what occurs in current computer models. These computer 'neural networks' have the ability, without further programming, to develop associations between stimuli and to categorize complex novel stimuli accurately based on previous exposure to a learning set (Churchland, 1995). Older computer models had to be given the rules for discrimination, however in the new network models 'rules' are learned as a result of being exposed to data. A potential account of recovery of function is that a process similar to the developmental process occurs following brain damage and that new neural networks develop to compensate for those which were damaged. There is however no current evidence supporting this hypothesis.

Behavioural compensation

Behavioural compensation is not a theory of neural plasticity but rather suggests that an individual, employing undamaged brain systems, adopts the use of strategies which were not used prior to injury. The use of this type of compensation has been demonstrated in animals as well as humans. Rats, for example, when deprived of sight may use their sense of smell to navigate a maze. The behavioural compensation hypothesis of recovery is not a theory of plasticity because it requires no changes in the existing functions of undamaged brain areas. Clearly this model often involves new learning and requires the individual to accommodate to the absence of cues and to make use of new cues. Some authors regard the vast majority of cases of recovery of function as the result of employing an alternate behavioural strategy (Gazzaniga, 1978). For example, a patient might be unable to translate visually presented material into language but is able to do so if he traces the outline of the image with his finger (Landis *et al.*, 1982).

There is increasing evidence that changes in the CNS take place normally as a response to changes in both the internal and external environment. For example, changes in dendritic arborization (new formation and loss) is part of a general process in all normal adults and not as a specific response to brain injury. As Laurence and Stein (1978) point out these types of structural changes may not indicate any fundamental change in the ground rules by which the brain operates. Some authors seem to regard any form of learning (or consistent behavioural change) as evidence of neural plasticity (Bach-y-Rita, 1980). With this type of definition the term is then no longer reserved for *abnormal* activity in the brain which underlies recovery of function. The view that all recovery of function after brain injury is by definition 'plasticity' fails to examine the role of normal learning in recovery of function (Yu, 1983) or expands the meaning of the term plasticity until it becomes meaningless. It is possible that the morphological changes seen in the brain after lesion underlie recovery (Illis, 1983). However, such changes may also impede recovery (Devor, 1982).

That the brain can compensate in some ways after loss of brain substance is clear. How it does so is a matter of conjecture. What is clear is that the efficacy of available techniques to assist the brain's regenerative ability is limited. Severe brain injury continues to leave patients with significant deficits. The amount of recovery possible may be related to the redundancy (spare capacity) in the brain and the way that the particular system is organized. Control of the motor system, for example, is widely distributed, involving among other areas the cerebral cortex, the basal ganglia and the cerebellum.

In terms of guidance that can be offered to the therapist, the most consistent suggestions from researchers into plasticity involve motivating, practical and repeated training in functional tasks (Bach-y-Rita, 1980; Finger and Stein, 1982; Yu, 1983). The theory of Neural Darwinism and current computer models suggests that exposure to multiple learning sets which include the potential for successful discrimination may be helpful. If we think of the injured brain as functioning as a damaged learning system then over-determining correct responses by saturating the environment with cues to the correct response may be indicated. This type of intervention is defensible in terms that do not require recourse to theories of neural plasticity.

IS REHABILITATION EFFECTIVE?

During the period immediately following injury it is clear that energetic management by an acute trauma team can improve outcome (Becker *et al.*, 1977;

Klauber *et al.*, 1985). After the acute trauma the role of therapeutic interventions in facilitating recovery is less clear. Large-scale prospective randomized studies of the effectiveness of brain-injury rehabilitation are unavailable. Support services for the mild to moderately injured do appear to positively affect outcome. Wade *et al.* (1998) report a prospective randomized control trial of support services offered to patients admitted to hospital for head injury. All patients 16–65 years ($N = 314$) admitted to hospital after a head injury of any severity were prospectively randomized into a trial group who received additional support services provided by a specialist team ($N = 184$) or a group who received the standard hospital management and no specialist follow-up services ($N = 130$). Patients were assessed at a 6-month follow-up with a measure of social disability and a measure of post-concussion symptoms. Each patient in the trial group was contacted 7–10 days after injury and offered assessment and intervention as needed, primarily information support and advice. Forty-six per cent of the trial group also received further out-patient intervention. At the 6-month follow-up the trial-group patients had significantly less social disability and significantly less severe post-concussion symptoms than the control-group patients. The study design requiring hospital admission excluded most patients with trivial or very minor trauma, although it is possible that it did not include all patients with head trauma efforts were made to ensure the inclusion of all patients with significant head injury. The majority of patients were in the mild to moderate severity categories (73%) and in only 10% of cases did PTA exceed 7 days. The main benefit of treatment appeared to be in the mild to moderate severity groups. The types of problems experienced by these patients are qualitatively different to those experienced by the more severely injured. The typical patterns of sequelae associated with the mild to moderate injury severity are described collectively as the post-concussive syndrome and include a range of symptoms such as headache, dizziness, fatigue, irritability, poor concentration, sleep and memory disturbance, anxiety and depression, sensitivity to noise and light, and blurred or double vision. It is these patients that this intervention appeared to assist, probably by minimizing the effect of a vicious cycle of anxiety exacerbating post-concussion symptoms and vice versa. Nonetheless significant percentages of patients continued to experience social disability (61%) and post-concussion symptoms (72%). The more severely injured appeared not to have benefited from the service. Since some patients do experience symptoms for a year and beyond it would be interesting to determine if the benefits of intervention continue.

No similarly well-controlled trials of severe brain-injury rehabilitation have been carried out. The studies that have been reported are so fraught with methodological difficulties that they are difficult to interpret (see Chestnut *et al.*, 1999; Giles and McMillan, in press). Prospective randomized control trials are unlikely to be carried out for ethical reasons. Treatment comparisons are a viable alternative to prospective randomized controlled trials. These types of studies have not yet been carried out in brain-injury rehabilitation although they have been performed in rehabilitation after cerebrovascular accident. Similar influences may operate on the recovery processes on patients with cerebrovascular accidents (CVA) and those with traumatic brain injury.

The evidence supporting the efficacy of physical and cognitive rehabilitation is discussed below. It is difficult to evaluate recovery after trauma to the CNS because, as noted above, patients make considerable natural recovery from brain trauma for the first 6 months after injury, and to a lesser degree thereafter. The actual recovery in any individual patient is not fully predictable, making the matching of patients for controlled trials difficult. A second complication is that factors relating to recovery (particularly initial severity) may determine how much therapy a patient receives (Brockleburst *et al.*, 1978; Wade *et al.*, 1984). In regard to physical rehabilitation, three major questions have been addressed: 'Does therapy affect outcome?', 'When should therapy be initiated?' and 'Is one form of therapy more effective than another?'.

Lind (1982) reviewed seven studies of stroke rehabilitation, concluding that improvements attributable to rehabilitation programmes are so slight as to be unreliable. As might be expected the greatest factor in improvement was spontaneous recovery. However, Lind concluded that patients with residual functional impairments may benefit from individually tailored retraining programmes to increase independence and to prevent (or reverse) institutionalization. Lind suggests that this approach could permit a substantial improvement in the quality of life for a limited number of patients (Lind, 1982). Tangman *et al.* (1990) found that 1 month of intensive intervention had a significant functional impact on patients who were at least 1 year post-CVA.

Studies comparing types of intervention have been more straightforward. In trials which compared the effectiveness of neurodevelopmental approaches such as those advocated by the Bobaths (Bobath, 1978), with the training of functional skills, no significant difference has been found between the two even when the neurodevelopmental treatment involved considerably more therapy hours (Stern *et al.*, 1970; Logigan *et al.*, 1983; Lord and Hall, 1986).

The results of a number of studies have indicated that early intervention is preferable to later intervention (Cope and Hall, 1982; Novak *et al.*, 1984). Novak and co-workers (1984) examined this question and found that time since injury had a small negative effect on response to treatment. However, they note that treatment has to be delayed by years rather than days before there is any appreciable effect. In Cope and Hall's study severely brain-injured patients in an acute rehabilitation setting were divided retrospectively into early and late rehabilitation admission groups (admitted before and after 35 days post-injury). Two groups of 16 and 20 patients were matched for length of coma, age, level of disability and neurosurgical procedures required. Findings indicated that late-admission patients required twice as much rehabilitation to reach a standard discharge criteria as did the early-admission group. Outcome at 2-year follow-up was comparable. Unfortunately no reasons are given as to why the later group were not admitted to rehabilitation sooner. Since there is a range of complications which can accompany severe brain injury it is possible that whatever caused the delay in admission to rehabilitation services also caused the slow response to these services (Cope and Hall, 1982). Similar methodological problems beset a study by Mackay *et al.* (1992). Mackay *et al.* (1992) compared the outcomes of 21 patients with severe brain injury who received acute care at ten different hospitals without a formal traumatic brain injury (TBI) programme (TBI-NF) to the outcomes of 17 patients who received acute services in a formal TBI programme (TBI-F). Criteria for inclusion in the study were GCS 3–8 indicating severe brain injury and discharge from the same rehabilitation facility. GCS, Injury Severity Score (ISS) and Rancho Los Amigos scale (RLAS) score did not differ significantly between the two groups. Treatment of the TBI-F rehabilitation group differed from the TBI-NF group in that the former consistently received interventions from all three rehabilitation disciplines (occupational therapy (OT), physical therapy (PT), speech therapy (SP)) and were involved in multisensory stimulation with a goal to increase both motor and cognitive skills. Comparisons of the outcome data for the two programmes revealed that the patients in TBI-F had shorter comas and rehabilitation stays were approximately one-third those of the TBI-NF group. Cognitive outcome was superior in the TBI-F group, with, as a result, a greater percentage from this group being discharged to home rather than long-term care facilities. These results seem to indicate that an early formal programme significantly reduces morbidity. However, this finding depends on treating coma duration as a dependent variable and not regarding it as evidence of failure to establish that the patient groups were truly comparable. GCS scores are available shortly after injury and have gained wide acceptance as a method of inferring severity of injury, however coma duration may be a more sensitive measure of injury. If we assume no treatment effect then the outcomes are readily explainable as a result of the more extended period of coma of the TBI-NF group. It is not that early formal programmes are not helpful it is only that this study cannot indicate either way. Spettell *et al.* (1991) examined the time of admission to rehabilitation and severity of trauma and the effect of these variables on brain-injury outcome. These authors found that severity of brain injury was correlated with acute hospital length of stay (LOS). Outcome of brain injury as measured by the GOS was correlated primarily with severity of brain injury. Duration of acute hospitalization explained only a small amount of the variance (i.e. 4%). However duration of acute hospitalization was a significant predictor of rehabilitation LOS. Degree of extracranial injury correlated with length of acute hospital stay. These findings suggest a possible reinterpretation of the results of Cope and Hall (1982) such that severity of brain injury and severity of other injuries and medical complications influence both length of acute hospitalization (and consequently the timing of rehabilitation admission) and rehabilitation LOS. Two years post-injury, only the severity of the brain injury influences outcome (Cope and Hall, 1982; Spettell *et al.*, 1991).

Other authors have cautioned against attempting to speed recovery by including the patient prematurely in an intensive rehabilitation programme (Long *et al.*, 1984). However, Bell and Tallman (1995) describe the problems of five patients admitted directly to skilled nursing facilities and not provided with rehabilitation. Each patient was at least 1 year post-injury when 'rescued' from the nursing home setting and provided with appropriate rehabilitation resulting in all patients resuming semi-independent community living (Bell and Tallman, 1995). Similar findings have been described by others (Shaw *et al.*, 1985).

Prigatano and co-workers (1984) report the effect of a 6-month intensive post-acute rehabilitation programme for severely traumatically brain-injured young adults (mean time post-injury 21.6 months). The study consisted of a comparison of 18 treated patients and 17 untreated controls. The treatment group showed a slightly greater improvement over controls on neuropsychological measures. Psychosocial adjustment was substantially improved in the treatment group versus the controls. In their discussion the authors suggest that patients most likely to benefit from the rehabilitation programme were those who had problems in coping with disability, had a good work history prior to brain injury and who could be taught strategies to overcome their problems (Prigatano *et al.*, 1984).

A large-scale analysis of the effectiveness of traumatic brain-injury interventions using conventional UK service provision methods concludes that although interventions can clearly positively affect outcomes in some individuals, others receive intensive interventions with limited positive impact. Unfortunately, given the cost of services which may be very high, it is very difficult to distinguish prospectively responders from non-responders (Stilwell *et al.*, 1998).

COGNITIVE REHABILITATION MODELS

Evidence relating to the efficacy of cognitive and perceptual training is extremely diverse and a full review will not be attempted here. Since the 1960s the association between cognitive impairments and functional loss has been recognized. Clinicians believed that increasing cognitive abilities would improve outcome. During the late 1960s, 1970s and early 1980s there was great interest in cognitive rehabilitation (Pattern, 1972; Gianutsos, 1980; Wilson and Moffat, 1984). The model of rehabilitation most widely advocated in the USA was a general stimulation model. It was thought that practice of impaired cognitive functions would lead to improved performance both on those skills and on functional behaviours. Initial work addressing neglect in individuals with right-sided CVA proved encouraging. Diller *et al.* (1974) found that perceptual retraining for neglect was effective and that generalization occurred from perceptual retraining tasks to functional (ADL) skills. Attempts to apply cognitive retraining to other areas of cognitive functioning proved disappointing. Lincoln *et al.* (1985) compared the response of a group of persons with brain injury or CVA to perceptual training versus conventional occupational therapy. Treatment lasted 4 h per week for 4 weeks. The perceptual retraining group engaged in the perceptual tasks commonly given to persons with brain injury at the time (activities included colour and shape matching and recognition games). The conventional group engaged in activities not designed to address perceptual functioning. At the end of treatment no significant differences were found between the groups on measures of visual perceptual skills or daily living skills.

Disillusionment with this approach led to the development of alternate models the most important of which is the process-specific approach. Process-specific approaches are theoretically driven and address a specific cognitive skill or set of skills. An example of a process-specific approach is that of Sohlberg and Mateer

(1987). Sohlberg and Mateer (1987) have stressed the importance of a theoretical model, comprehensive assessment, a process approach (that basic cognitive components are addressed before complex components or functional skills), repetition, knowledge of results (feedback) and use of probes to evaluate efficacy (Sohlberg and Mateer, 1986).

More recently approaches based on theories of metacognition have been developed. The term metacognition has been used to describe a person's understanding and use of his or her own basic cognitive and perceptual processes. Nelson and Narens (1994) describe a two-level, two-process model of cognitive functioning. The two levels are the basic object level and the meta level, and the two processes are monitoring, in which the flow of information is from the object level to the meta level, and control in which the flow of information is from the meta level to the object level. The meta level contains an imperfect model of how the object level works. If, following neurological damage, there is no change in the model of object-level functioning, then the individual will have no ability to adjust his or her control functions to compensate for impairment. A readjustment of the model would however give the person the opportunity to engage in new object-level regulatory behaviours, which could significantly improve performance (by, for example, the development of a strategy to write things down). From this perspective the two models of cognitive retraining attempt to remediate object-level performance whereas metacognitive rehabilitation attempts to change how the person *uses* retained object-level skills. Programmes involving the verbal regulation of behaviour and the use of prosthetic devices (such as electronic memory aids) require the individual to change their metacognitive model of themselves (or they will not use the aids).

The use of computers in cognitive rehabilitation

During the mid 1980s the microcomputer was embraced as a way to provide appropriate stimulation/retraining in basic cognitive activities. Microcomputers provided immediate feedback on performance and excellent data collection capabilities. The computer tasks were designed to remediate neuropsychological processes by the use of game-like programs in a manner analogous to the types of non-computer cognitive retraining advocated at the time. Patients with brain injury were able to improve on the computer tasks. However, it was soon recognized that the improvements were predominantly task specific, i.e. a person who practised a computer task improved on the computer task but not on other, apparently related, activities (Fussey and Giles, 1988). Currently three types of cognitive rehabilitation using computers can be identified, the general stimulation approach and the process-specific approaches described above and a third approach that uses computers to teach domain-specific information or skills. Controlled trials examining patient improvement with a generalized stimulation approach with and without computer-augmented cognitive retraining have failed to find improved outcome with the use of computers (Batchelor et al., 1988; Chen et al., 1997). Evidence relating to the process-specific skills approach has been mixed. Positive effects for retraining of attentional skills have been found by some (Sohlberg and Mateer, 1987; Gray and Robertson, 1989) but not by others (Ponsford and Kinsella, 1988). Wood and Fussey (1987) found that behavioural aspects of attention improved with computer-augmented cognitive retraining but not neuropsychological aspects. Evidence relating to the third approach, the use of computers to assist in the learning of domain-specific information or skills has been more consistently positive (Glisky *et al.*, 1986; Clark-Wilson, 1988; Glisky and Schacter, 1988). As a general rule the generalized hierarchical approach whether computer augmented or not has not been shown to be effective whereas more focused efforts have been more encouraging. The more concrete the task the more positive the outcome of a training approach leading to a move away from isolated cognitive rehabilitation towards functionally oriented intervention strategies (Giles, 1994a).

MODELS OF THERAPY

As in cognitive rehabilitation, using 'stimulation' as a model of treatment therapists have developed hierarchical programmes designed to move the patient towards improved functional performance (Rothi and Horner, 1983). This 'stimulation' model suggests that by asking the individual to perform to the limits of his or her ability the therapist will facilitate recovery. There are two possible arguments for this approach (or they might be considered strong and weak versions of the same argument). The first argument best applies to the period early in recovery when it is thought that attempts to call upon a damaged system may increase changes in the brain's structure by, for example, neural regrowth. The second argument does not require changes in brain structure, and suggests that impaired functions must be maximally stimulated in order to redevelop and be maintained.

As noted above, there is no firm evidence that neuronal regeneration underlies recovery of function in the CNS. Nor is there evidence that a patient's performance of tasks requiring cognitive skills assists neurological regeneration. Although practising a task usually improves performance (Newell and Rosenbloom, 1981), there is no evidence for a generalized effect on cognitive skills. Such a model implies the belief that cognitive skills are analogous to 'mental muscles' which become stronger with practice.

Despite limited verbal-learning capacity (Levin *et al.*, 1988) patients are learning throughout the period of spontaneous recovery. Patients may learn early on that they cannot perform tasks which later in the recovery process they achieve. A patient may develop a type of learned helplessness (Seligman, 1975) and have a capacity which considerably outstrips performance. For instance, early in treatment when the patient is extremely motivated to walk, the patient learns a wide-based, shuffling gait. Over the next few months the patient overlearns this walking pattern, despite being capable – because of improved motor coordination, posture and balance reaction – of a more normal gait. Only specific gait training will enable the patient to perform at the level of their increased potential.

Early in rehabilitation a major role of the therapist is to help the patient perform maximally as his condition improves. Cope (1985) describes the course of recovery of an 18-year-old man who was in a coma for nearly 6 months. The course of recovery was charted closely and continued for 5 years after the resolution of the coma. The patient was provided with active rehabilitation. Although it is not demonstrated that the rehabilitation was causally related to the recovery, it is realistically suggested that alternative management could have impeded the functional gains shown by this patient. Providing unnecessary assistance has been shown to reduce the independence of other institutionalized patients (Avorn and Langer, 1982) and similar considerations apply to the brain injured. In many senses the early rehabilitation process can be seen as an attempt to avoid complications (Giles and Clark-Wilson, 1993), not only the physical complications of soft tissue contractures, heterotopic ossification or decubiti, but also avoiding creating or accentuating inappropriate behaviour patterns.

The emphasis on stimulation has led to treatment approaches being adopted which are unlikely to have a specific treatment effect. Poor memory and reduced attentional capacity indicate that if the patient is to learn, information provided must be small in amount, frequently repeated and highly motivating. Instead, therapeutic interventions have tended to be non-specific and not focused on practical tasks. Therapists have used concepts such as 'judgement', 'abstraction' and 'flexibility', and patients who show deficits relating to these constructs have been given tasks that are believed to provide practice in these 'skills'. The idea that judgement or abstraction can be practiced is extremely problematic: no evidence is available to suggest that tasks constructed to develop them show any therapeutic effect. Many tasks used have been irrelevant to normal life outside the rehabilitation setting. Although some workers have claimed to be able to rehabilitate frontal lobe impairments these attempts have typically involved the routinization of hitherto frontally mediated behaviours. Practising a task by necessity reduces its novelty and consequently the need for judgement and abstraction.

Over recent years it has been recognized that brain-injured patients can develop alternative cognitive strategies to help them overcome both cognitive and functional deficits. Most clinicians will have seen patients who painstakingly examined objects most people would just glance at, or perform functional behaviours in a set routine which would previously have been more spontaneous and random in execution. Therapists have developed programmes designed to facilitate the development of metacognitive control strategies or to teach strategies to overcome deficits where patients have been unable to generate such compensatory strategies themselves. However the model is limited in application to the severely brain injured for a number reasons:

1 *Relevance.* The skill trained must be relevant to the individual's needs and be sufficiently useful to the patient to warrant the effort needed to acquire it (the more impaired the individuals the more difficulty there is to acquire the skill). Most internal strategies used in memory retraining do not meet this criterion. Where patients have a poor memory to start with, some of the methods may be extremely difficult to teach. Many of the techniques of imagery are limited in their usefulness to shopping lists or other highly

structured situations. Some of the elaborate methods described to help patients remember faces are absurdly time-consuming with respect to the possible advantages.

2 *Generalization.* By generalization we mean the ability to transfer a skill learned in one situation to other novel situations. A vast amount of evidence is available which suggests that individuals with severe deficits after brain injury have great difficulty in generalizing skills (Glisky *et al.*, 1986). Practice of a task leads to improvement (Newell and Rosenbloom, 1981). Improvement in a particular task should not be taken to imply improvement in an underlying process. Patients have improved with practice in recalling a single shopping list or in finding their way in a new environment, but this does not imply their memory has improved. When teaching the use of a mental routine the individual has to be able to recognize their current circumstances as necessitating the use of the skill and the natural environment has to be sufficient to prompt the use of the procedure.

3 *Initiation.* Brain-injured patients can often learn information or routines but be unable to apply them (e.g. they may learn that they should write down important information but not recognize when they need to do so). Individuals with cognitive processing deficits may find compensatory techniques can be difficult to use because they are too demanding. Patients are most likely to use techniques if they are overlearned and require the least effort (Giles and Clark-Wilson, 1993). Both the task itself and the mental processes required for its initiation need to be overlearned. Put another way both the object-level task and the meta level cognitive initiation strategy need to be trained to the point of overlearning. If it is possible to help the patient create a habit in both domains the demands on the patient's capacity to initiate the behaviour are reduced.

Rather than view the patient's deficits from the perspective of the cognitive impairments, and attempt to address these directly, it is possible to address the patient's problems from the perspective of functional skills or behavioural change. This is particularly important when a specific functional deficit impedes further progress in rehabilitation. It is often possible to train individuals in compensation habits that they have not been able to develop themselves. It is also possible to alter the environment, to increase the individual's functional capacity (Giles and Clark-Wilson, 1993).

Successful outcomes have been reported when: (a) training has addressed functional deficits, i.e. difficulty in washing and dressing is addressed directly, taking into account the memory problem but not treating the memory problem and ignoring the ADL deficit; (b) training has been highly structured; (c) training has been based on behavioural-learning principles; and (d) the meaning of the behaviour and the behavioural change is addressed. It is therefore necessary to stress the importance of specificity and function rather than non-specific approaches.

By adopting a functional-learning perspective the range of problems that can be addressed is vastly increased. Patients with severe brain injuries can display behaviour disorders which make them extremely unpopular with therapy staff. In some cases behaviour disorders may completely sabotage attempts at rehabilitation. Therapists may feel that they expend more time and energy in attempting to 'deal' with the patient's behaviour disorder than in the practice of rehabilitation. Often the behaviour disorder is never directly addressed. Adopting a functional behavioural approach vastly expands the types of behaviours that can be addressed, and there is now a wealth of evidence supporting its use (Eames and Wood, 1985a, b; Burke *et al.*, 1988; Giles and Clark-Wilson, 1993; Lloyd and Cuvo, 1994).

A FUNCTIONAL BEHAVIOURAL-LEARNING APPROACH TO BRAIN-INJURY REHABILITATION

A functional behavioural-learning approach offers clear advantages over other available methods in brain-injury rehabilitation. Learning theory offers a structure for rehabilitation with emphasis placed on measurable and reproducible techniques. Behavioural assessment and behaviour therapy look at real-life situations and state goals with clear criteria for success and failure. Brain-injured patients frequently undergo neurological and neuropsychological tests, but there is no clear way to relate test performance to functional deficits (Bennett-Levy and Powell, 1980). Behavioural assessment (more fully described in Chapter 5) can help pinpoint how adaptive behaviours break down, examine how environmental factors maintain unwanted behaviours and evaluate the functional consequences of organic damage. The form of recording will vary depending on level of impairment and areas of deficit.

Naturalistic observations are the most valuable in describing the patient's normal and habitual unconstrained behaviours. Recording of antecedent, behaviour and consequence (ABC) allows assessment of the environmental precipitants of a behaviour and the factors maintaining a behaviour. Observations need to be undertaken in a wide range of settings and include periods where the patient is under stress. Areas examined may include social interaction, self-care, leisure and family interaction. Some extremely significant behaviour disorders may only become evident in response to a limited range of cues. For example, aggressive behaviour might only be displayed with family members after drinking alcohol. A behavioural approach helps in the selection of appropriate goals and in assessing the patient's response to treatment. The discipline of establishing a baseline, designing an intervention strategy and operationally assessing the patient response to treatment helps clinicians avoid such vague goals as 'improve safety awareness'. Behavioural techniques cover a wide range of possible strategies and are problem orientated. Behavioural interventions can be seen as lying on an antecedent control–conditioning–cognitive behaviour therapy continuum. The more severely or acutely impaired an individual the more likely they are to require antecedent control, and the more intact they are the more they are likely to be able to make use of cognitive behavioural interventions. Training approaches, however, remain central to the rehabilitative endeavour. Antecedent control can often be combined with a training approach to produce lasting change with the minimum of distress for the patient (see, for example, Slifer *et al.*, 1997). Training approaches reduce the cognitive demands on higher-functioning patients and facilitate the integration of new skills.

Conditioning methods may not at first sight seem appropriate for use with the severely impaired brain-injured person since many of their deficits are organic in origin and these patients usually have problems with new learning. Optimal treatments for many conditions with organic origins (e.g. depression, panic disorder) involve a combination of pharmacological and behavioural intervention. It is widely recognized that other groups who have impaired learning ability have benefited from behavioural methodology (e.g. individuals with mental retardation and pervasive developmental disorders). A number of studies have demonstrated the similar learning characteristics of the mentally retarded and the brain injured (Miller, 1980; Giles *et al.*, 1997). Among the most significant methods of learning in this group are:

1 *Associative learning.* Both classical (Pavlov, 1927) and operant (Skinner, 1938) learning are concerned with the causal relationships between events in the organism's environment. This type of learning is thought to be mediated by subcortical brain structures, much of this type of learning can be implicit (without awareness) and can be contrasted with:

2 *Cognitive learning.* This involves the formation of representations (often linguistic in humans) which are apparently dependent on the neocortex and hippocampus to establish rules and regularities about the environment (Goldstein and Oakley, 1983; Vargha-Khadem *et al.*, 1997). Cognitive deficits can hamper the severely brain-injured individual's ability to benefit from cognitive learning but, by consistently presenting the information, and by making this process rewarding, the individual's chances of learning can be maximized. One of the most important roles of the therapist is to highlight the central features of a skill so as to facilitate the patient's learning (Giles and Clark-Wilson, 1993).

A complex interaction of different types of learning probably underlies most acquisition of behaviour in man. Although the specifics of a therapeutic intervention will depend on the type of learning thought to predominate, in general terms behavioural techniques aid in the mapping of relationships between events occurring in the environment. The key to this is reinforcement, being an event following a behaviour which increases the rate of recurrence of the behaviour.

The state of the damaged brain is of fundamental importance in assessing how to facilitate learning. Powell (1981) has emphasized the importance of considering the triad of behaviour, cognition and neurophysiology. This is a return to the views of Hull (1952) where an 'O' for organism is incorporated into the S–R chain (S–O–R). Attempts can be made to modify the internal environment both pharmacologically and by cognitive behavioural intervention just as the external environment can be adapted. Both types of intervention can increase the receptivity of the patient to other types of treatment.

In examining the capacity of the injured brain for learning new or more adaptive behaviour neuropsychiatric and neuropsychological limitation should be recognized. The first of these limitations involves organic disorders arising from the brain injury, such as thought disorder, anxiety states, obsessive–compulsive disorders and affective disorders. These disorders can be thought of as active disruptive factors that impede learning and behavioural regulation. Episodic dyscontrol syndromes should also be included in this category and have been implicated in a range of bizarre behaviours and aggressive outbursts (Blumer, 1970; Hoshmand and Brawley, 1970; Bear, 1983).

Many of these disorders are treated pharmacologically. Evaluation by an experienced specialist in neuropsychiatry is essential, as some of these disorders can present as apparently pure behaviour disorders; temporal lobe epilepsy as aggressive outbursts or a depressive illness as poor motivation. Alternatively behavioural deficits can be misdiagnosed as psychiatric illness (Shaw *et al.*, 1985).

The second category refers to limitations of learning arising from brain injury. The neuropsychological disorders are impairments in the learning processes themselves and include disorders of arousal and attention, perceptual deficits, impaired memory, or frontal lobe dysfunction.

For instance, attentional deficit has been noted to be one of the most frequent consequences of brain injury (Van Zomeren and Deelman, 1978; Gronwall and Wrightson, 1981) and if patients do not attend to regularities in their environment they may have more difficulty learning from them. By pairing the naturally occurring environmental consequences with additional consequences it is possible to make the effects of a particular behaviour more salient to the patient (adding new controlling variables). Giles *et al.* (1997) suggest that the need for additional reinforcers in functional retraining programmes depends on the level of motivation towards what is to be taught: where the subject is highly motivated tangible rewards may be irrelevant.

Many individuals with brain injury are under-motivated or motivate towards unrealistic or inappropriate goals. Behavioural techniques, whilst not solving the problem, can help therapists manipulate the environment to help overcome motivational problems. Patients with frontal lobe disorders may have difficulty grasping their true circumstances. The shifting nature of reality for some of the most severely affected patients makes it difficult to establish effective learning programmes (see below) partially because they have difficulty learning from the social consequences of their behaviour.

The problems functional behavioural interventions can address in the brain-injured population can be divided into three types (Eames and Wood, 1985a): positive behaviour disorder, negative behaviour disorder and specific skill deficit. Behavioural interventions attempt to modify established automatic behaviour via practice and reinforcement of alternative thoughts and behaviours. Cognitive behavioural interventions reviewed in detail in other chapters of this book can help patients focus positively on changing inappropriate behaviours and on learning adaptive ones.

Stern and his co-workers (1985) have examined behaviour disturbance as a function of severity of cerebral damage. The authors attempted to examine four areas of symptomatology: behaviour, personality, affect and cognition. The authors do not establish the separate identities of these symptom complexes but their research does indicate that the more severe the diffuse injury the less behaviour the individual is likely to produce. Their results suggest a complex inter-relation between disinhibition, ability to initiate behaviour and arousal in determining positive and negative behaviour disorder. With extremely severe damage the degree of disinhibition may be masked by a generalized paucity of behaviour characterized by Lishman (1998) as slowing, inertia and aspontaneity. In an analysis of personality and behavioural change after severe blunt head injury, Brooks and McKinlay (1983) found that most patients were rated as showing increased temper and irritability and decreased energy and enthusiasm. The authors suggest that these changes are a very common consequence of severe brain injury (Brooks and McKinlay, 1983). Our clinical impression is that the more severe the diffuse injury the more the individual has difficulty in initiating behaviour and that these 'negative' behaviour problems are more difficult to address therapeutically than positive disorders.

Only a few attempts have been made to relate site of lesion with response to behavioural techniques and research has focused on response flexibility rather than skill learning. Petrides (1985) has reported that patients with damage to parts of the frontal cortex may have problems with conditional associative learning. Rolls *et al.* (1994) found that patients with damage to the ventral part of the frontal lobes had difficulty suppressing previously rewarded responses. Clinically patients with profound ventral frontal disorders may be fatuous, confabulatory, labile and irritable but may nonetheless demonstrate behavioural learning if the therapist can help the patient to practise and attend to the to-be-learned behaviour. The capacity of severely brain-injured persons to develop automaticity – an important component of behavioural skills acquisition – has been confirmed experimentally (Schmitter-Edgecombe and Rogers, 1997). Patients however developed automaticity far more slowly than a control group (Schmitter-Edgecombe and Rogers, 1997). No predictive test of behavioural learning has been reported, although the work of Miller (1980) represents a useful beginning. Behavioural training with the patient with memory impairment (which may imply damage to specific brain structures) is not only possible but definitely indicated in the development of both behavioural control and specific skill development (Glisky *et al.*, 1986; Giles and Clark-Wilson, 1993).

Eames and Wood (1985b) described the first use of a token economy for patients with severe brain injury whose disturbed behaviours prevented them from benefiting from standard therapy aimed at reducing their physical, behavioural and functional skills deficits. The methods used are similar to those used in the management of severe behaviour disorders in other populations, but had not been used with this population.

The behavioural treatment is based on positive reinforcement of appropriate behaviours (social reinforcement, attention and praise plus tangible reinforcement, e.g. chocolate, soft drinks, cigarettes or other privileges). In order not to support inappropriate behaviour by social interaction a 'time-out on the spot' (TOOTS) procedure is used. TOOTS is an extinction method based on removing from the subject the opportunity of gaining positive reinforcement contingent upon the subject producing an unwanted behaviour, and is adapted from the behavioural procedure of time-out (Ullmann and Krasner, 1969). Episodes of physical aggression led to a time-out for 5 min in a time-out room. These methods are more fully described elsewhere (Eames and Wood, 1985b). Within this context patients were taught positive behaviour and skills to increase their performance and quality of life.

A follow-up study examined a consecutive series of 24 patients treated on this unit. Time since discharge ranged from 6 to 39 months with a mean of 18.8 months. The principal outcome measure used was a hierarchical scale of placements ranked in terms of quality of life for the patient (Eames and Wood, 1985b). The results of the study show improvement in behaviour and subsequent placement. There was no trend towards relapse as time from discharge increased, nor was length of time since treatment a factor which reduced response to treatment.

Mean interval between injury and admission to the unit was 4 years, and the condition of all patients on admission was considered static in that it was highly unlikely that they would make further improvement. This report suggests that even years after injury highly structured, directed and persistent rehabilitation can achieve changes significant enough to make valuable improvements in quality of life. In practice length of stay in this kind of programme needs be considerable. Although this kind of intervention is costly it would appear justified if it leads to greater independence from long periods of unnecessary institutional care.

CONCLUSION

Since the early 1980s there has been considerable progress in the understanding of the nature and consequences of severe brain injury. Currently the pattern of service provision to the brain-injured population is changing. It is important to keep in mind what we have learned. Acute medical management has advanced and there are more brain-injured individuals surviving. Most rehabilitation workers are convinced of the importance of energetic management in the acute recovery period. Despite the lack of strong evidence of a positive treatment effect from early acute rehabilitation we do know that the effects of not intervening are disastrous both for the patient and the family. New behavioural methods have been developed to manage the behaviours often seen at this stage of recovery. In the late acute and post-acute phase of treatment we know that services should be functionally, behaviourally and socially oriented. Specific task training, behaviourally oriented social-skills retraining and behavioural control retraining, when carefully selected and obsessively applied can meaningfully affect real world functioning. Patients are moving out of acute rehabilitation hospitals and into community re-entry programmes earlier. Lengths of stay in these programmes are also becoming shorter (Jones and Evans, 1992). Many of these patients are still on what we might consider the acute stage of the curve of recovery. Also critical is the transfer of relearned function into real-life performance. Relapse or deterioration may be a very significant issue for a significant minority of individuals following brain injury (Brooks *et al.*, 1986). At the post-acute stage piecemeal behavioural engineering can significantly improve placement opportunities and quality of life. Finally, we know that many brain-injured people require very long-term treatment and support. We know that psychosocial outcome for brain-injured people is often terrible and the fact that the patient is neurologically damaged does not prevent them from having a significant psychological response to injury. Families also require long-term support. Although much more needs to be learned about how to help people recover from brain injury, keeping in mind what we have learned can help us be informed advocates for the needs of brain-injured people.

SUMMARY

Following severe brain injury many patients have cognitive deficits which are likely to interfere with their ability to make use of standard rehabilitation approaches. After the initial stages of recovery patients are often left with cognitive, behavioural and physical deficits. The more severe the deficits the more likely the individual is to be dependent, often putting great stress on family or care staff. Without appropriate intervention patients often deteriorate in self-help skills and social behaviour. Functional behavioural-learning programmes are particularly flexible in meeting the patient's needs, and can be used to present information in a way which maximizes the individual's chances for learning. The fact that even very handicapped patients have retained some capacity for new learning means that it is possible to teach patients new skills which increase their independence and reduce their unacceptable behaviour.

2 MEDICAL CONSIDERATIONS IN BRAIN-INJURY REHABILITATION

Martyn J. Rose

INTRODUCTION

In the USA and in the UK early rehabilitation usually follows the medical (illness) model. This model continues in the UK with a consultant physician to head the team and to wield the power, making many of the important decisions (for example about admission, treatment, targets and discharge). Unfortunately there is no career path that provides a sufficient source of appropriately qualified and experienced consultants, and many are still associated with rheumatology for reasons of history rather than good practice.

Doctors with a background in neurological or neurosurgical conditions are expected to cope with the whole range of neurological rehabilitation so that they are dealing with a difficult mix of progressive disease and traumatically acquired damage. The medical model ensures that many rehabilitation teams are similarly handicapped.

Individuals with acquired brain injury are often sufficiently different from those with other neurological conditions to make a dedicated service necessary. More Health Authorities are appearing to recognize this need, especially since the UK government injected a modest amount of money in 1994 (£5 million divided between 12 centres). However, financial constraints often mean that a very limited (and therefore inadequate) service is provided at best.

Rehabilitation aims to help the brain-damaged individual to minimize loss (handicap) and maximize function (independence). This active process may need to last for the life-time of the individual and must extend to involve the family.

Brain injury does not affect a representative cross-section of the population. There is over-representation of young, extrovert males, whilst people with a range of other problems (e.g. psychiatric illness, substance abuse) show an increased incidence (Ritzo and Tranell, 1996; Lishman, 1998). Every rehabilitation team needs to be aware of the pre-existing problems as they try to draw-out 'normal' function and behaviour from their group.

The brain-damaged adult has different management requirements at each stage of recovery. In the early stages supportive and preventative measures assume primary importance. Subsequently re-education (supplied by 'physical' therapists and others) is needed and later there is a need for a combination of some support and replacement or substitution for the abilities that have been totally lost.

Brain injury can be expected to produce physical, cognitive, communication, psychiatric, behavioural, social and other problems in varying combination and degree. It is generally accepted that the neuropsychological and neuropsychiatric sequelae produce the greatest handicap (Levin *et al.*, 1979a).

The severity of an injury is still best judged by the length of the period of post-traumatic amnesia (PTA – the time between injury and the return of *continuous* day-to-day memory). Many doctors still wrongly regard the first memory to indicate the end of PTA. Many appear not to know the agreed classification which is:

PTA up to 1 h → mild injury
PTA 1–24 h → moderate injury
PTA 24 h or more → severe injury

Other indicators are the length of coma, the Glasgow Coma Scale (GCS) (Teasdale and Jennett, 1974) score, or the time spent in hospital. However, often there is little useful correlation between the severity of injury and outcome although combining information presumed to reflect severity can increase predictive ability (Klonoff *et al.*, 1986).

Brain injury is sometimes missed in Accident and Emergency Departments and orthopaedic wards, or its severity underestimated with detriment to the individual outcome.

Follow-up services are patchy and often unhelpfully undertaken by the doctors who assume the role of primary carers – orthopaedic surgeons, general surgeons, or general physicians. All too often if the victim can walk and talk, they are considered to have made a good recovery.

Those with severe injury can show recovery extending over years rather than months and the belief that improvement ceases at 2 years (or less) should have been extinguished by now but, unfortunately and in some cases disastrously, this is not so.

Significant numbers of people with mild to moderate injury continue to show symptoms which are attributable to the injury more than 2 years after the accident whether or not litigation is involved. The majority of those with severe injury are reported to make a 'good recovery' (often by doctors or therapists with strong leanings to the disciplines of physical medicine), although that can include significant residual physical problems and may take little or no account of neuropsychological and neuropsychiatric problems.

There is a general assumption that the earlier 'active' therapy starts the better, but this may not be entirely true. However it is essential that 'passive' management in the earlier phases will have attempted to prevent the development of problems with, for example, posture/spasticity or behaviour.

Rehabilitation facilities demanding highly trained and motivated staff are still in lamentably short supply or even non-existent depending on the area of the country. On the positive side there are many more services available now than 10 years ago, but the picture is still patchy and inadequate with little apparent understanding of the life-long effects that brain injury can have on individuals and families.

There has been a laudable move towards better community-based rehabilitation, but resources remain impoverished (Freeman, 1997). In the USA services may or may not be available, depending on the state, but truly adequate care is available only to those with private health insurance.

There is still little evidence to show that rehabilitation works, although this is mainly because of the difficulties in carrying-out adequate research in this area (Eames and Wood, 1985a; Cope, 1995; Eames *et al.*, 1995; Freeman *et al.*, 1996). In recent years single case studies – a valid means of assessment – have appeared in increasing numbers (Alderman and Knight, 1997; Manchester *et al.*, 1997a).

Long-term management is commonly provided on an *ad hoc* basis and leaves much to be desired, especially in those cases with the greatest need. Many of the most severely handicapped people still face the prospect of placement – long term or short term – in hospitals or homes for those with learning disability or the elderly. As these hospitals are progressively closed, placement problems for the most vulnerable continue. An unknown proportion of individuals with brain injury in the UK are in prison, special hospital (secure hospitals for serious criminal offenders), or homeless.

MECHANISMS OF INJURY

Most brain injuries are acquired as a result of an acceleration/deceleration injury, in a road traffic accident (RTA), during sport or following a fall. Important rotational forces are also generated, and produce diffuse axonal damage (DAD) (Strick, 1956, 1969; Graham and Adams, 1971; Adams *et al.*, 1977). There is usually contusion to frontal and temporal poles, and to brain-stem pathways and centres, whatever the site of impact.

Secondary damage follows if the complications of raised intracranial pressure (RICP) and hypoxia/anoxia occur. Brain injury is associated with important changes to cerebral blood flow and cerebral perfusion (Teasdale and Mendelow, 1984), and there are important changes in neurochemistry which can affect the whole brain (Novak *et al.*, 1996). If the injury involves a skull fracture and scalp laceration, infection can produce further problems, although the problems of raised intracranial pressure may be reduced. Injuries involving a compound skull fracture (when brain may be visible through the wound) can look more frightening and serious, but may be associated with good outcome.

Focal damage may be produced by, for example, a blow with a blunt instrument and the prognosis in such a case can be good. Contrecoup (damage to the brain at a site opposite to the point of impact) injury may on occasion be more pronounced than the site of impact.

Rehabilitation teams are sometimes asked to deal with individuals whose brain damage results from subarachnoid haemorrhage, infection (such as herpes simplex encephalitis) or anoxia after cardiac arrest or insulin-coma.

Anoxic damage is still thought to carry the worst prognosis with major cognitive loss (especially memory) and handicapping behavioural change. However, some people with unequivocal primary anoxic damage have much less cognitive loss than would be expected despite major physical impairment. Sometimes there is a latent period between recovery from coma and the onset of profound neurological or mental disorder – classically in cases of carbon monoxide poisoning, but also reported after anaesthesia and cardiac arrest. No satisfactory explanation has been found (Richardson *et al.*, 1959; Bour *et al.*, 1967). In people with very severe injury neuropsychological assessment (which can provide essential information for physicians) can be extremely difficult (Wilson, 1996; McMillan, 1997)

The prognosis of acquired brain injury varies dramatically from case to case, sometimes depending upon the underlying cause of the damage or pre-morbid traits and problems but often for no predictable reason. Every individual must be assessed individually, without preconception, and reassessed as appropriate. Bizarre-sounding symptoms should not be dismissed out of hand. It is generally better to take the complaint at face-value.

WHAT GOES WRONG?

The human brain consists of an astronomically large number of neurons (10^{14}) and twice as many vital support cells. Each neuron can make up to 10 000 communications with neighbouring or more distant cells via synapses.

The neurons work by generating and passing minute electric currents from dendrites through cell body to axons whilst specific neurochemicals are released into each synapse when sufficient current flows in the cell. These chemicals (neurotransmitters) are made within the cell and transported to the site of use. Other chemicals (neuromodulators) influence cell responses. There is an efficient re-cycling process to enable neurons to respond regularly and reliably and to maximize the use of neurotransmitters.

The processes of the brain demand high energy expenditure. It has been estimated that 20% of the cardiac output goes to the brain, and about 20% of the body's energy demands are made by the brain.

Trauma triggers changes in brain structure and function, some of which may be permanent. Some of the processes of recovery (for example, collateral sprouting) may produce some of the complications seen later (for example, spasticity).

There is often debate about the presence of 'organic' brain damage – often in courts of law. The work of, for example, Gennarelli (Gennarelli *et al.*, 1982) is often cited by those who support the hypothesis that even mild injury can produce important organic damage. Disbelievers comment (reasonably) on the problems which arise from attempts to correlate research work on animals with humans. Nonetheless it is interesting to know that Gennarelli was able to demonstrate actual neuronal death in experimental animals subjected to relatively low velocity acceleration/deceleration injuries – even without head impact. Recent human research using SPECT (single photon emission computed tomography) scanning gives support to these animal studies (Kant *et al.*, 1997).

Many individuals with major neuropsychological and/or neuropsychiatric problems appear to show disorders of the mechanisms of arousal/alerting. They can show problems of reduced drive (apathy) or excessive drive (rages, hypomania, disinhibition) or may vary unpredictably and quickly between the two. These problems provide a major barrier to rehabilitation.

Patients with brain injury commonly do not have symptoms which fit conventional neuropsychological or psychiatric diagnosis (which is predicated on the existence of a circumscribed lesion, or probable discrete neurochemical dysfunction, or particular psychiatric diagnosis). Treatment teams must expect to find problems with arousal, perception, memory, emotion, organization, insight and self-monitoring (among others) (Dombovy and Olek, 1996; Hillier and Metzet, 1997).

NATURAL HISTORY OF RECOVERY

Once the life-threatening situations have been controlled, progressive recovery is the most common pattern. In broad terms, a brain-injured individual can be expected to be worse at the start (or at the height of any cerebral complication) with progressive improvement thereafter although there are important caveats. A very small percentage of individuals (often those with apparently mild, or even trivial injury) progressively deteriorate without clear reason. Individuals known to have been only briefly unconscious may ultimately report a PTA of many months and become physically, cognitively and emotionally dependent. Whilst such cases may have a degree of organic brain damage, such 'illness behaviour' requires psychiatric as well as physical therapy (Giles, 1994b).

Individuals who develop problems of 'confusion' leading to agitation and wandering or even aggression may be prescribed (inappropriate) neuroleptic medication which will compound the cognitive and behavioural problems. Such treatment may do nothing to reduce the 'confusion', and may well worsen the problem.

Improvement is often seen to proceed at a variable rate with a tendency to slow down as time passes. Recovery may be in a series of steps with periods of unpredictable consolidation in between. No-one can predict the rate or the degree of recovery. After some time has elapsed, the past rate of recovery may give some clues to the likely future rate but caution in giving prognosis, and a readiness to admit ignorance is the best policy.

Severe communication problems often form a very high barrier to rehabilitation, whatever techniques are employed. Occasionally individuals with near-complete aphasia may show flashes of normal communication (which are hard to explain) and the unwary or inexperienced rehabilitation worker may not readily realize how much communication depends on body language and tone of voice. Some physically well-recovered individuals who appear alert and attentive may not have their language problems fully appreciated in the absence of expert assessment.

Improvement in most areas of cerebral function (including physical change) has been clearly observed to continue for many years after injury, both with and without therapy. Complications such as hydrocephalus and epilepsy may slow, stop or reverse improvements and demand treatment in their own right.

The great majority of traumatically brain-injured people make good but incomplete physical recovery whilst large numbers are left with varying degrees of neuropsychological, neuropsychiatric and consequent behavioural impairment. These problems produce major handicap.

The effects of age on recovery are unclear. It had long been assumed that youth protected to a variable and unpredictable extent but this may not be true beyond the age of perhaps 9 or 10 years. More recent studies have suggested that the outcome for those under 21 with severe brain injury may be worse than the older group, perhaps because (in part) of the relative lack of important stored memories (Thomsen, 1974, 1989). The prognosis for those over about 60 may be poorer than those under 60. It is worth remembering that prognosis is commonly better than most 'experts' allow.

The work of Anthony Roberts (1979) remains one of the small numbers of long-term studies to consider life expectancy. Whilst an important study in its time, its relevance to the 1990s and beyond is questionable. The study accepted as cases individuals with brain injury from 1948 to 1961 and none received rehabilitation. Many will not have received the benefits of expert intensive care. Only a small number died young and many from infections which, almost certainly, would now be more vigorously treated. The ready use of gastrostomy-feeding now, which prevents much nutritional deficiency, may lead to less risk of infection as well. It is unlikely that such a detailed and comprehensive study will ever be repeated.

There is no generally accepted recent evidence to suggest that life expectancy is reduced for any but the most dependent group. Individuals who remain completely wheelchair bound or are very obese may have a shortened life expectancy. The same may be true for those with significant dysphagia (associated with inhalation of food and chest-infection – sometimes missed for surprisingly long periods) and urinary-tract problems (for example, the complications of urethral stricture) may also lead to a reduced life expectancy.

Studies have shown quite clearly that those with uncontrolled epilepsy (from any cause) may die suddenly and for no clear reason.

Dementia may appear earlier although clear evidence is still emerging. It is of course accepted that the 'punch-drunk syndrome' associated with repeated head-injury seen in boxers, footballers and other athletes is a real entity (Roberts, 1969). The influence of an individual's genetic make-up may be of much greater importance in the development of dementia.

The quality and quantity of care provided for individuals with severe impairment will often be the critical factor in determining life expectancy as well as quality of life.

A proportion of those with partial recovery (and the retention of the ability to understand their loss) commit suicide. They may not communicate their distress or intentions clearly in advance, and vigilance on the part of carers is the most important preventative measure. The increased risk of suicide has been estimated at 10–15%.

Grief affects a majority of the injured and the grieving process is lengthy – certainly taking years rather than months. The grieving process is complex and compounded by the fact that many losses occur some time after the injury. Thus relationships may break down after a number of years and the fact that unemployment will be the 'norm' rather than employment may not be appreciated for some length of time. Whilst the individual mourns the loss of physical and mental abilities as well as relationships, employment and financial loss, the family are also undergoing their own grieving reactions (Wood and Yurdakul, 1997).

Post-traumatic migraine is relatively common, possibly more so in those with better overall outcome. Prophylaxis with propranolol is often effective whilst antimigraine preparations should also be tried. Individuals with headache may also have mechanical problems with their cervical spine or their jaws whilst 'tension' may well add to the problems. Post-traumatic migraine may spontaneously resolve over 2–3 years, and some children may lose the symptom at puberty. Previously existing migraine has been recorded to be 'cured' by head injury.

Post-traumatic epilepsy affects a proportion of individuals with brain injury and most authorities accept an overall incidence of about 5% whilst the population 'norm' is accepted to be between 0.5% and 1%.

Jennett's (1975) work identifying high-risk factors is still quoted but further studies using computerized tomography (CT) and magnetic resonance imaging (MRI) brain scans are needed.

It is almost certainly the case that prophylactic anti-convulsants are of no value but anything up to 50% of neurosurgeons continue to use them. Many neurologists in the UK would still not treat one seizure but debate about the need to gain early and complete control if seizures continue.

Carbamazepine remains the ideal drug of first choice with sodium valproate a close second. Phenytoin (which must be used in individuals who cannot swallow in the early stages) has many unhelpful side-effects. Newer anti-convulsants may be of value but experience is limited (Childers and Holland, 1997). Vigabatrin probably should not be used, especially where there is a history of psychosis or behavioural disturbance (British National Formulary).

MECHANISMS OF RECOVERY

Initial recovery follows the resolution of brain-swelling, hypoxia, cerebral perfusion, electrolyte imbalance and neurotransmitter depletion. Later changes may be associated with axonal re-growth, collateral sprouting and neuronal additions. Other mechanisms which may account for the restoration of function in large tracts of neurons include substitution, compensation, redundancy, inter-hemispheric transfer and restitution (Robinson, 1986) – see Chapter 1 for a more detailed discussion.

ORGANIZATION OF SERVICES

Patients and their families benefit from the care and advice of experts at every stage of the treatment and recovery process. This is true whether the injury is mild, moderate or severe. The ideal brain trauma service would provide appropriate care for all at the right time, in the right place, and for as long as is necessary. The resources for such a service will almost certainly never be available. However all health-care workers should be given a greater knowledge and awareness of the problems that may occur.

The members of the rehabilitation team need to have a range of professional training and relevant personal qualities. The patients' needs range from the management of life-threatening situations through to physical and mental well-being; from total dependence to total independence. In practice it is very difficult to cope with ebb and flow of referrals.

The rehabilitation services to be provided should be based on three main levels of recovery, irrespective of time from injury – early, intermediate and late. The requirements at each stage are very different and need staff of differing training and ability. The brain-damaged person has lost far more function than any other traumatized patient whether or not there is multiple injury. Initially the 'medical model' of treatment is necessary, if not essential, but too often this leads too many people to assume that brain injury will be of little more problem than a broken leg. Treatment is made more difficult because of the inevitable interference with perception, learning, memory, communication and often 'executive' function (when drive, judgement, self-monitoring and awareness are diminished or lost).

GENERAL PRINCIPLES OF MANAGEMENT

Rest has long been recognized to be an important aspect of the management of all disease and trauma. Cerebral trauma is no exception. It is impossible to rest the brain totally but it is essential that all physical and mental activity is appropriately targeted.

Early recovery is characterized by the need for supportive, preventative and protective management. The management of the unconscious patient is well described in other texts and will not be detailed here (Teasdale, 1995). Respiration is controlled to ensure optimal levels of oxygen and carbon dioxide and to allow some control of intracranial pressure. Steroids are increasingly thought to be of little value in the control of brain-swelling after head injury, and there is no indication for prophylactic antibiotics or anti-convulsants.

Recently there has been an upsurge of interest in techniques involving cooling (hypothermia) although these techniques were abandoned in the UK in the late 1960s.

Interest has also been aroused by work (much of it in China) in the use of hyperbaric oxygen. In the USA Neubauer has written a number of papers strongly advocating the use of hyperbaric oxygen in brain injury – even many years post-injury (Neubauer *et al.*, 1990). As with all recommended treatments in brain injury further work is needed before these approaches should be uncritically accepted.

The background environment in which the person is nursed should be simple and uncluttered, with good lighting and a minimum of staff and visitors passing through. This approach ensures that stimuli reaching the brain-damaged patient are controlled at least to some extent.

Regular and careful observation of the recovery of function needs to be made to avoid the possibility of, for example, patients emerging from coma or mis-diagnosed vegetative state being under-treated or patients with well-recovered swallowing reflexes and adequate nutritional status receiving continued nasogastric or gastrostomy-feeding.

The more widespread and much earlier use of gastrostomy-feeding has produced very significant improvements in levels of nutrition which should reduce morbidity in the longer term. Efforts to establish swallowing and to retrain movements of lips, tongue and palate should start early with the speech therapist using techniques of icing and other stimulatory methods.

Anyone who is slow to emerge from coma or 'confusion' should at least undergo CT brain-scanning. MRI scanning should also be considered. Intra-cranial pathology is sometimes surprisingly severe in such people, yet may not leave any detectable structural deficit.

In the early stages, even simple and essential nursing procedures (such as turning the patient) will produce significant rises in intracranial pressure (ICP). The effect of these rises can be assumed to be potentially damaging to the recovering but vulnerable brain no longer adequately protected by automatic control mechanisms. These facts should urge caution to those who believe in 'maximal stimulation' of even comatose patients.

The effects of other forms of stimulation (especially sound, but also touch) is probably minimal. The benefits of early stimulation remain a matter of debate amongst practitioners (Wilson *et al.*, 1996).

Individuals commonly experience problems of impaired concentration and fatigue throughout their recovery. These problems can be expected to be maximal in the early stages.

When it is considered reasonable to start stimulation, it is better to use stimuli that are clear, familiar and given in short sequences with rest in between. The timing of the introduction of 'therapeutic' stimuli remains empirical. However, as there is evidence of depletion of neurotransmitter substances in the early stages of recovery, this alone probably argues for the restriction of early intensive treatment. There is the theoretical concern that under-stimulation at critical periods will lead to a continuing deficiency of neurotransmitters and neuromodulators, but no evidence is available.

There is still interest in the use of neuronal growth regulators but the 'window of opportunity' for their use may be short and very soon after injury.

MEDICAL ASSESSMENT

The doctor in rehabilitation medicine needs to reappraise all that has gone before. Some physical problems – sometimes of great importance – may have been missed and may require urgent treatment.

Prolonged bladder catheterization is associated with a 10–15% incidence of urethral stricture which can then produce complications of incontinence, infection, stone or renal failure. Be aware of the patient with dribbling incontinence and/or recurrent urinary-tract infection.

All patients should be known to have a good stream of urine. Expert urological review should be requested if in doubt.

Dysphagia requires assessment by experienced speech and language therapists and dieticians. If in doubt video-fluoroscopy should be undertaken. Be aware of the patient with recurrent chest infections.

Other complications of previous treatment (for example, tracheal stenosis or vocal-cord paralysis) are uncommon but usually more readily apparent. Treatment may be needed by otolaryngologists or thoracic surgeons.

Epilepsy can be difficult to diagnose and the clinician needs to retain a high degree of awareness of the possibility of the presence of some form of epilepsy.

Epilepsy remains a clinical diagnosis with EEG (electroencephalogram) as a supportive investigation. On rare occasions EEG, if undertaken routinely, will reveal grossly unstable 'epileptic-type' patterns in the absence of any clinical history. The clinician must decide whether it is ever reasonable to treat an EEG rather than actual epilepsy?

Hydrocephalus may produce a deterioration after initial improvement or simply a failure to improve. The classical symptom triad is reduced response level (or failure to continue to improve), developing ataxia and urinary incontinence. A CT brain scan is usually sufficient to confirm the diagnosis although intracranial pressure-monitoring may sometimes be required.

Mobility

Therapy aims to promote control of position and posture whilst continuing to minimize spasticity and tremor if present. The 'bilateral' neurodevelopmental (Bobath) approach to improving function is most commonly adopted and is probably best even if patients fail to continue to use it. However, there is still no evidence for the efficacy of any particular treatment method, and eclecticism is necessary. Claims have been made for the value of electro-acupuncture in the management of spasticity but it is probably only of use when there is also pain. In this and other treatment areas there is room for more controlled studies.

Tremor – sometimes in a relatively pure form of basal-ganglia dysfunction or cerebellar dysfunction but occasionally of mixed origins – is, if severe, disabling by itself and hard to treat. There is every reason to use medication to try to reduce tremor. The approach to use of medication is usually empirical, starting with the drugs least likely to cause additional problems, and progressing in an orderly fashion from propranolol through to tetrabenazine. Relaxation and biofeedback may help (Guerco *et al.*, 1997).

Thalamotomy is sometimes considered necessary for extra pyramidal-type tremors and also on rare occasions where tremor is so disabling. However there are perils to thalamotomy in people with brain injury who will have diffuse brain damage. The response to thalamotomy is much less predictable in such cases, and there may be unfortunate complications with regard to intellectual performance and behaviour.

Disorders of function of the hypothalamic–pituitary axis may become apparent. In the rare cases of a pituitary-stalk trans-section, the situation is relatively readily diagnosed and treatment successful directed by endocrinologists.

Debate continues about the likely symptoms from insufficiency of the hypothalamic–pituitary axis with some doctors believing that disorders of attention can result from insufficiency of (posterior) pituitary hormones with others considering that the almost ubiquitous complaint of fatigue may represent some insufficiency of adult growth hormone (Weingartner *et al.*, 1981). Most recently it has been suggested that the relatively common complaint of always feeling cold can be successfully treated using vasopressin (Eames, 1997). This is an area of neuroendocrinology which is in need of evaluation and research.

Neuropsychiatric assessment is essential – in conjunction with expert neuro-psychological assessment. Brain injury can produce any of the psychiatric symptoms seen in other conditions. It is now well recognized that all forms of psychiatric syndromes can be seen more commonly after brain injury than occur naturally. It has been estimated that schizophreniform illness, obsessive–compulsive disorders and bipolar affective disorders are at least twice as common after brain injury – sometimes following the less severe rather than the more severe injury.

It is always important to enquire about the possibility of even mild brain injury and to diagnose and treat the individual presenting with perhaps unusual psychiatric symptoms accordingly. However, as Gualtieri has stated

Physicians have little difficulty in diagnosing ABI [acquired brain injury] if the victim has a well-defined syndrome (hemiplegia, aphasia, topagnosia or cortical blindness) but seem less likely to recognize ABI manifested by symptoms involving arousal, attention, self-regulation, memory and initiative. When such problems are compounded by symptoms of anxiety, depression, emotional instability, somatic pre-occupation, and cognitive disorganization, physicians are much more likely to attribute the patient's difficulties to a functional or psychiatric disorder rather than to appreciate the link to neuropathic injury.

Gualtieri (1990)

The use of the membrane-stabilizing drugs such as carbamazepine may be much more efficacious than the more usual neuroleptics.

Brain injury creates problems in many of the basic areas of brain function so that there can be a disturbance of:

- arousal and alertness
- perception and perceptual integration
- memory
- mood-state and mood-control
- insight.

Any recognition of loss is complicated by complex grieving whilst an absence of insight produces all of its own problems.

As a result of underlying neuropsychological deficits a range of neuropsychiatric conditions can be seen. Major difficulty is produced by both problems of reduced drive (apathy) and over-activity/disinhibition. High-impact behaviour (aggression, sexual disinhibition) is common. Alcohol (ab)use to control 'tension' adds greater difficulty (Kreutzer *et al.*, 1995; Kelly *et al.*, 1997). In addition, and despite the accuracy of the comment by Thomas Gualtieri, some individuals do present with symptoms of predominant anxiety or depression or psychosis. In all cases of disturbed mental state the use of psycho-active medication is to be considered, whilst recognizing that environmental factors are of very great importance and that successful manipulation can be of great benefit (Hornsdean *et al.*, 1996; Powell *et al.*, 1996; Kraus and Mackie, 1997). Remembering the diffuse neuropathic cause underlying the symptoms may indicate the reasons for using drugs such as carbamazepine earlier rather than later, and in preference to the major tranquillizers (Anderson *et al.*, 1995).

Frontal lobe dysfunction affects many people with brain injury producing the dysexecutive syndrome. An individual may retain a veneer of social ability – sometimes for quite long periods – whilst having significant problems with, for instance

- ability to persevere with goal-directed activities (especially involving postponed gratification)
- shallow affect
- self-centredness (or exclusive self-awareness)
- altered rate of flow of language production producing loquaciousness, circumstantiability or over-inclusiveness.

These changes, sometimes hard to detect, may reduce significantly the individual's ability to use retained intellect.

Apart from the intensive care unit where claims are made for the use of intra-venous haloperidol and/or lorazepam in the control of acute agitation, the weight of clinical experience would be that major tranquillizers, even in small doses, worsen cognition and behaviour (Santos *et al.*, 1982; Garza-Trevino *et al.*, 1989; McShane *et al.*, 1997). The diffuse nature of the underlying causation may indicate that less selective (i.e. older) drugs may be of benefit when newer ones fail. It may also lead to the need for more polypharmacy than most doctors would wish to use.

The treatment of unusual problems, e.g. hyperphagia/pica has yet to be shown to be amenable to drugs (Read *et al.*, 1996). People with brain injury may respond to the usual doses of medication but on occasion are exceedingly sensitive or under-reactive. There is, for instance, evidence that some individuals achieve 'therapeutic levels' of carbamazepine on as little as 100 mg twice-daily while others may need 8–16 times that dosage before there is either therapeutic response or evidence of an appropriate serum level.

In some individuals drugs such as propranolol can reduce levels of over-arousal and thereby reduce the risk of paranoid ideation, and the need for a major tranquillizer, such as haloperidol.

CONCLUSION

The doctor in rehabilitation medicine works best when he or she recognizes the therapeutic limitations of medicine and medicines. The brain is a dynamic organ, exquisitely responsive to the (external) environment. Most drugs should be used sparingly, but important disorders of mental state should not be left untreated. Someone from the rehabilitation team may need to remain involved in patient and family care over many years if the best outcomes are to be achieved. Care is costly but probably cost effective, whilst lack of care ultimately kills.

3 THE PHARMACOTHERAPEUTIC MANAGEMENT OF BEHAVIOURAL AND EMOTIONAL DISTURBANCES FOLLOWING BRAIN INJURY

Tom W. Freeman

A pharmacological intervention directed at the complete eradication of an unwanted behaviour in a brain-injured individual is usually characterized by partial or complete failure. This is because, as a rule, behavioural and emotional disorders in severely brain-injured individuals do not occur in isolation, but exist as a portion of an entire picture of cognitive and functional skills deficits, so these attempts may fail because no pharmacological intervention can completely improve all areas of impairment simultaneously. The prescribing physician cannot hope to isolate an unwanted behaviour and exterminate it. This approach will fail and this failure is most often followed by frustration and disappointment on the part of the prescribing physician, the individual, and the individual's family. This frustration and disappointment may lead the physician to shy away from the use of medications of any kind in the case of less intrusive or less severe behaviours, or it may lead to polypharmacy (multiple medications used simultaneously) or high drug doses that impair function in the case of more severely disturbed behaviours.

At best, pharmacotherapeutic intervention in the management of brain-injured patients can improve learning and performance by enhancing existing abilities or decreasing the interference of unwanted behaviours. At its worst, pharmacotherapy can lead to worsening of unwanted behaviours and interfere with acquisition of new skills, retention, and performance. Occasionally, well-intentioned pharmacotherapeutic intervention may even precipitate new undesirable behaviours. However, even at their best, the most successful pharmacotherapeutic interventions are useless in a therapeutic vacuum. Since virtually no behavioural disorders in brain-damaged individuals exist detached from both a background of cognitive and functional skills deficits or from the surrounding environment, one cannot expect an isolated pharmacotherapeutic intervention to be successful. In short, one does not expect an elixir or pill to teach a patient anything, but one can expect rational pharmacotherapy to facilitate patient learning and improve overall outcome.

Behavioural and emotional disturbances are a frequent sequelae of brain injury (Brooks *et al.*, 1986a). When present, they may be the most significant obstacle to a good outcome. In order to rationally intervene into these behaviours, the prescribing physician must have access to and an appreciation of a variety of factors that contribute to the patient's overall care. These include the potential ill effects of medications on the function of the damaged brain, the time course needed for an adequate pharmacologic trial, the cognitive abilities of the patient at the initiation of pharmacotherapy, and a method of determining whether a targeted behaviour is in fact changed by intervention.

A certain degree of therapeutic pessimism is required in order to properly initiate and maintain a trial of a medication, since all medications offer both potential risks and benefits. Unless a medication is started on an emergency basis, the prescribing physician should fully inform the patient and their families or guardians of these potential risks and benefits before a therapeutic trial is begun so that all parties can weigh the possible advantages and anticipate potential hazards. The physician should be watchful for any suggestion of drug toxicity. This is particularly complicated in the brain-damaged patient, since these patients are often quite sensitive to subtle drug effects. For example, brain-damaged patients treated with low-potency neuroleptics such as chlorpromazine may manifest severe impairments in memory and arousal at relatively low dosages due to the high anticholinergic effects of the drug. On the other hand, similar patients treated with high-potency neuroleptics such as haloperidol may exhibit severe restlessness or akasthisia – a common adverse effect of this medication – and be given more of the offending medication in order to decrease their 'agitation'.

In addition to their sensitivity to drug effects, brain-damaged patients often require multiple medications for the treatment of various medical conditions. These medications may alter the absorption, blood concentrations, or breakdown of medications given for behavioural syndromes and lead to toxicity. In short, a full knowledge of potential ill effects and interactions for all prescribed medications is required for the physician working with the brain-injured population.

The time course for full pharmacotherapeutic effect of a given drug may be different for brain-damaged patients than non-neurologically impaired subjects. In general, it is longer. Patience on the part of the physician, the patient, and the patient's family is required for proper medication trials.

Prior to starting a medication, the physician needs an appreciation of the baseline cognitive/mental status of the patient. This allows for later comparison for evidence of improvement or decline. In addition, this allows the physician to appreciate the patient's cognitive strengths and deficits. For example, the aprosodic patient will usually appear emotionally depressed or blunted, although he may verbally relate that his mood is actually much improved. Another example would be the dysphasic or aphasic patient who may have great difficulty verbally relating his emotional state, but exhibits improved sleep, less fatigue, and improved appetite after a trial of antidepressants. The minimum (and most readily available) form of evaluation needed for this purpose are bedside evaluations such as those found in Mesulam (1985) and Ovsiew (1992), as well as other sources. If available, neuropsychological testing and structured observations of functional abilities prior to pharmacologic trials and at regular intervals thereafter are invaluable in giving the physician objective measures of a patient's overall status.

Last, the physician must have a method of integrating the myriad of signs and symptoms presented by brain-damaged patients into recognizable and coherent behavioural syndromes, which then can be targeted for pharmacotherapeutic intervention. In other words, the physician must have a strategy and a goal. To accomplish this, the physician must be fluent in behavioural abnormalities and have an objective means available to quantify behavioural changes. The latter requirement is needed because the patient is typically not able to give reliable, objective data. The physician should have available a charting system for recording specific target signs to be completed by trained staff; examples might include number of hours slept or number of verbal or physical assaults in a 24 h period. This can even be done with outpatients by enlisting the patient's family or guardian as a recorder of specific observations. The key word in both cases is 'specific' – broad, subjective impressions are simply not useful to the physician.

Behavioural syndromes manifest themselves as changes in patterns of behaviour. These patterns may be chronic or episodic in duration, 'positive' or 'negative' in nature, and since we are discussing pharmacotherapy, amenable to or resistant to pharmacotherapeutic intervention. The concept of positive and negative symptoms may require some explanation. 'Positive' symptoms are behavioural excesses, usually secondary to disinhibition, in brain-damaged patients. 'Negative' behavioural symptoms are deficit conditions – such as apathy, anhedonia, and motor impersistence – symptoms manifested by the absence of various behaviours. Of course, one can always confuse the issue by arguing that many disinhibited positive symptoms are actually the result of a deficit of higher cortical inhibitive functions, but it is usually more practical to consider symptoms such as aggression and sexual disinhibition as positive symptoms. As a rule, pharmacotherapy is more successful at decreasing the frequency and severity of positive symptoms than decreasing negative symptoms by augmenting brain function.

The following are a listing of some recognized behavioural syndromes. The reader should keep in mind that nearly every type of known behavioural disturbance has been reported as occurring after brain damage, so this listing is far from complete. Included here are the more commonly encountered and described behavioural syndromes associated with brain injury.

BEHAVIOURAL SYNDROMES

Apathy/amotivation

Apathy as a neuropsychiatric syndrome is a frequent sequelae of brain damage, in particular damage to the frontal lobes and subcortical areas. In an excellent recent review, Mann (1991) discusses the criteria for a syndrome of apathy and possible aetiologies for this syndrome. Apathy should be considered as a negative behavioural syndrome.

Apathetic individuals exhibit both a lack of internal drive and reduced responsiveness to external environmental stimuli relative to their previous state. This manifests itself in decreased goal-directed behaviour and decreased interest in previous activities, lack of initiative, decreased socialization, and lack of interest in new activities.

Apathy ranges widely in severity from simply exhibiting less interest in new learning or recreation to exhibiting no interest in maintaining critical functions, such as eating. As a rule, less severely affected patients rarely seek the advice of a physician. However, since this syndrome is so commonly encountered in brain-damaged patients, its recognition is vital. Immediate recognition is essential because apathetic patients cannot fully engage in necessary therapeutic activities. Since these patients are not well motivated by internal or external factors, their rehabilitative course is usually protracted and often a source of frustration to therapists.

Like all the behavioural syndromes listed here, the syndrome of apathy has a differential diagnosis. One must not include those individuals suffering from aprosodias or disturbances of movement alone. As Mann (1991) points out, a patient with Parkinson's disease may be physically inactive and appear emotionally blunted, but may be appropriately concerned with their usual responsibilities and goals in life and therefore would not qualify as apathetic. Probably the most difficult differential diagnosis to be made in these patients is between depression and apathy, since depressed patients are generally apathetic. These diagnoses differ in that in addition to inertia and lack of initiative, depressed patients frequently exhibit neurovegetative signs such as insomnia, depressed mood, constant fatigue, thoughts of suicide, and tearfulness.

Apathy may also be iatrogenic in aetiology. Various medications (for example, neuroleptics and some anticonvulsants) may induce this syndrome.

The neuroanatomic basis of apathy is poorly defined. As mentioned above, damage to the frontal lobes (common in traumatic brain injury) and subcortical structures such as the basal ganglia and thalamus are frequently associated with apathy, but damage to the non-dominant hemisphere and bilateral temporal lobe structures has also been cited as associated with this syndrome, supporting the contention that there is no unique structural lesion associated with apathy.

Neurochemically, dopamine deficiency is often associated with apathy. This is in part due to the presence of dopamine deficiency in several illnesses associated with apathy – such as neuroleptic-induced akinesia – and in part due to the improvement of some apathetic patients on dopamine-stimulating drugs such as amantadine, levodopa, and bromocriptine (Lal, 1988; Barret, 1991).

Disturbance of mood

Affective disorders are common in the brain-damaged population. These present in three forms: depression, mania, and mixed states. Depression is probably the most common mood disturbance associated with brain damage (Jorge *et al.*, 1993), with mixed states and pure mania seen less frequently. When these conditions occur as a clear result of brain damage, they are termed 'organic' in aetiology to distinguish them from similar conditions not associated with known damage termed 'functional' in the psychiatric nomenclature. Organic affective disturbances should be considered as positive syndromes, usually episodic in duration, and frequently amenable to pharmacotherapy. More has been written about depression after stroke than as a consequence of traumatic brain injury, but in general, depression after brain damage resembles 'functional' depression in clinical presentation. The diagnosis of depression in brain-damaged patients is complicated by several factors. First, the patient may not be able to offer a good history. Since much of the diagnosis of depression is based on a history from the patient, the diagnosis must then be made on the presence or absence of signs of depression such as changes in appetite, insomnia, fatigue, decreased socialization, thoughts of suicide, slowing of thought and activity ('psychomotor retardation'), and crying episodes. A second complicating factor for proper diagnosis is the similarity of depressive features to other common behavioural changes seen in brain-damaged patients such as the blunting of affect seen in aprosodic patients and the lack of drive seen in apathetic patients. This leads to confusion on the part of therapists, but a practical strategy is to look for depressive signs, target these signs, and follow these signs for improvement with antidepressant therapy.

A final complicating factor is the 'depressive' effect of many medications used to treat brain-damaged patients. Examples of these would be the antihypertensive propranolol frequently used to manage aggressive patients and the anticonvulsant phenobarbital.

Many medications can elicit depressive symptoms and it is the responsibility of the prescribing physician to determine whether a depressive illness or a medication effect is responsible for the patient's mood disturbance. Often a judicious discontinuation or change of medication can eliminate a 'depression'.

Mixed affective states (conditions in which depressive and manic signs and symptoms commingle) and mania are also frequent consequences of brain damage. Again, the diagnosis of these affective syndromes are susceptible to the same complicating factors mentioned regarding depression. Patients may not be capable of giving a good verbal history and so one must rely on vegetative signs such as sleep, appetite and physical activity; other common behavioural changes in brain-damaged patients can mimic these signs, so one must be cautious with the diagnosis; and these syndromes can be due to iatrogenic causes.

The literature on affective changes after stroke suggests that depression is more frequent in association with left-sided and anterior damage to the brain, while mania is more common after combined lesions to the right hemisphere and subcortex (Robinson and Starkstein, 1990). Neurochemically, while much has been written in the past regarding the catecholamines norepinephrine and serotonin in affective disorders, there is no clear consensus at present regarding a direct association between these neurotransmitters and affective disorders.

Aggression

When psychiatrists discuss speech, they differentiate between the form of speech and the content of speech. The form of speech is comprised of the patterns in which the patient expresses their thoughts. The content is what is actually said. Psychiatrists glean more from the form of speech than from the content of speech, since content is more or less unique to the individual patient. In a similar fashion, aggression has form and content. Brain-damaged patients may exhibit a variety of aggressive acts, but more can be gleaned from the precipitating circumstances and manner in which the aggression was played out than whether the act was verbal or physical or who was struck. When obtaining a history of aggression, it is important to ask the following questions so that proper intervention can be initiated.

1 Was the aggressive act premeditated? Premeditation implies planning and therefore intact memory and executive skills, which would be inconsistent with most severely brain-damaged patient's abilities.

2 Was the aggressive act precipitated by some environmental stimulus? Most aggression by brain-damaged patients is precipitated by environmental events which are small in proportion to the violent response elicited. For example, a frequent stimulus is touching the patient to change their clothing. In these patients, generalized apathy may be punctuated with brief episodes of severe verbal and physical attacks on staff, suggesting extreme defensiveness and stimulus misinterpretation on the part of the patient. Much more rare is completely spontaneous aggression.

3 Was the aggressive act preceded by a period of altered levels of physical activity, and do the acts of aggression follow a cyclic course or are the incidences of aggressive episodes fairly constant over time? Levels of varying activity with an increase noted in violent acts at the heights or depths of this activity may suggest an underlying affective disorder if accompanied by vegetative signs. Observation of patterns of violence over weeks or months may be required to answer this question.

4 Is the aggression goal directed? In the case of patients reacting defensively to touch, the aggressive act is directed at ceasing the unwanted touching. When the touching stops, the aggression stops. Alternatively, brain-damaged patients may simply physically attack the first object in their paths, animate or inanimate. For example, a patient may suddenly attack a chair or doorway in a fit of rage.

5 Is the aggression usually preceded by a brief period of physiologic arousal in the form of tremor, sweating, pupillary dilation, or flushing of the skin?

6 Is the aggression associated with sexual disinhibition? In many cases, male patients will assault only female staff and do so with clear sexual intent.

These features aid the therapist in determining the overall form of aggression exhibited by the patient. Physicians may be able to elicit these features by questioning staff regarding whether or not they can tell when a patient is 'getting ready' to be violent, and if they can, what is it exactly that they see?

Aggression that is predominantly or exclusively stimulus bound is usually exhibited by brain-damaged patients who are overtly disinhibited and may be generally apathetic. Although they lack initiative, their aggressive behaviour is usually goal directed. There is usually no form of autonomic arousal preceding the aggression and no vegetative features of an affective disorder are present. The violence is usually short lived, but occasionally these patients will escalate their behaviour in a perseverative, almost self-stimulating fashion. In patients where stimulus-bound aggression is common, evidence of frontal lobe damage is nearly always present. Sexual aggression is a form of stimulus-bound aggression, but treatment of the patient with predominant sexual aggression differs from other types of aggressive patients and will be discussed separately below. Another frequently encountered form of stimulus-bound aggression is territorial in nature, where the eliciting stimulus is entering the patient's self-defined 'territory' or perhaps even making eye contact with the patient. In these cases, defensive 'zones' are extended beyond the individual's body.

Spontaneous aggression – that is, aggression occurring in the absence of any possible stimulus – is rare. In these patients, aggression usually follows autonomic arousal, can be relatively long lived, and is later poorly recalled by the patient. Patients exhibiting this form of aggression may also relate a number of paroxysmal psychomotor symptoms in their histories such as olfactory hallucinations, rapid shifts in affect, and perceptual distortions and frequently have evidence of damage to the limbic areas of the brain.

Psychosis

Psychosis has been reported in subjects after a variety of neurological insults including traumatic brain injury, encephalitis, stroke, and even migraine headaches (Cummings, 1985; Fuller *et al.*, 1993). Psychotic symptoms secondary to brain damage may or may not differ dramatically from psychotic symptoms exhibited by patients with so-called 'functional' psychoses such as the schizophrenias. Therapists should note that some delusional states are typical of certain neurological damage (for example, the association of denial of hemiparesis with parietal lobe damage). Therapists must also keep in mind that there is significant evidence for neuropathological variance in schizophrenic brains, but unlike injuries from cerebral insults, neuropathological examination of schizophrenic brains suggests defects in normal maturation.

When symptoms such as delusions and hallucinations present after brain damage, they are designated as 'organic' in the current psychiatric nomenclature, just as affective disorders presenting after damage are termed organic affective disorders. Unlike typical 'functional' delusions, delusions in severely brain-damaged individuals are poorly organized as a rule and tend to be short-lived, lacking stability and consistency over extended periods of time. In fact, it is often difficult to discriminate between confabulation and delusions in severely brain-damaged or demented patients (Flint, 1991). More common among these patients is extreme suspiciousness that is stable and consistent over extended periods of time and may lead to episodes of aggression. However, some brain-damaged individuals present with very stable delusions as well as other symptoms typical of schizophrenia (Cummings, 1985).

In a similar fashion to non-brain-damaged patients, delusions may occur in combination with affective symptoms, and when they do they are congruent with the expressed mood state; for example, manic patients will present with grandiose delusions while depressed patients will present with delusions of illness or guilt. When present, these affective features greatly influence the physician's plan for treatment.

Hallucinations occurring in brain-damaged patients should not immediately be interpreted as psychotic symptoms. Hallucinations are defined as sensory perceptions without the presence of sensory stimuli and are common among brain-damaged patients as are sensory illusions – defined as misinterpretations of existing sensory stimuli. Before labelling a hallucination or illusion a symptom of psychosis and initiating some form of pharmacotherapy, the treating physician must consider several other possibilities. Could the hallucinations be a symptom of drug toxicity?

Is the patient merely misinterpreting an actual event, such as intercom communications? Could the hallucination be a manifestation of continuing or worsening cerebral insult? These questions must be addressed in the physician's mind prior to initiating treatment.

Self-injurious behaviour

Reports of self-injurious behaviours are more common in patients with developmental disorders such as mental retardation and severe personality disorders than in patients with brain damage due to trauma or stroke (Winchel and Stanley, 1991). When present in brain-damaged patients, it seldom takes the form of the 'delicate self-cutting' described in patients with personality disorders and frequently takes the form of head-banging or biting. Patients exhibiting self-injurious behaviour will often also exhibit externally-directed aggression.

Assessment of these patients should include a report of the frequency and severity of the self-injurious acts, as well as responses to attempted intervention, whether the patient exhibits any depressive symptoms, and whether the patient relates any obsessions or ritualistic acts that are not associated with self-injury.

STRATEGIES FOR INTERVENTION

Proper patient assessment is the most important component of a successful pharmacotherapeutic intervention. Communication between all involved parties, appropriate patience on the part of the physician and staff, and an adequate monitoring of target symptoms are the other necessary components to success. Assessment is a dynamic process, based on consistent observation of the patient over time. Proper assessment relies on the following components:

1 A history of the patient's pre-morbid condition, an objective history of events leading to brain damage and any complications of treatment, a history of the evolution of the patient's symptoms, family psychiatric history, and social history. Is the patient responsible for taking his or her own medications? Does the patient have history of substance abuse?

2 A history of any previous interventions (pharmacological or otherwise) to address the patient's behaviours.

3 Complete neuropsychiatric mental status exam, neurological and neuropsychological evaluation if warranted, and appropriate laboratory studies.

4 Assessment of all of the patient's current medications for possible untoward effects.

5 Ideally, assessment should also include a period of observation by the physician and staff in a controlled environment. This allows for an assessment of the responses of the patient to known environmental cues and a thorough assessment of the patient in terms of functional deficits.

The purpose of assessment is to define treatment goals. When assessment is complete, the physician and staff must define their goals. Any severely impaired patient will probably present with a number of behavioural disturbances, but pharmacological intervention must be directed at behaviours that are most likely to respond to this mode of treatment. An approach with a single target syndrome, a defined goal, and adequate monitoring is much more likely to be safely and successfully accomplished than targeting several behaviours simultaneously with poorly defined goals.

Once a target for pharmacotherapeutic intervention is established, it is usually helpful to measure the frequency of the behaviour in its unmodified state for later comparison. This may not be possible in the case of severe aggression or self-mutilation, which require immediate intervention. In the case of apathetic patients, one monitors the level of patient interaction and initiative.

Treatment

Instead of lengthy and technical discourses on treatment, the following case reports are offered for examples of pharmacological treatment of the behavioural syndromes discussed above. Unlike treatment of behavioural syndromes not associated with brain damage, i.e. 'functional' illnesses, the literature on pharmacological treatment of 'organic' behavioural disturbances is very sparse, containing few controlled studies, a great deal of extrapolation from animal data, and a wealth of unsupported opinion. Even so, one must start somewhere. References to useful supporting studies are made when this material is available.

CASE STUDY 3.1 Severe apathy

A 25-year-old female presents with a 7-month history of impaired self-care, poor concentration, and markedly decreased socialization after recovering from an episode of carbon monoxide poisoning and hypoxia after an unsuccessful suicide attempt. The patient shows little involvement in therapies, and reacts passively to feeding and toileting. If not passively engaged in an activity, she will remain seated and nearly motionless. She is on no medications. Mental status examination reveals gross verbal and motor perseveration, bilateral grasp°reflexes, and markedly aprosodic speech. Questions are answered with one or two words if at all. Staff observe no difficulties sleeping and no lack of appetite, although the patient does not initiate feeding. The patient's family comment on her speech as being 'robotlike' and her activity as being 'like she's empty – not really there'.

In the case of this apathetic patient presenting with no clear vegetative symptoms of depression, the literature would support a trial of a stimulant such as methylphenidate or antiparkinsonian agents such as levodopa/carbidopa combinations, bromocriptine, or amantadine (Barrett, 1991). Monitoring might include staff observations of altered mobility and initiative in self-care. Monitoring should also include possible untoward effects such as weight loss, insomnia, agitation, motor tics, or psychosis. These effects are less frequent if the physician is cautious, gradually increasing the dose to maximum beneficial effect and carefully watching for any unwanted complications.

CASE STUDY 3.2 Iatrogenic 'depression'

A 22-year-old male presents for a 2-year history of dysphoria, memory impairment, poor concentration, lethargy, increased sleep, and recent suicidal thoughts. He relates that his suicidal thoughts stem from the fact that he 'can't take being so tired and useless all the time'. He suffered a severe closed-head injury and developed a seizure disorder 2.5 years ago, for which he was treated with phenobarbital and phenytoin. Neither family nor patient can be specific as to either injury severity or length of coma. At the onset of his depressive symptoms his physician added amitriptyline, and more recently chlorpromazine for his 'agitation'.

CASE STUDY 3.3 Depression after stroke

A 56-year-old male presents for a 2-month history of decreased appetite, weight loss, lethargy, social isolation, and resistance to participating in rehabilitation after a left hemisphere cerebral infarction that also left the patient with a mild right hemiparesis and dysphasia. The patient currently takes no medications other than antihypertensives.

CASE STUDY 3.4 Mixed affective symptoms

A 25-year-old male presents with a 3-week history of decreased sleep without complaint of fatigue, increased physical activity to the point of agitation, and rapid speech. Although his physical activity and arousal have increased, he complains of dysphoria, feelings of worthlessness, and vague suicidal thoughts. He suffered a severe closed-head injury at the age of 18 years in a motorcycle accident (GCS unknown, according to his parents he was hospitalized for 3 months after the initial accident, length of coma unknown) recovered without complications, and had been in a good state of health until the gradual onset of symptoms over the last 3 weeks. Family psychiatric history is significant for recurrent depression and alcohol abuse in the patient's father and paternal grandfather.

Case Study 3.2 illustrates the role medications can play in the production of unwanted behavioural symptoms. In this case, phenytoin and phenobarbital – both known to adversely affect cognition – have been followed by the initiation of amitriptyline, an antidepressant with intense anticholinergic and antihistaminic effects, and chlorpromazine, a neuroleptic with a high degree of anticholinergic effects. The patient's 'agitation' following the initiation of amitriptyline was very probably an adverse effect of this medication. Medications with intense anticholinergic effects should be avoided for the most part in treatment of brain-damaged patients, since adverse effects are common. These adverse effects include dry mouth and eyes, blurring of vision, constipation, and, most important for brain-damaged patients, memory impairment and delirium at high doses. In addition, Case Study 3.2 illustrates the dangers of multiple drug interactions. Overall, it is wisest to use medications for which there are readily available serum levels, since many medications (such as phenobarbital) can alter the metabolism and serum concentrations of other drugs. For this man, it is wisest to attempt weaning from amitriptyline and chlorpromazine under controlled conditions and consider other less impairing anticonvulsants such as carbamazepine or sodium valproate if possible. If depressive symptoms persist, a trial of an antidepressant with fewer anticholinergic effects such as desipramine or an SSRI (selective serotonin reuptake inhibitor) should be considered.

Case Study 3.3 is typical of a patient presenting with depression after brain damage. In the past, depression after stroke was regarded as an understandable reaction to the loss of physical and cognitive abilities. Current research (Robinson and Starkstein, 1990) suggests that post-stroke depression is common (about 40% of patients experience depression in the first month after stroke and another 30% of patients may develop depression in the first 2 years after a stroke), associated with the site of infarction (depression is more common with anterior than posterior lesions and left-sided rather than right-sided lesions), and treatable. Depression after traumatic brain injury is also common (Jorge *et al.*, 1993), but less work is available on this subject. Pharmacotherapy for depression in brain-injured patients should be initiated once the physician has ascertained the depressive symptoms are not secondary to other medical problems (such as thyroid disease) or other medications. Tricyclic antidepressants are the most carefully studied interventions in post-stroke depression, but this is not saying much, since only one or two controlled studies exist. Again, it is best to initiate a medication for which serum levels are readily available (to monitor toxicity and compliance), and to be cautious, since the anticholinergic effects of many typical antidepressants can impair cardiac conduction. ECT (electroconvulsive therapy) has been shown to be effective for treating post-stroke depression (Murray, 1987) if pharmacotherapy is not an option.

The young man in Case Study 3.4 presents with symptoms of depression and mania. When faced with this collection of symptoms, as with any behavioural disturbance, the physician must consider the possibility of substance abuse as aetiology. If this has been ruled out, treatment can begin with a variety of medications, including lithium carbonate, carbamazepine, or sodium valproate. In addition, medications such as clonidine (Bakchine *et al.*, 1989) have been shown to be effective in treating brain-damaged patients with mania. Physicians may wish to consider the anticonvulsants carbamazepine or sodium valproate first in treating these patients due to the relatively low therapeutic index of lithium (memory-impaired patients may accidentally overdose if they self-administer their medications) and the overall efficacy of these drugs in treating patients with brain injuries (Pope *et al.*, 1988).

Physicians must also consider the potential for suicide or accidental overdose in any brain-damaged patient suffering from depression. Tricyclic antidepressants can be lethal in doses only slightly higher than regular daily doses, and physicians must be cautious in prescribing large amounts of these medications to patients.

CASE STUDY 3.5 Aggression and apathy

A 32-year-old female presents for a 2-year history of generalized apathy with episodes of physical aggression described as being brief, goal-directed, and almost always associated with toileting or clothing changes. The patient sustained a severe head injury (GCS unknown) and skull fracture in a hang-gliding accident that also left the patient with a mild left-sided hemiparesis. When not involved in therapies, the patient shows little animation and virtually no initiative. Acts of aggression cease completely after the patient is left alone. The patient exhibits no vegetative signs of depression except psychomotor slowing.

CASE STUDY 3.6 Spontaneous aggression

A 20-year-old male presents for a 10-month history of severe episodic aggression after a bout of viral encephalitis. Aggression is sometimes associated with environmental stimuli, but more often is completely independent of any discernible environmental 'trigger'. Episodes of aggression last for seconds to minutes, and are usually not goal directed. The patient often appears confused during and after the episodes and attempts to 'talk him down' nearly always result in an increase in violence. Leaving the patient alone does not decrease the level of aggression displayed by the patient.

CASE STUDY 3.7 Sexual disinhibition and aggression

A 24-year-old male presents for a 3-year history of aggression directed almost exclusively at females. The behavioural disturbance followed a severe traumatic brain injury (GCS and length of coma unknown). In addition to aggression, the patient frequently disrobes and masturbates in public.

Although aggression is not the most common behavioural sequelae of brain damage, it receives considerable attention in the literature. Unfortunately, aggression is often regarded as a unitary phenomenon. As noted above and in the preceding case reports, there are many forms of aggression, and by differentiating each patient's aggression profile physicians may begin to create a strategy for intervention.

The most commonly cited pharmacological interventions for the treatment of aggression are the antihypertensive propranolol, the anticonvulsant carbamazepine, and serotonergic agents such as buspirone, trazadone, and fluoxetine (Corrigan *et al.*, 1993). These medications have been reported to be effective and safe in the treatment of aggressive, brain-damaged patients. However, the most commonly used pharmacological interventions are probably neuroleptics and benzodiazapines. This is due to their ability to be given parenterally and their relatively rapid sedating effect. Unfortunately, these medications may exact a price in the form of long-lived increases in cognitive impairment with both benzodiazapines and neuroleptics, and potentially very severe adverse effects in the form of acute dystonia and tardive dyskinesia with neuroleptics. While neuroleptics and benzodiazapines may be a short-term intervention, their adverse effects often make them very poor long-term interventions.

Case Study 3.5 illustrates what is probably the most common form of aggression encountered in brain-damaged patients: aggression in the form of exaggerated defensiveness from a generally apathetic and under-aroused patient. Frontal lobe damage is very common in this group. Violent acts in these patients are almost entirely environmentally dependent. In fact, in severely impaired apathetic patients, essentially all activity is environmentally dependent. If left without environmental stimuli, these patients become inert. These patient's aggressive acts may be secondary to an inability to properly interpret their environment. Pharmacological intervention in these cases may be aimed at improving the patient's level of arousal, thus improving the patient's ability to properly interpret their environment and decreasing 'defensive' aggression. This intervention may take the form of removing various medications, or it may take the form of initiating antiparkinsonian medications or stimulants in hopes of improving arousal. Obviously, starting an aggressive patient on stimulant medication should be a task undertaken only with extreme caution. In addition, there is very little support for this approach in the literature (Allen *et al.*, 1975).

Stimulant medications may also be considered in patients who are impulsive, hyperactive, and aggressive but without vegetative symptoms of mania. In either under-aroused or over-aroused patients stimulants must be used with caution, always keeping in mind that these medications may increase agitation and irritability.

Case Study 3.6 is an example of a less frequently encountered, more spontaneous form of aggression. Evidence of damage to the limbic areas of the brain is typical for these patients. In fact, this form of aggression is frequently referred to as 'limbic dyscontrol'. Anticonvulsants such as carbamazepine, the beta-blocker propranolol, or both agents are often successful in the treatment of this form of aggression (Corrigan *et al.*, 1993). Propranolol is used in high doses (60 mg to more than 300 mg a day), and physicians should be aware of contraindications to the use of this medication before initiation. Another antihypertensive agent that has been cited as useful in the treatment of a wide range of behavioural disturbances such as aggression, anxiety, and affective disorders is clonidine, and this medication may be of use if propranolol is contraindicated. Again, the physician must be aware of the contraindications for use of these drugs alone and in combination before initiating therapy.

Case Study 3.7 briefly illustrates aggression associated with sexual arousal. Medroxyprogesterone acetate in depot form has been shown to reduce both sexually motivated and non-sexually motivated aggression in male patients (Blumer and Migeon, 1975). Dosages range from 100 mg per week to 300 mg per week (the latter dose being used in 'chemical castration'). Improved control of aggression with limited effects on sexual activities were reported with the lower doses. Physicians should take particular care to inform patients and families of the risk of adverse effects of this medication (for example, feminization) prior to initiation.

CASE STUDY 3.8   Psychosis

A 27-year-old female presents with a history of delusions for 5 years after the second severe head injury she sustained in a motorcycle accident (GCS = 7, duration of coma = 8 days). The patient's delusions are usually fragmented in nature and short lived, based on a misinterpretation of actual events. For example, the patient related to staff that her father had taken the job of radio announcer at a local radio station and she demanded to see him immediately (her father was an attorney living several hundred miles away). This delusion was based on the similarity of her father's voice to the voice of the radio announcer.

Despite the usually transient nature of her delusions, the patient also exhibited a few well-entrenched delusions; for example, she consistently explained to staff that her father was coming to visit her 'this weekend' even though the patient was not oriented to time on a regular basis. The patient displayed no vegetative signs or symptoms of an affective disorder.

As noted many years ago by Roth and Myers (1969), delusions in brain-damaged subjects may be delusions in the technical sense (false convictions in the face of clear evidence to the contrary), but these delusions are not usually outright rejections of reality. Instead these delusions usually represent failure to understand or properly integrate actual events.

Treatment of these patients is difficult. Once it has been established that there is no treatable affective disorder present, pharmacotherapeutic intervention is usually limited to neuroleptics. Neuroleptics are usually effective in the control of psychotic symptoms in brain-injured patients, but may have numerous adverse effects in this population, including cognitive and memory impairment, seizures, bone marrow suppression, and extra-pyramidal effects such as tardive dyskinesia, dystonias, akasthisia, and drug-induced parkinsonian symptoms. In general, the low-potency neuroleptics (such as chlorpromazine) will interfere with arousal, cognition, and memory to a greater degree than the high-potency neuroleptics (such as haloperidol), but the high-potency drugs will produce more extra-pyramidal effects such as akasthisia and dystonia. Newer neuroleptics such as clozapine have different risk profiles, but using neuroleptics for long-term treatment of the brain-damaged population with chronic psychotic disorders is frequently a no-win situation. Neuroleptics should always be used at the lowest possible dose to control psychotic symptoms

CASE STUDY 3.9 Self-injurious behaviour

A 16-year-old male presents 4 years after a severe closed-head injury sustained in a bicycle accident (GCS unknown, parents relate patient was in the hospital for 4 months) For the last 2 years he has exhibited gradually increasing episodes of self-mutilation and depressive symptoms. His self-mutilation takes the form of biting his fingers, tongue, and lips 20–30 times a day. Further self-mutilation is limited by the patient's lack of mobility. In addition to self-mutilation, the patient complains of fatigue, lack of appetite, insomnia, frequent bouts of crying, and suicidal ideations. He relates that the episodes of self-mutilation are prefaced by an urge to harm himself that is impossible to resist. He also relates that the mutilation does not hurt at the time it is done and that the sensation at that time is actually pleasurable. Immediately after the mutilation he feels both pain and guilt.

Self-injurious behaviour is certainly one of the most disturbing behavioural syndromes therapists may encounter. As mentioned above, self-injurious behaviours are more commonly described in mentally retarded, psychotic, and personality-disordered populations, but a fair number of reports exist regarding the incidence of this phenomenon secondary to various types of brain damage (Winchel and Stanley, 1991). Animal data and case studies suggest a role for serotonin agonists, opiate antagonists, and dopamine receptor antagonists in the treatment of this syndrome (Winchel and Stanley, 1991; Criswell, 1992). Specifically, D1 (dopamine one)-receptor antagonists are reported to be effective, but fluphenazine (a dopamine-receptor antagonist with mixed D1- and D2-activity) is also reportedly effective. Serotonergic agents such as fluoxetine and trazadone, shown to be effective in externally directed aggression, have also been reported to be effective in treating self-injurious behaviours. These will also be effective in the treatment of depressive illness that may accompany self-injurious behaviour. Opiate antagonists such as naloxone and naltrexone are reportedly useful in decreasing self-injurious acts, but the need for parenteral administration and short half-life of naloxone limit its usefulness.

In conclusion, pharmacotherapeutic management of behavioural disturbances following brain injury can be a difficult task, but it becomes an impossible task if attempted by a physician in isolation from the remainder of the treatment team. Although a poorly planned pharmacotherapeutic intervention almost always ends in failure, a well-considered pharmacotherapeutic intervention can be a tremendous boon to a patient's care. Planning, patience, good communication, careful monitoring, and appropriate expectations are the keys to therapeutic success.

4 THE PRACTICE OF BEHAVIOURAL TREATMENT IN THE ACUTE REHABILITATION SETTING

James C. Wilson, William Dailey

Over the past 20 years advances in medical management and early post-injury intervention have led to a remarkable increase in the survival rate from traumatic brain injury (Morgan, 1994). The improved survival rate may be attributed to improved pre-hospital care delivered by paramedics, the emergence of trauma centres, and improved coma management. In parallel with this improvement in the outcome of the injured person, has been the increased demand for acute rehabilitation services. The value of early rehabilitation in treatment of brain injury has been demonstrated (Carey *et al.*, 1988; Sahgal and Heinemann, 1989). The growth of brain-injury rehabilitation settings (Cope and O'Lear, 1993), while in itself astonishing, has also increased the demand for professionally trained and educated staff familiar with the intricacies of brain-injury rehabilitation. Current approaches require highly trained staff who can work in an interdisciplinary team (Cowley *et al.*, 1994). The rehabilitation team process involves the delivery of services with the aim of improving the overall health and functional capacity of the injured person. The rehabilitation of the brain-injured person is itself, in essence, a medical-behavioural process, guided through the expertise of an interdisciplinary team (Muir *et al.*, 1983)

The recent trend toward managed care in the USA has threatened many health-care delivery models. This trend has created a challenge to the quality of health care and poses a threat to the existence of centres of excellence in brain-injury rehabilitation that have developed over the past 20 years.

The provision of adequate and experienced rehabilitation staffing poses new difficulties for programme administrators and directors, who must bow to the new health-care economics. It is our assertion that the conceptualization of the rehabilitation process *as a behavioural approach*, may enable services to be coordinated by the treatment team around common functional objectives, while at the same time managing costs most effectively. In this chapter we explore the benefits of implementing a behavioural approach in the acute rehabilitation unit.

Unlike the rehabilitation of patients with other types of trauma, brain-injury rehabilitation encompasses a wide array of unique and critical issues. The implementation of treatments in the acute rehabilitation setting involves skills and knowledge in more than the traditional areas of physical medicine. The treatments require an integrated approach, weaving the knowledge of many professional domains into patient care (Muir *et al.*, 1983).

Of particular importance is the need for the integration of behavioural management strategies and techniques.

The need for systematic application of behaviour-modification procedures is especially critical in the rehabilitation of head-injured patients. Given their cognitive deficits, these individuals often cannot comprehend the connection between a therapeutic exercise regimen and long-term goals.

(Muir *et al.*, 1983, p. 382)

When a brain-injured person is entering the rehabilitation phase of recovery a number of cognitive disorders can impede, limit or block progress. These cognitive disorders include perceptual and sensory deficits; impaired concentration, attention, and memory; language dysfunction; and processing and executive problems. These problems can reduce the capacity of the injured person to use abstract thinking, and engage in meaningful problem solving (Muir *et al.*, 1983).

This chapter describes the use of behavioural approaches in the acute setting and factors that can affect the delivery of behavioural services. We examine medical acuity, behavioural assessment and monitoring, medical management issues, patient treatment history, the nature of cognitive impairments, the influence of pre-morbid personality, the rate of recovery, the significance of environmental factors, the types of behaviour problems, the timing of behavioural interventions, the types of reinforcement, the use of structure, the significance of family education and counselling, the generalization of behavioural gains to the discharge setting, the team approach, and the important issue of cost management. Brief case examples are used to illustrate these issues and, finally, a comprehensive case study which touches on many of these topics is presented.

ACUTE REHABILITATION

In the acute rehabilitation setting medical management is supplanted by rehabilitative treatments, and the brain-injured individual begins the difficult and arduous process of redefining the changed sense of self (Cope and Hall, 1982; Ragnarsson *et al.*, 1993). The acute rehabilitation process begins when the brain-injured person is medically stable, and able to benefit from rehabilitative treatments. Patients may range from the minimally responsive (those emerging from a coma or vegetative state) to the maximally responsive (aware of his or her limitations and motivated to pursue treatment). Although the acute rehabilitation setting is focused on treatment and recovery, this does not imply that patients are without significant medical problems, many of which were formerly managed in the acute hospital setting.

INITIAL ASSESSMENT AND PHILOSOPHY

The complexities of the early phase of acute rehabilitation necessitate a careful balancing of different treatment modalities, medical, behavioural, and physical. Each treating discipline conducts important initial or baseline evaluations, which form the basis for guiding the individual's functional recovery in ambulation, in activities of daily living, and in cognitive and linguistic functioning. The integration of these assessments, the timing of interventions and the management of medical complications including hydrocephalus, seizures, and heterotopic ossification, require teamwork, communication, and careful coordination as attention cannot be paid to one issue at the neglect of another (Ragnarsson *et al.*, 1993).

Brain-injured patients at the acute level frequently receive numerous medications all of which can affect behaviour (Cope, 1994). It is important to assess changes in medication when evaluating changes in behaviour. Close cooperation between medical and other treatment staff is critical to monitor the side-effects and other consequences of the use of medication. However, it is also important not to treat 'learned behaviour' only through medication. One of the most common causes of behavioural outbursts in the acute setting is pain. Rigorous range of motion is often indicated early in brain-injury rehabilitation, when cognitive limitations and medical condition inhibit motoric functioning. Range of motion is frequently painful due to a high degree of muscular tone and in some cases the presence of heterotopic ossification. Difficulties in integrating stimulation by the patient can also compound this effect. Range of motion and many nursing procedures, can be invasive for the patient and are often the cause of the first aggressive behaviours exhibited. Medications to address pain are problematic at this point, because the patient is also cognitively impaired and pain medication that further impairs cognitive processes and slows learning is contraindicated. Patients in this phase of recovery often have little capacity to suppress reactions to noxious stimuli, and may be easily irritated and act or respond vigorously to try to remove the source of irritant, such as a feeding tube.

There are other medical procedures in the acute phase of brain-injury rehabilitation that may trigger behavioural outbursts or agitation. Assessing, monitoring and treating patients for a variety of medical risks such as seizures can be a difficult task. Transporting patients to off-site facilities, and requiring them to be calm and remain still through a lengthy process, is difficult and frequently requires the use of sedating medications. Staff at non-specialist centres are ill-equipped to deal with this type of patient. It is important to develop a relationship with non-specialist settings used for evaluation or treatment, in order that proper training may be provided for staff who will interact with the brain-injured patient so that they understand the difficulties being faced in assessing these patients. If not located in the same building, the acute rehabilitation unit will need to work with the local general hospital to schedule multiple procedures to occur at the same time whenever possible. Once medicated, the patient would be transported, the procedures completed, and upon return to the rehabilitation unit, the staff would complete many other difficult activities such as nail cutting, blood drawing, etc. In this manner, only 1 day of treatment is lost to the completion of many necessary tasks and procedures, further episodes of sedation are avoided, the staff face fewer scheduling problems, and information is gathered more rapidly.

Another problem that must constantly be addressed on the acute rehabilitation unit is the question of how restrictive to make the environment for reasons of safety. Safety must always be maintained, and yet there is a fear of litigation that can at times clash with the rehabilitation needs of the patient. It is important to monitor safety throughout the entire rehabilitation process, but also to strive for the least restrictive environment that will still keep the patient and others safe. A quality assurance or quality improvement committee in the acute rehabilitation hospital, composed of multidisciplinary staff, is highly recommended. The function of this committee is to discuss specific incidents of harmful or unsafe behaviour (e.g. falls, assaults, 'AWOL' attempts, etc.), and to devise corrective plans, keeping in mind treatment goals, safety and facility regulations.

SPECIALIZED MANAGEMENT OF BEHAVIOURS RELATED TO MEDICAL COMPLICATIONS

The types of medical problems encountered in the rehabilitation setting dictate that behavioural approaches be altered to accommodate medical needs. These include: the use of IVs, nasogastric and gastric feeding tubes, tracheotomies and respiratory care problems, positioning and skin-care concerns, blood pressure problems (postural hypotension), seizures, abnormal muscle tone and contractures. Additionally, the risk of heterotopic ossification (periarticular calcium deposits), may be a concern in some cases. Each of these medical issues may complicate behavioural interventions, and require specialized management strategies. It is not uncommon to see a brain-injured patient attempt to pull out or remove a feeding or tracheotomy tube. Behavioural interventions should, in such instances, be geared to patient safety, and cognitive level. The Rancho Los Amigos Scale of Cognitive Functioning provides a schema for cognitive recovery that is useful in judging what intervention may be used, based on the individual's level of cognitive/behavioural functioning (Hagen *et al.*, 1977) (Table 9.2). With an agitated and confused patient, the use of soft-restraints, mitts, and/or an abdominal binder is sometimes helpful in preventing tube pulling. Due to the severe limitation of the Rancho level III–IV patient, mitts allow the patient to localize and rub, but prevent grabbing. Abdominal binders put the tube out of site and add one more layer to be dealt with before being able to remove a gastrostomy tube. Both the mitts and the binder allow the patient to move without the use of more restrictive restraints.

Range of motion is often prescribed for heterotopic ossification to prevent 'locking' of joints due to calcification (Garland, 1980; Berrol, 1983). While critical medically, this procedure has a high degree of associated pain and discomfort. In a confused and agitated patient, tolerance for pain is limited and so behavioural management strategies are needed to assist them in tolerating range of motion. Such strategies may include 'counting', mental distraction, and brief treatments with immediate reinforcements. Counting allows the patient to be involved in the process and have some control over its completion. For example, the therapist can cue the patient, 'I want you to count to five with me. At five, we will stop and rest'. Invariably the patient will attempt to count to five at an extremely accelerated rate so therapy staff should either have the patient count with them, or change to a target number that will last for approximately five seconds. If painful procedures are not structured in a therapeutic manner, the patient can become conditioned to respond with aggressive behaviours (Watson, 1924).

When orthopedic procedures are required they should be timed, if at all possible, to coincide with the decline of agitated and combative behaviours, due to the negative impact of protracted pain on the recovery process when agitated behaviours are present.

An example of the timing of interventions can be seen in the following case study.

CASE STUDY 4.1

The patient was a 20-year-old male injured in a motorcycle versus automobile accident 2 years prior to admission to the unit (Rancho level IV–V). Following his accident he was in a coma for approximately 2.5 months, and was treated unsuccessfully in a prior facility. On arrival at our unit he required a specialized behavioural programme consisting of initial desensitization and token economy. The frequency of negative behaviour (e.g. hitting and biting) dropped precipitously with the success of these interventions and improved medication management. Surgical interventions were carried out at the end of the period of stabilized behaviour, several weeks prior to his discharge to a community setting (see Fig. 4.1).

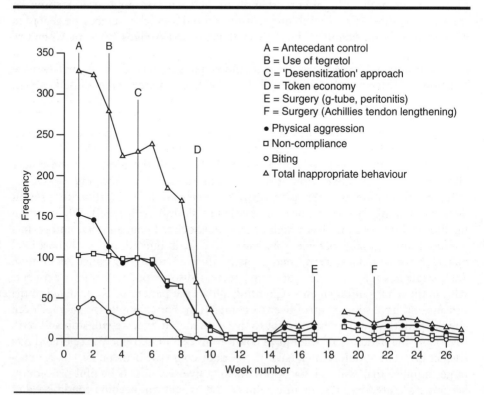

A = Antecedant control
B = Use of tegretol
C = 'Desensitization' approach
D = Token economy
E = Surgery (g-tube, peritonitis)
F = Surgery (Achillies tendon lengthening)

• Physical aggression
□ Non-compliance
o Biting
△ Total inappropriate behaviour

Figure 4.1

COGNITIVE IMPAIRMENTS

The nature of brain damage

The consequences of brain injury depend on the location and extent of the lesion and vary greatly from person to person (Miller, 1984). No two brain injuries have the same consequence, given the presence of interindividual differences, different aetiologies, and, in some cases, multiple aetiologies. Many approaches are available in classifying injuries and aid an understanding of their overall cognitive and behavioural significance:

- primary versus secondary injury
- focal versus diffuse injury
- subcortical versus cortical injury
- polar injury versus intracerebral damage
- grey matter versus white matter injury
- axonal versus neuronal injury
- right hemisphere versus left hemisphere injury
- traumatic, anoxic, metabolic, infectious, vascular
- frontal, occipital, parietal, and temporal lobe foci.

Behaviour following brain injury may vary greatly from one person to the next, with the functional impact expressing itself in different ways (Miller, 1984). A frontal lobe injury (i.e. pre-frontal cortex), expresses itself in ways very different from an occipital cortex injury. In the case of the former, judgement, reasoning, insight and ability to self-regulate or monitor behaviour may be greatly impaired. In the case of the latter, the individual may experience 'cortical blindness', leading to anxious and disoriented behaviour secondary to failure to see patterns or objects accurately or at all.

Aside from the primary lesion or injury, secondary damage to the brain often occurs as a result of oedema, elevated intracerebral pressure, intracranial infection, hypoxic or ischaemic injury, uncontrolled seizures and brain herniation. In some instances the effect of the secondary damage to the brain may be more devastating than the primary lesion itself (Jennett, 1983).

Sensory impairment and sensory integration difficulties

Sensory loss, involving more than one modality, is not unusual following brain trauma. Alterations in the senses of vision, hearing, touch, temperature, position, pressure, and awareness of pain, may occur in varying degrees. Such deficits may impact, not only the behaviours associated with activities of daily living, but may also interfere with the provision of treatments. A careful assessment of the role of these deficits is essential in managing problematic behaviour.

Language processing deficits

Like sensory impairments, language-related brain dysfunction poses special problems in the acute rehabilitation setting. The traumatically brain-injured person is often unable to process the normal cadence and rhythm of speech, may persever-ate on responses, have difficulty retrieving a specific word, and be unable to articulate a personal need effectively (see Chapter 9).

Memory and learning deficits

Memory impairments usually follow significant brain injury, although the nature of the memory impairment may vary greatly from one individual to the next. In some cases the person's memory problem stems from impairments in the person's arousal or attentional processes, which makes the complete and accurate encoding of infor-mation difficult. The distinction between attentional processing and retrieval is important in determining why there is memory dysfunction. Accurate, timely and repeated (serial) neuropsychological screening, i.e. the Galveston Orientation and Amnesia Test (GOAT) (Levin *et al.*, 1979b) or the Barry Rehabilitation Inpatient Screening of Cognition (BRISC) (Barry *et al.*, 1989), may be the best means through which memory functioning is explored, and an appropriately tailored treatment approach developed. Repeated, simple cueing to tasks (or task elements) in the early stages of recovery and integration of self-employed strategies in the later stages (e.g. therapy log or notebook), coupled with behavioural reinforcement (praise or recognition) for completed or self-initiated tasks, are ways of structuring treatment to accommodate memory loss.

Executive dysfunction/higher level deficits

Higher level impairments are major issues in the assessment and treatment of persons with traumatic brain injury (Lezak, 1993). Neuropsychologists have strug-gled with the development of adequate and reliable means through which these deficits and their impact on functional living can be assessed (Hart and Jacobs, 1993). While formal standardized assessment is often problematic, the behaviours associated with the dysexecutive syndrome can determine the patient's overall outcome. The frontal lobes are primarily associated with disorders of executive function. Common brain-injury-related behavioural symptoms of frontal lobe disorders include: disinhibition, loss of social restraint, poor impulse control, lack of self-monitoring ability, decreased insight (see Chapter 10), altered pacing or regulation of sequence-dependent tasks, poor planning and organization, impaired reasoning and abstraction, and the absence of an 'overview' in thought (loss of the 'abstract attitude'). Such executive functions are critical in the development of an accurate sense of self, post-injury, and in the person's motivation and follow-through with treatment. Because frontal lobe injury may alter the self-initiating and drive components of personality, the behavioural implications are profound. Social, interpersonal, and vocational aspects of adjustment are negatively impacted (Schwartz *et al.*, 1993).

Integration of neuropsychological data

The role of neuropsychological assessment in brain-injury rehabilitation is critical in providing information to the treatment providers or team members on the degree of cognitive impairment and improvement, the rate of improvement, and

residual problems. Serial neuropsychological testing is widely practised in rehabilitation of brain-injured patients, and involves repeated testing at set time
intervals. Although practice effects may occur with repeated testing, memory
impairments following brain injury limit the confounding effects of repeated trials.
Whenever possible utilizing alternative forms of tests, or tests less easily influenced
by practice is recommended. GOAT (Levin *et al.*, 1979b), is a test of basic
orientation to self, setting and circumstances. The return of continuous memory
with emergence from post-traumatic amnesia may be assessed with this test, which
can be administered on a serial basis.

Serial testing can demonstrate patterns in recovery of function following brain
trauma. Figure 4.2 shows GOAT scores contrasted with the total frequency of physical and verbal aggression in a single patients and demonstrates the inverse correlation between cognitive impairment and negative behaviours. Figure 4.3 illustrates
the same phenomena using the BRISC (Barry *et al.*, 1989). In this case, the cognitive
improvement occurred following the patient's emergence from coma, and the
negative behaviours peaked and then began to decline with further cognitive gains.

Types of problem

Behavioural problems which may follow brain injury can be described as positive
or negative disorders. Positive disorders are behaviours that are outwardly focused
or active behaviours (i.e. aggression, abusive language), whereas negative disorders
refer, typically, to an absence of behaviour (aspontineity or behaviour lacking drive
or initiative). Behavioural treatment of positive disorders has been more

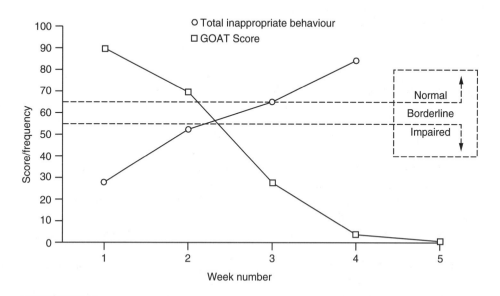

Figure 4.2

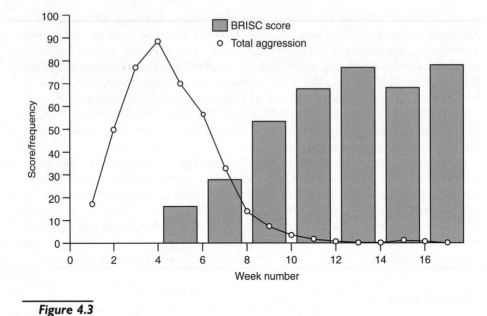

Figure 4.3

researched, and these disorders, in some respects, are easier to get a 'handle on' than the disorders of initiation. Positive disorders, being outwardly focused, are readily apparent and generally problematic at earlier stages of recovery. Negative disorders may be overlooked in a structured setting, due to the prompting and support provided by the staff and the environment. Drive disorders may not be fully realized until the patient has moved to a post-acute setting or to the home environment.

Agitation

Agitation is an early sign of emergence from coma. Initially the agitation may be non-specific associated with severe confusion, disorientation, and sensory-motor impairment. Later, agitation may occur only in specific circumstances and is typically a product of overstimulation or lack of ability to manage stimulation in the immediate environment. Agitation can lead to inappropriate behaviours such as biting, hitting, grabbing, and scratching at or toward anyone who comes within reach. The aggressive behaviours at this time are non-discriminating and will be directed toward others, objects, or even the patient himself or herself. When learned behaviour (conditioned responses or operant learning) increases, the agitated behaviour may give way to more specific aggression (see Fig. 4.4). Agitated and confused behaviour should be treated with the least restrictive approach possible. For example, allowing the patient to move about freely in a floor bed, or bed enclosure, as opposed to restraining the patient in a standard bed, may help facilitate better management of the agitation, and provide more restful sleep for the patient.

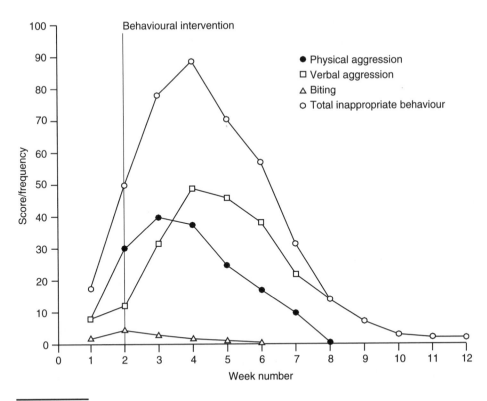

Figure 4.4

Physical aggression

Physical aggression is frequently a major impediment to rehabilitation. The aggressive patient can significantly limit his or her own recovery by attempting to physically assault others, reducing treatment time, preventing therapists from performing needed procedures due to the danger to the therapists or the patient. Adequate staff preparation, training in the safe management of aggressive behaviours, and behavioural interventions, can make the difference between success and failure in the treatment of an aggressive patient. Standard psychiatric interventions in the physical management of aggressive behaviour, however, may not be appropriate in brain-injury rehabilitation, due to the aversive and potentially injurious nature of this type of protocol with medically compromised individuals. The cognitive contraindications of neuroleptic medications, particularly pheno thiazines, in the management of aggressive behaviour following brain injury have been described (Cope, 1994).

Verbal aggression

Verbal aggression is not as problematic as physical aggression, except to the degree that staff, visitors or family may become uncomfortable, alarmed, resistant, or over respond while interacting with the brain-injured patient. Distressing as it may be, verbal aggression can usually be managed or modified through a number of approaches, including redirection, non-reinforcement, and situational time-out.

Non-participation

Non-participation can usually be addressed through a graduated approach, and through preferred reinforcers, shorter sessions of increasing length (shaping and chaining) (i.e. nap time following physical therapy). Non-participation (or refusal to participate) is usually amenable to operant approaches. Manipulative behaviours such as scheming to avoid therapy by deliberate self-soiling, however, require a far more active and unified team approach, with consequences and rules (sometimes taking the form of contracts), spelled out clearly, along with positive incentives for appropriate behaviour. Manipulative behaviour is often the result of pre-morbid tendencies which, in the presence of less social restraint and self-awareness, become more pronounced.

Apathetic behaviours

Apathetic behaviours pose special challenges for the rehabilitation team. When severe frontal lobe injury limits the patient's motivational state, including initiation, problem-solving skills, and the ability to self-monitor, and operant approaches fail (i.e. chaining and shaping), then medical interventions need to be entertained, including the use of medication trials that may improve the degree of arousal in the brain-injured patient (e.g. stimulants and some antidepressants). If behavioural and pharmacological interventions fail over time, maximum structure and external cueing may be required within the living environment on an ongoing basis. Such a condition unfortunately imposes a greater degree of institutional dependency and may significantly limit discharge options.

Structure

The term structured living environment is used often to describe interventions with combative brain-injured patients. What exactly does this structure entail? The first priority in providing structure is consistency, both in staffing and approach to interaction, without it, therapeutic progress through learning may not be possible due to the patient's cognitive deficits. Development of a programme structure takes time and considerable effort from staff and administration but with persistence, what, at first seems artificial, can become routine and make life easier for both patients and staff. The concept of reinforcement, becomes practised within the level of structure provided by all staff. Reinforcement programmes must be general enough to be able to be reinforced by all treatment staff in the facility and yet must be individual enough to motivate and meet the needs of each resident.

Environment

The management of the environment on the brain injury unit is a form of antecedent control (see also Chapters 5 and 6). The creation of a therapeutic environment is the first goal in brain-injury rehabilitation, with attention to managing such things as lighting, sound and noise, extraneous or unnecessary contact with others, activity availability, and accessibility to fixtures in the patient's room. Careful assessment at all phases of rehabilitation, in regard to environmental influences or hazards, is always indicated. Initially staff must anticipate the needs and difficulties that may arise for each patient and intervene as necessary. As the patient improves, there is a shift toward a greater degree of independence, and 'shadowing' (the assignment of a one-to-one observer or nursing assistant) is frequently warranted, especially where safety considerations, wandering or elopement may be concerns. Shadowing should never be intrusive, but provide a line of sight on patient behaviour, yet still be close enough for intervention, when necessary. This allows for the patient to continue to explore his or her environment in a safe manner with the minimal use of restraints.

Data collection

Behavioural data collection facilitates the understanding of recovery processes through the use of objective, quantifiable measurement and tracking, and the increased ability to correlate events or alterations in the environment with that data. The advantages of standard behavioural methodology has been well documented in the clinical setting (Kazdin, 1994). In brain-injury rehabilitation, the ability to carry out controlled behavioural planning is more limited than it is in traditional psychiatric or institutional settings, due to the acute treatment process, the inability to control medical variables, and because of the unknown factors influencing recovery. Nonetheless, behavioural monitoring plays an important role. In addition to measuring targeted or specific behaviours (i.e. physical aggression, verbal abuse, unsafe standing), behavioural measurement is a cornerstone in overall treatment. For example, the efficacy of treatment regimens, including medication protocols, requires an objective data collection system, so that interventions can be systematically and carefully examined, and where the contributions of single factors can be weighed against the background of overall change.

The collection of data is an ongoing process that can require many adjustments to ensure accurate and reliable results. The system of data gathering must be simple, quick, and painless for staff in order to achieve maximum staff compliance. Recording forms can either be kept in a central location or given to specific team members to be completed and returned weekly. One of the most efficient and effective ways to collect data is a grid listing specific behaviours. Staff need only record simple hashmarks to indicate incidents. This method also allows staff to indicate when the recording was done, to allow for further investigation, and staff can enter a zero to show the difference between no incidents and a failure to record. Involving all treatment team members in deciding where to locate recording sheets and what to record, improves participation, communication, and the accuracy of the entire process. A designated team member needs to be responsible to collect completed data sheets and provide new ones, tabulate data, and graph the results. This team member must also encourage staff involvement and reinforce participation. Target behaviours should be clear and concrete to avoid different interpretations (Giles and Clark-Wilson, 1993). This process should be further clarified through team discussions and observation and feedback during therapy sessions. For example if the goal was to track the effectiveness of interventions and/or medications with a negative drive disorder, the number of requests for toileting, or the number of completed meals could be counted and recorded.

The baseline period

The baseline period is the period of observation prior to the implementation of interventions. Baseline periods are helpful for gathering information on base rates of response and to track normal fluctuations in the frequency of behaviours. If an intervention is to be employed, even a brief period of data collection prior to the implementation of the behaviour plan may be helpful. Of course, in ideal circumstances, multiple interventions and baselines would be preferable, especially when a number of approaches must, for whatever reason, be tried. Unfortunately, in the acute rehabilitation setting, it is often not possible to delay the use of an intervention even for a few days of baseline recording. The emphasis on cost containment and the well-being and safety of the patient (and others) dictate immediate response. In our acute rehabilitation setting, baseline periods are, at best, very brief. Information gathering must accompany, simultaneously, the provision of treatment, without any delay of service.

Timing of interventions

Effective behaviour programming at the acute rehabilitation setting is characterized by the careful, considered and timely use of interventions. The right approach, employed at the wrong time, may be ineffective in changing behaviour. A behavioural approach should be considered from the standpoint of its learning requirements (how much operant responding is required), its complexity (how many steps or repetitions), its rewards or consequences (what the patient derives from it), and the likelihood it will facilitate a desired outcome. If the intervention cannot be performed because the patient is unable to process the steps involved (i.e. severe memory or other marked cognitive limitation), the intervention should be re-examined and an alternative approach attempted. The potential benefit of some interventions may be lost because the patient has not recovered sufficiently to be able to make use of them. Approaches involving antecedent control, habituation or classical conditioning may need to be substituted where operant approaches are not effective.

Management vs modification

The terms 'behaviour management' and 'behaviour modification' have been used interchangeably by many in the rehabilitation community. However, there is an important distinction between these two terms. A patient who is at a lower level of cognitive functioning, such as Rancho level IV, 'confused/agitated' (Hagen *et al.*, 1977), is frequently overstimulated and agitated, and is 'managed' by having his environment altered, with the responsibility lying solely on the staff to modify their behaviours in order to facilitate the rehabilitation process. These approaches are common in brain-injury programmes, yet could hardly be considered a modification of the patient's behaviour. Management approaches frequently involve altera- tions in the environment such as controlling stimuli, and regulation of inter- personal interaction.

Although the frequency of aggressive behaviours may increase during the initial period of recovery, the approach described below is important to limit rein- forcement of inappropriate behaviours, thereby decreasing maladaptive learning. Maladaptive learning can occur when inappropriate behaviours are reinforced by unknowing staff who have good intentions, but whose actions generate unintended behavioural consequences. A modification approach, to change or alter these learned behaviours, is often required.

BEHAVIOUR-MANAGEMENT APPROACHES

The following 'do and don't' approaches are suggested ways of interacting with the brain-injured person to manage the environment, improve treatment compliance and limit the acquisition of maladaptive behaviours.

Do:
- Remain calm and pleasant, ask for assistance from other staff when needed.
- Work in a quiet room. Remove stimuli when the patient is agitated (see stimulus control).
- Use simple words and sentences. Repeat if necessary.
- Reassure and orient the patient frequently.
- Attempt to involve the patient in basic motor routines and daily care activities.
- Provide consistent staff, environment, and schedule.

Don't:
- Show anger towards the patient or take patient responses personally.
- Use restraints unless absolutely necessary.
- Punish, reprimand, or make demands.
- Overwhelm with many staff or visitors at one time.
- Expect attention of more than a few seconds, participation in tasks, or carryover of information.

For better control of stimuli (be aware of the following):
- The number of people present, no more than two people at a time.
- The presence of external stimulation (television/radio).
- The noise levels in the room and nearby hallway.
- Voices:
  – speak only to the patient, one person at a time
  – speak slowly and calmly
  – allow for delayed response.

Once cognitive improvement occurs, the patient becomes able to learn, and reinforcement contingencies can be used to modify behaviour to allow for discharge to a less restrictive setting. Whether a behaviour must be managed or can be modified depends the patient's level of cognitive functioning. A less impaired person may benefit more from the implementation of an approach that is based on the learning of new behaviours, whereas the regaining and practising of formerly learned behaviours may be a more effective approach with the severely impaired person (see Fig. 4.5).

Rehabilitation staff must decide how severe the neurological impairment is, incorporate current testing data and use operant approaches gradually, while managing the environment carefully. Some operant learning may be possible, but the rate of acquisition of learned behaviours is much slower than desired. Therefore accurate and reliable data collection is required as the means of making these important determinations. With recent injuries, particularly severe closed brain trauma, the Rancho Los Amigos Level of Cognitive Functioning is a useful scale for assessing recovery from coma, and for describing neurological, cognitive and behavioural improvement. This scale should be employed as a guide for families who may inquire about the recovery process.

Levels of patient involvement

Another useful way of conceiving learning for the agitated and confused patient,

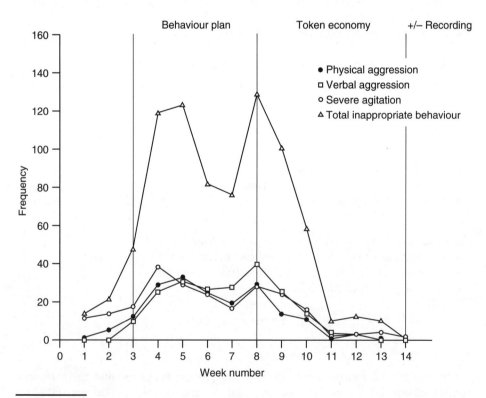

Figure 4.5

who is having difficulty with task completion, utilizes the shaping of patient involvement. These levels are described in the following conceptualization:

- toleration (guided performance in unwilling situations)
- participation (limited willing involvement)
- cooperation (increased compliance and initiation)
- independent completion (self-generated activity).

A graduated approach to task completion provides a means of judging the level of initiation of which the patient is capable, and prevents 'judgements' from being made about 'motivation' in the absence of a standardized approach. In other words, behavioural modelling, shaping, and task approximation become the means toward achieving goals, without the use of labels referring to ambiguous or projected mental states.

INTERVENTIONS

Reinforcement is any event that strengthens a behaviour and therefore makes it more likely to occur (Skinner, 1976). Traditionally, reinforcement has been divided into the categories of 'positive' and 'negative' types. Positive reinforcement can be either primary or secondary in nature. Primary reinforcers can be social (attention or praise), or an item or object that the person desires. Primary reinforcers are very useful in the acute setting for several reasons. Reinforcement strategies are frequently critical in the success or failure of brain-injury programming (Dolan and Norton, 1977). The effectiveness of the intervention may rest on whether genuine reinforcers (i.e. reinforcers that have a high preferential value to the person) have been utilized (Bandura, 1986). Attention and praise are reinforcing to most individuals on a basic level and are readily available and inexpensive. The difficulty with social reinforcement with this population is that brain injury can cause impairments of social cognition (e.g. awareness of social boundaries), which must be carefully considered in the use of socially based reinforcers.

Primary reinforcement is also useful with brain-injured patients because many are unable to make a connection to reinforcing behaviours after a delay. One common primary reinforcer is food. Many clients, at this stage, are on very restricted diets, such as pureéd food, or are unable to take any food by mouth due to a combination of attention deficits and swallowing difficulties (see Chapter 9). There may be disagreement among team members about using particular food items or even whether food should be used as a reinforcer at all. The resolution of this issue is decided by the treatment, team members, the patient, and their family, in consideration to both safety and behavioural goals.

If the patient can delay gratification and still make the connection between the target behaviour and the reinforcer, a secondary reinforcer can be used. Secondary reinforcers, such as tokens or stickers, can be exchanged for rewards and increase the number of options for reinforcement due to fact that the actual reinforcers do not have to be carried and supplied immediately by treatment staff.

Another type of secondary reinforcement are self-monitoring systems which include 'Plus–Minus' (+/–) recording notations actually done by the patient during or immediately following therapy sessions (see Chapter 9). An established percentage for the day is equated to a preferred reinforcer. Alternatively, graphs can be used, in which the patient shades a square each time the target behaviour is exhibited. Target behaviours can be either appropriate or inappropriate in nature, and goal thresholds can be set during a discussion with the patient at the beginning of the session. Self-monitoring systems are generally useful for higher-level patients who have the ability to become more aware of the disruptive nature of a particular behaviour and who are able to play a more active role in their treatment. The patient can then be reinforced for setting goals for a particular behaviour and achieving it.

One critical factor in setting up an effective secondary reinforcement system is that the system needs to be both active and interactive. Active, in the sense that adaptations can be made to the system – as a patient at this level of recovery can change at a rapid pace – and interactive, in the sense that the patient and staff need to be involved in contracting together, for the target behaviours and the reinforcers.

Negative reinforcement also increases the likelihood that a behaviour will occur again, but does so by removing, or reducing, typically aversive stimuli (Bandura, 1986). On the brain-injury unit, this is commonly achieved through the reduction of aversive stimuli such as pain, fear, or even confusion. The repositioning of an immobilized patient in discomfort and the orientation of a confused patient are two examples of appropriate negative reinforcement (i.e. the removal of painful or aversive stimuli). Another example can be seen in the following case study.

CASE STUDY 4.2

The patient was a 29-year-old male injured in a bicycle versus automobile accident 3 weeks prior to admission to the rehabilitation unit (Rancho Level V–VI, coma duration I week). He exhibited profound short-term memory deficits due to anoxia following cardiac arrest. Over the first 3 weeks of his stay on the rehabilitation unit, he became increasingly non-compliant with requests to attend therapy. Upon interview, following refusal to attend therapy, he stated that he was very upset because everyone knew who he was and he didn't know them or what they wanted him to do. Intervention focused on every interaction beginning with an introduction and a reason for why the patient should assist with that particular activity. Over the next few weeks, participation in therapy and nursing activities improved from 52% to 100% in all interactions. Intervention continued for 6 weeks and then was gradually phased out without an increase in non-compliance (see Fig. 4.6).

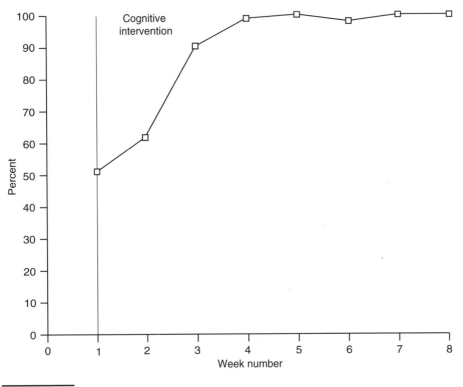

Figure 4.6

Non-reinforcement of behaviours includes the interventions of ignoring, time-out, and the structuring of interventions to allow certain behaviours to have only a limited impact. These processes can be very powerful and yet much more difficult to implement than first appears. When choosing to ignore a particular behaviour, a process termed time-out-on-the-spot (TOOTS) has been effective (Wood and Burgess, 1988). However, staff must be trained and able to implement the concept of ignoring the particular behaviour and not the person. The targeted behaviour must be attention seeking (and not related to the attention used by the patient to gain needed assistance, e.g. to change soiled clothing). Furthermore, the brain-injured person must have the social cognition to benefit from the fact that a particular behaviour has been ignored. Many patients at the acute setting do not have this level of cognition, and may not be trying to gain attention with it. They may not even understand that there is anything inappropriate about that particular behaviour. Frequently, cueing must occur first, to assist the patient in learning that a behaviour is 'not okay' and what substitute behaviour others feel should occur, such as 'John, it's not okay to spit on the floor, could you please use this towel? Thank you'. Once the connection has been made, then spitting can be ignored and John can be positively reinforced for using the towel, either socially or with something more tangible.

Time-out is another intervention that can be difficult to implement effectively. The process can be reinforcing in itself and remove the expectation that led to the inappropriate behaviour to begin with. If the patient is removed from an aversive activity and then receives reinforcement because the time-out procedure is difficult, the process may actually increase the frequency of inappropriate behaviours.

CASE STUDY 4.3

The patient was a 22-year-old female injured when her car struck a tree. She was in a coma for approximately 6 weeks and was admitted to the unit at Rancho level IV–V. She was hemiparetic, and prone to verbal tantrums that would escalate into physical assault of others. The treatment team decided to use time-out in a time-out room, an intervention that increased the frequency of the behaviour steadily over the next several weeks. The process of time-out turned out to be reinforcing to the patient. She was taken out of an activity which was frustrating and led to the outburst, and taken down the hallway. She then had to be lifted out of her wheelchair, as she would attempt to tip it over while in the time-out room. At the completion of the time-out procedure (5 min), she was then assisted back into her chair, repositioned and taken back down the hallway to rejoin the group. Once the intervention was determined to be ineffective (and reinforcing), the approach was shifted to non-reinforcement and a token economy, and the frequency of physical and verbal aggression decreased rapidly. (see Fig. 4.7)

Time-out can be an effective treatment, when used with patients at the acute care setting, primarily with agitated patients who are beginning to be transitioned into a more regular therapy programme. Patients in the earlier stages of Rancho level IV can become easily overstimulated and exhibit agitation and aggressive behaviours. A time-out can be used effectively to decrease reinforcement and surrounding stimuli which cannot yet be readily processed. The removal of stimuli, the therapy session, takes place without going anywhere and is negatively reinforcing because it removes stimulation that the patient cannot tolerate. It can be used as an effective form of desensitization to assist the patient in becoming more aware when he is 'saturated' and needs to take a break, and in gradually increasing his tolerance to physical activities. The patient can be taught to request a break or to stop himself from escalating when situations become overwhelming.

There are those in the rehabilitation community who believe that having a consequence that takes away reinforcers that have been earned is itself a punishment (Kazdin, 1994). It is easy to see where this type of intervention could be misused and become a form of punishment when people are faced with difficult or frustrating situations. Response cost is an intervention that is only rarely indicated for brain-injured adults. However, it is valuable for altering patterns of

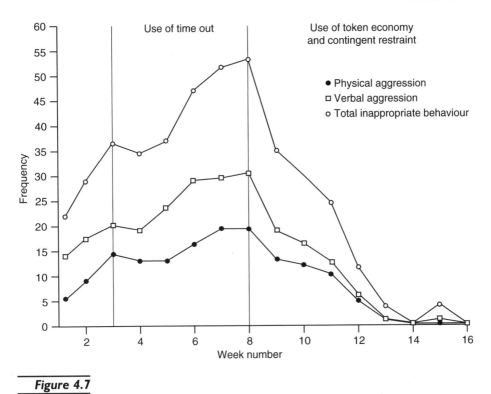

Figure 4.7

behaviour which are dangerous, self-reinforcing, and disruptive of the therapy process (Giles and Clark-Wilson, 1988b). Punishment is also commonly confused with negative reinforcement, but punishment is designed to extinguish behaviour and negative reinforcement generates it (Skinner, 1976). Punishment is a violation of the patient's rights and should not be used in rehabilitation settings. Punishment generates avoidance or escape responses both of which are undesirable in the context of rehabilitation. The following case study illustrates the appropriate use of response cost.

CASE STUDY 4.4

The patient was a 20-year-old male who was injured when his car went off the road over an embankment 2 weeks prior to admission. He was in a coma for approximately 10 days. Upon admission he exhibited behaviours corresponding to Rancho level IV. He went through several days of intense agitation but improved rapidly. He began to exhibit manipulative verbal abuse and physical assaults. He was unable to perform any self-care activities and refused most therapy sessions. A system of positive reinforcement, using tokens, was implemented with very little success. The patient

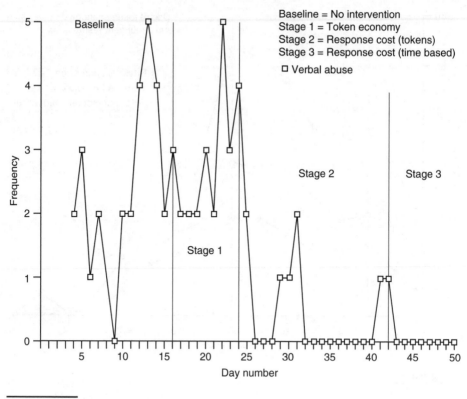

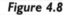

Figure 4.8

was then placed on a programme of response cost, with the consequence for assaultive behaviour being the loss of the token he could have earned and one that he already had. Within 2 days, the incidents of assaultive behaviour were nearly extinguished with very few incidents occurring after that. At that point the patient was participating in all therapy sessions and became independent in all self-care activities. The programme of response cost was phased out gradually over the next few weeks and the patient was able to be discharged home with outpatient therapy (see Fig. 4.8).

Pre-morbid personality

In working with the behavioural consequences of brain injury, the treating clinician must determine the influence of prior personality on current behaviour. This can be accomplished by a comprehensive psychosocial history, collateral interviews with family members, and a review of school and work records where available. In one sense, a brain injury both magnifies and diminishes some of the traits that define a person. Many traits stand out more clearly or are more pronounced with damage to frontal lobe inhibitory and executive functions. Behaviour becomes more stereotyped, rigid and reactive. These qualities may lead to serious social and interpersonal conflicts which, while having a remote similarity to past personality features, are actually not consistent with the former self (Varney and Menefee, 1993). The level of social functioning, and typical pre-injury interpersonal traits must be accurately ascertained in work with brain-injured patients. Individuals with impulsive and risk-taking characteristics have an increased incidence of closed-head injury (Rimel and Jane, 1983). While the extent and severity of the injury will shape the outcome significantly, the role of pre-morbid traits, personality char-acteristics, or personality disorders cannot be minimized. There is also a high incidence of substance abuse among closed-head injury survivors. Inpatient rehabilitation, while often inducing enforced sobriety, must include individual and family counselling directed at the ultimate goal of eliminating or substantially reducing the future impact of alcohol or drug abuse. Alcohol and drug usage may lower the seizure threshold, create or enhance socially inappropriate behaviours in otherwise disinhibited individuals, decrease or impair brain functioning even further, and contribute to the potential for another brain injury.

A history of prior psychiatric problems such as depression or psychosis, greatly alter patient prognosis. In some situations, prior psychiatric problems will require simultaneous monitoring and treatment during the process of brain-injury rehabilitation. Psychiatric consultation is essential, and the use of psychiatric medications should be evaluated carefully in light of the cognitive impairments fol-lowing brain trauma. Anticholinergic antidepressants may further decrease memory functioning, antipsychotic medications may decrease seizure threshold and lead paradoxically to less cognitive control and impaired processing ability (Cope, 1994; Boyeson and Harmon, 1994).

Lastly, academic and vocational history provide valuable information on overall goal-directed behaviour, adjustment, motivation and intellectual and personal accomplishments. This information is essential in tailoring a meaningful program-me of treatment. Behavioural reinforcement is most successful for those individuals who have an identified set of preferences and whose goals, though changed, remain a vital part of their lives. In the rehabilitation setting, pre-morbid personality should be assessed as soon as treatment begins or before, especially, when the individual is unable to accurately provide any sense of their own history.

Treatment history

It is important to review prior hospitalization records and the course of treatment (when patients have been treated in more than one rehabilitation setting) particularly with patients who have maladaptive behaviour. The clinician should in particular evaluate not only what interventions were attempted but when they were attempted. Patients following brain injury can change very rapidly and an intervention that failed at a prior setting or time, may now, in a new setting, be an effective method of modifying a problematic behaviour, as illustrated by the following case study.

CASE STUDY 4.5

The patient was an 11-year-old male who was involved in a bicycle versus automobile accident. He had been at a local general hospital, which had its own rehabilitation unit, for 10 weeks and had also failed a 2-week home trial prior to admission. On admission he was incontinent, combative, continually agitated, and unable to perform self-care activities. In 6 weeks of intense rehabilitation, he improved considerably and was fully continent, free from assaultive behaviour, occasionally verbally aggressive (two times/week), and able to perform all self-care activities with cueing. Following his discharge, staff from the general hospital contacted us and were perplexed to learn that the bulk of the intervention covered things that they had attempted. It was then probably too early in his recovery for the patient to benefit. The successful intervention also focused on working with the patient's parents to increase their compliance. This allowed discharge home at an earlier date than expected, as his parents had already had 6 weeks of training.

Previous failure of an intervention should not preclude subsequent efforts using similar methods. The patient's level of functioning should be assessed carefully, particularly assessing for changes in cognitive status.

Discharge goals

At the acute rehabilitation level of care, it is frequently difficult to predict discharge status with certainty. Once initial goals for improvement have been established, the team must continuously evaluate the patient and the availability of resources to transition to the least restrictive environment.

The patient's quality of life and the containment of costs are the two primary factors in long-term discharge planning. Family proximity and level of involvement also play a major role in determining where the patient should be discharged following the end of the acute rehabilitation stay. It is not uncommon to hear a brain-injured person state, 'I am ready to go home and back to work if I could just get out of this place', despite severe cognitive and physical deficits that prohibit this from happening. Decreased insight is due largely to neurologically based problems following the brain injury (see Chapter 10). In situations where the patient's remaining problems may be chronic and prohibit him or her from independent living, the family plays an even greater role and may be under a great deal of stress. The brain-injured person may need prompting and supervision throughout his day and may not be able to be left alone safely at all, or may need only periodic prompts for activities such as meals and medications. The process of discharge has two major components if it is to be successful. The first is matching the goals and expectations of the acute phase of treatment to the anticipated level of discharge, and the second is the generalization of these gains to the next setting, or the setting where long-term care will occur. It may be important to spend time helping the patient to become acclimatized to his or her new home. This step not only allows for a better transfer of information, but can help with the generalization of the gains made previously in treatment. Staff training and behavioural modelling of interventions can make the difference between a successful or failed placement.

Family involvement and counselling

The involvement of family members in brain-injury rehabilitation is essential. In regard to behavioural treatment, families should be equal participants in the process of shaping behaviours in positive directions. For this purpose, their full and informed consent, concerning interventions, must be obtained. Once they have been educated on the rationale for behavioural strategies, they can become powerful participants in the process. The absence of the family's participation and education poses great risks in regard to outcome. The dangers lie in the potential for dependent relationships developing and the creation of impediments to further levels of independent functioning (Eames *et al.*, 1995). Ongoing family counselling, dealing with alteration in roles, changes in the personality of the brain-injured family member, and other personal realities, is a requirement for good treatment. Families play a pivotal role in treatment, placement and future care, and, as such, they should become early allies in this process.

Rate of recovery

Brain-injury recovery follows no particular nor universal timetable. Various attempts have been made to ascribe limits to the recovery process within '6 months', or '2 years', or '5 years'. In reality, little is known about the long-term recovery of brain tissue from traumatic injury (Miller, 1984). There is some evidence to suggest that brain tissue may undergo a limited 'repair', through the process of reassignment of function to intact neurons, and the process of dendritic rebranching. However, the magnitude of both processes is usually less significant than the overwhelming limitations posed by the traumatic injury.

The integration of behavioural treatment in rehabilitation, pre-morbid personality variables, rate of recovery, and cognitive factors are illustrated in the case study described below.

CASE STUDY 4.6

The patient was a 27-year-old man, who had suffered a severe closed-head trauma from a pedestrian versus bus accident during military service. He remained comatose for several weeks and was admitted to the acute rehabilitation unit at a Rancho level III–IV. When he emerged from his coma, his sensory losses, as well as visual imperception (unilateral neglect), and tactile processing problems marked by tactile defensiveness, necessitated a gradual programme of sensory management (a stimulus controlled or regulated environment).

A programme of behavioural desensitization to once basic and familiar activities (e.g. toileting and dressing) was instituted. This programme of desensitization involved learning and conditioning over an extended period of time, using shaping and chaining multiple task components, to achieve a desired goal, while managing the occurrence of negative behaviours.

The patient also had limited expressive language ability. However, through a combination of gestures, visual reminders, and staff training, an effective communication protocol was created. Even when discharged from the acute rehabilitation setting, 5 months later, he was significantly impaired in expressive capability, but he had acquired the ability to communicate basic needs more effectively, and, more importantly, had a marked decrease (near extinction) in the incidence of negative behaviours (e.g. physical and verbal aggression). He was able to be discharged to a home environment, as opposed to placement in a locked institutional setting, due to the absence of these negative behaviours. Communication, although a problem, was not as limiting a concern as his behaviour had been.

Memory impairments were profound, and included both attentional deficits and retrieval problems. Much of the patient's early recovery could be attributed to the slow conditioning and shaping of desired behaviours over a very slow learning curve. The patient's learning, could be classified as non-declarative or procedural learning. That is, his improvement involved the performance of familiar routines, which were repeated over and over. He had difficulty expressing, verbalizing or recalling sequences, but could more readily perform a sequence (i.e. toothbrushing), when cued to the right environment (setup and prompting).

The patient had been diagnosed with severe bilateral pre-frontal cortex contusions and showed virtually all of the associated frontal lobe-related behaviours, and required a highly structured regimen to pace his routine, to enable feedback (his therapists assumed the job of providing accurate feedback, to enhance self-monitoring), and to promote the timely (although at first limited) completion of tasks or task components. Because of the severity of his injury it was not expected that he would ever be able to work again, but it was hoped that through increased feedback and generalization of learned behaviours to the home environment, he would acquire some self-regulatory and self-motivating capability.

Pre-morbidly, he was estimated to be of average intelligence and was described by his family as 'stubborn, independent, and prone to getting his way'. What the treating staff encountered in his rehabilitation, mirrored this personal style. The trait associated with 'getting his way', emerged in the negative behaviours (e.g. non-compliance and verbal abuse) associated with conflicts over tasks. He would often insist on doing tasks the way he wanted, and without regard to the concerns of others. Staff members feared for his safety when he would impulsively try to perform an action in his activities of daily living, such as toileting. While limits had to be prescribed to deal with these behaviours the limits were not 'imposed' arbitrarily. His history provided a clue to the type of structure he responded to most favourably. The regimentation and structure of his schedule corresponded to the structure he had been accustomed to before in the army. More important for his outcome was the drive he had, which could be channelled as his rehabilitation programme progressed.

Conclusion

To summarize the significance of behavioural approaches in the acute setting, several important aspects should be re-emphasized and are considered essential to a successful implementation of behavioural interventions.

Interdisciplinary team approach in behavioural intervention

The behavioural plan is a common denominator for all the treatment staff but team members will relate to the behavioural plan from the unique perspectives of their respective professions. Regular team meetings should focus on the patient's responses in the various therapy sessions. The information gleaned from this approach will provide clues to the greater issue of post-treatment adjustment (i.e. generalization of learned behaviour to different environments and different people). Behavioural data should be reviewed in these meetings and behavioural planning conducted so all members have an opportunity to make suggestions. This behavioural treatment planning process, in essence, becomes a patient quality assurance method, with periodic reviews occurring at regular intervals.

Staff education and training

Ongoing staff education and training is essential in brain-injury rehabilitation (Mozzoni and Bailey, 1996). And, given the complexities of behavioural intervention with the brain-injured patient, staff education should incorporate training in many areas, including the neural basis of behaviour, and the use of behavioural interventions in brain-injury rehabilitation. A well-trained staff, who have learned how to monitor behaviours, manage aggressive patients safely, and utilize consistent behavioural approaches, are a valuable asset. Training opportunities should be frequent, recognizing staff attributes and accomplishments, and providing a means for training in 'hands-on' demonstrations (e.g. dealing safely with aggressive or assaultive behaviour).

Integration of medical and behavioural treatments

The complexity of medical issues in the care of the inpatient acute rehabilitation patient requires a close coordination of treatments and providers. As described earlier, the range of complex medical issues necessitates a behavioural treatment approach. The benefits of including behavioural interventions are improved management of pain and discomfort, improved compliance with treatment, and increased progress toward treatment goals.

Cost-effectiveness in behavioural interventions

The issue of cost management is now reaching all levels of medical care. Medical cost management will remain a potent force in the economics of patient care. While patients' lengths of stay in the acute hospital setting have shortened, it is even more important that rehabilitation treatment approaches have justification and good documentation of effectiveness. The integration of systems of behavioural data collection and behaviour planning provide an empirical and scientific approach to measuring these treatment contributions, improving quality of patient care, and providing better projections concerning treatment outcome (Schmidt, 1997). The rehabilitation process is at its heart a behavioural process, and when it is viewed in that context, treatment will be most successful and cost effective.

5 MANAGEMENT OF BEHAVIOURAL DISREGULATION AND NON-COMPLIANCE IN THE POST-ACUTE SEVERELY BRAIN-INJURED ADULT

Gordon Muir Giles

A significant proportion of traumatically brain-injured people display continuing behavioural disturbance well past the acute phase of recovery (Brooks and McKinlay, 1983; Brooks *et al.*, 1986a). The behaviour disturbance may become worse as time since injury increases and may result in continuing stress on the patient's family. Serious behavioural disorders may result in significant social isolation or in more severe instances in prolonged periods of hospitalization. Appropriate social behaviour is a prerequisite for successful community reintegration.

Following the first edition of this book numerous single case and small series design papers have been published describing behavioural intervention for behaviour disorder in individuals with brain injury. At first interventions were usually based on the operant-conditioning paradigm (described below) but more recently there has been a trend for interventions based on other aspects of learning theory to be utilized. The range of inappropriate behaviours which may be demonstrated following brain injury is vast and a variety of behavioural management techniques are needed to deal with these different types of behaviour (Wood and Burgess, 1988). This chapter describes the theoretical principles derived from learning theory used in the development of intervention programmes and types of intervention programmes. Behaviour disorders may occur in the absence of obvious precipitants but are often demonstrated when the brain-injured person is asked to do something. Emphasis is therefore placed on how to incorporate behavioural principles in the development of rehabilitation programmes aimed at the development of functional skills.

TYPES OF BEHAVIOUR DISORDER

Periods of behavioural dysregulation are a normal part of the process of recovery from acute brain injury. Most, if not all, severely injured patients go through a period of acute agitation characterized by repetitive movements, self-stimulation and behaviours such as pinching, hitting, biting and scratching. During this period patients are acutely confused and present significant management problems (these issues are a central focus of Chapters 4 and 9). In this chapter the focus is on behaviour disorder which continues past or emerges following the delirium that may occur after brain trauma.

It is important to distinguish behaviour disorder which is a reaction to the injury from behaviour disorder which is a direct consequence of the injury. The former is a psychologically driven attempt by the individual to manage events after the injury or results from frustration with current limitations and demands. The latter results from damage to the brain itself and as such is not under the direct volitional control of the individual (e.g. aggression associated with seizure disorder). Having said this it must be admitted that most behaviour disorder following brain injury can be considered as lying on a continuum somewhere between the poles of completely volitional and completely organic. For example, patients may have exaggerated responses due to damage to frontal brain structures (the area of the brain which is normally able to inhibit behaviour). Patients with brain injury may have organically mediated disorders and continue to display behaviours despite neurological recovery, as a result of being reinforced for the behaviour. Pre-existing personality factors may also contribute to behavioural presentation after injury. Individuals who were impulsive and aggressive prior to injury and who had a limited behavioural repertoire available to them are particularly prone to learning that the only effective way for them to meet their needs following injury is to be aggressive.

Assessing the relative contributions of learned versus organic factors to behaviour disorders is important because learned behaviours are more likely to respond to learning-based interventions and organically based disorders are more likely to respond to combined learning and pharmacological intervention (see Chapter 3). In general terms it is possible to talk about patterns which distinguish the two ends of the continuum. Psychologically motivated aggression tends to be intermittent (it is not constant and repetitive), purposeful, and predictable based on motivation or avoidance (it appears to follow a pattern of self-interest). Organically mediated aggression is often characterized by rapidity of onset and frequency, behaviours are often highly repetitive, are not clearly goal directed and there appears to be no gratification. Individuals with organic behaviour disorder are often either remorseful for the incident or amnestic about the incident frequently denying that it ever happened (making statements such as 'I do not behave that way'). For example, a profoundly impaired patient (coma duration 8 weeks) was requiring total care. Most of the time he was pleasant and cooperative smiling at staff but primarily passive. Four to five times a week, for periods of approximately 20 min he would become enraged charging around the unit, overturning furniture and medication carts and attempting to assault staff who tried to interrupt the behaviour. The period of episodic dyscontrol would abate rapidly and within a few minutes he returned to his normal sunny disposition with no memory of the period of agitation.

Within the category of organically mediated behaviour disorder it is possible to make some useful distinctions. Cassidy (1990a, b) has suggested a typology for considering organically mediated aggression. Cassidy describes three types of aggressive behaviour: predatory aggression, affective aggression and non-directed aggression. Predatory aggression does not involve increased irritability or autonomic arousal. It is sudden and goal directed. Individuals (or objects) entering the patient's visual field are at risk of attack (often with lunging or biting behaviours). Affective aggression is accompanied by autonomic arousal and characteristically escalates in relation to some form of provocation. Individuals who know the patient well can predict the occurrence of the aggressive outburst. Non-directed aggression may involve a brief period of autonomic arousal. The behaviour is generally short lived.

Another major distinction within the category of organically mediated disorders is that between positive and negative behaviour disorder. Positive behaviour disorders are those of aggression, irritability and are marked by increased activity. At its extreme patients may be constantly in motion and be apparently compelled to engage with other people or objects in the environment. Areas of brain damage tend to include medial and basal frontal lobe structures. Patients with negative behaviour disorder are those whose behaviour is marked by apathy, aspontaneity and lack of drive. Patients tend to respond to stimuli and then lapse into inactivity. Patients with negative behaviour disorders are difficult to rehabilitate as they do not exhibit enough behaviour to be modified by learning-based interventions (Giles *et al.*, 1997). Negative behaviour disorders may follow diffuse or brain-stem injury. Pharmacological interventions in conjunction with persistent retraining efforts may prove effective in some cases (Pulaski and Emmett, 1994).

Finally, as noted by Lishman (1972), the range of psychiatric disturbances which may follow brain injury embraces most of what can be found in psychiatric symptomatology. Psychiatric impairments may contribute to behaviour disorder. Psychotic and paranoid states are common following brain injury (Thomsen, 1984) and misperceptions of reality may contribute to aggressive behaviour. Patients may fear that they will be harmed and attempt to strike out first. Delusions which may occur following brain injury may be less fixed than in psychotic states with other aetiologies but nonetheless do respond to antipsychotic medications. Mood disorders are commonly associated with brain injury. Contemporary studies suggest that brain injury may be a far more common cause of affective disorders than has been realized hitherto (Fujikawa *et al.*, 1995). Mania can lead to increased activity, irritability and belligerence. Depression may present as a negative behaviour disorder with resistance during care. Pharmacological interventions may have dramatic effects on patients with these disorders.

Eames and Wood (1981) have pointed to the existence of a syndrome which may follow brain injury characterized by hysterical, dissociative and ahedonic behaviours. Eames (1992) reviewed 167 patients referred to a unit treating severe behaviour disorder following brain injury for symptoms of some form of hysteria. Fifty-four patients showed symptoms of hysteria which were associated with diffuse insults such as hypoxia but not with severity of injury. There was no increased family or social history of psychiatric disorder amongst the group with hysteria. Eames suggests that damage to the basal ganglia and diencepahlon is implicated in the origin of the disorder (Eames, 1992). For some reason these patients reject demands to change, and may work very hard to maintain the status quo, they also have difficulty in developing true interpersonal relatedness, and may be very frustrating to treat.

The literature suggests that the majority of patients who are physically aggressive following brain injury are treated pharmacologically (Alderman *et al.*, 1997). Most brain-injured people are treated in non-specialist centres and the technical expertise and personnel resources to manage very severely brain-injured individuals continue to be in short supply. Manchester *et al.* (1997b) describe the vast amount of resources which may be needed to bring the behaviour of even a single patient under control. It is therefore not surprising that pharmacological intervention may be used as a 'quick fix' approach to get patients and staff through an acute crisis. More general availability of behavioural management expertise would enable decisions to be based on patient needs.

BASIC PRINCIPLES OF LEARNING THEORY

In this section basic principles of learning theory are described. The remainder of the chapter describes how to apply these principles to the rehabilitation of patients with behaviour disorder following brain injury.

Fundamental to the behaviourists understanding of behaviour is the law of effect. The law of effect, first formulated by Thorndike in 1932, states that if an organism's response to a given stimulus is followed by a pleasant event (a satisfier) the association formed between the stimulus and the response is further strengthened. If the response is followed by an aversive event (an annoyer) the association is weakened. Skinner (1938) refined the definitions and attempted to make them more objective.

Classes of behaviour are identified by reference to their origins. In classical (Pavlovian) conditioning, responses originate with the stimuli that elicit them and are called *respondents*. This class of response is illustrated by the stimulus–response (S–R) relationships called reflexes. Through respondent conditioning, responses prepared in advance by natural selection can come under the influence of new stimuli. Recent research suggests that classical conditioning is more complex and less easily defined than suggested by standard definitions. Pavlovian conditioning may be best considered a mechanism by which organisms map important regularities in their environment (Rescorla, 1988). It underlies important human emotions, such as anxiety and anger.

Other types of behaviours called operants develop as a result of their effect on the environment. These behaviours are said to be *emitted* because they do not require an eliciting stimulus. The consequences of operants influence the rate at which they are emitted either raising or lowering subsequent responding. Events which follow an operant which raise the frequency of responding are called reinforcers and events which lower the frequency of responding are called punishers. Mapping the relationships between responses and their consequences establishes the contingencies of reinforcement or punishment.

Although operants do not require an antecedent stimulus the likelihood that a response will be reinforced or punished often depends on other aspects of the environment which may then act as a cue to the emission of an operant. When a stimulus sets the occasion on which responding will have a particular consequence then that stimulus is said to be discriminative.

Antecedent stimuli are important both for discriminative operants and in classical Pavlovian conditioning but there is an important distinction between them. A response that only requires the presentation of the stimulus as in a reflex is a respondent. A response elicited by a stimulus but which is also influenced by its consequence is a discriminated operant. The discriminated operant is said to be defined by a three term contingency (discriminant stimulus, response, reinforcement).

Once a behaviour has been established it is possible to influence the likelihood that it will continue to be emitted despite little or no continuation of the reinforcement. The tendency for a behaviour not to be produced if it is no longer reinforced is called extinction. A one-to-one correspondence between stimulus and response is often not necessary for behaviour to be maintained. Intermittent reinforcement can be very effective at maintaining behaviour – and in fact is often more effective in maintaining certain classes of behaviour. A third type of learning is observational or vicarious learning. Vicarious learning occurs when an individual observes another person engage in a behaviour. The other person need not engage in the behaviour or be reinforced to later emit the behaviour, however whether and how often the behaviour is emitted may depend on its consequences.

BEHAVIOURAL INTERVENTIONS

First principles

Behaviour management principles can be applied in many different settings from acute hospitals to nursing homes and the community, however the types of behaviours which can be managed will vary. Physical aggression either towards self or others is the most difficult to manage because the response must be effective and immediate. The facility must be able to provide containment and safety for the patient, other patients and staff. If these criteria are not met the patient must be transferred to a facility which can assure safety and containment.

Most interventions for aggression are designed to strip the aggression of its reinforcing consequences for the patient. Failure to receive expected reinforcement is functionally equivalent to punishment so staff must expect that patients' behaviour will deteriorate when a behaviour programme is first applied (a positive reinforcement extinction effect). Staff must therefore be reasonably confident that they can manage any behaviour which the patient is able to produce. Physical contact to an agitated patient is likely to produce escalation of aggression. Physically unimpaired individuals who are unpredictably physically aggressive are the most difficult to care for which is why until recently these individuals have been managed in acute psychiatric facilities. Many aggressive individuals also have profound physical impairments and may therefore require management in facilities which can provide for intensive medical management. Judgements about acceptability for a specific programme include both knowledge of the programme's strengths and limitations but also an understanding of how an individual's combination of impairments will affect the manifestation of their behaviour disorder. For example a patient with severe episodic dyscontrol might be managed in a facility for mild neurobehavioural disorders because the nature of his physical impairments limits his ability to harm himself and others.

The physical setting of the programme must be conducive to its purpose. The physical environment can be thought of as a type of antecedent control. A patient was failing at a placement due to repeated destruction of televisions. The patient had a destructive utilization behaviour – he was unable to resist grabbing and pulling at attention-getting objects and had destroyed four televisions. The new facility to which he was admitted had ceiling-mounted televisions that he could not reach obviating the problem. If the programme is designed for people who wander and are frequently agitated some foolproof system must be designed to keep them contained. If the programme is designed primarily to work with patients who are being prepared for community integration, an open facility in an appropriate community setting must be used.

The organization of a behaviour-management programme

Staff must be reasonably and accurately confident that they have the resources to manage the most difficult behaviours patients are likely to demonstrate. Staff must feel that a system is in place which supports them and gives them the tools to carry out their work. Responses to the most severe disorders seen in the programme must become second nature to staff. The established system must be up to the task, staffing must be adequate (even at night and on weekends), and staff must be trained. Individuals responsible for the management of behaviour programmes should actively engage in the development of a culture which supports staff and helps communicate the basic principles used in caring for patients at the facility.

Staff training

Staff may have a variety of explanatory models which they use to account for behaviour. These explanatory models may be tenacious in the face of evidence and may significantly help or hinder the development of a behavioural approach to helping patients. Staff who secretly (or not so secretly) believe that the patient's problems are due to moral weakness are in danger of developing a punitive attitude towards patients which can undermine the quality of treatment and staff–patient relationships. Ross (1977) has described an attributional error fundamental to understanding how human beings interpret the interpersonal environment. People tend to underestimate the impact of situational factors and to overestimate the role of dispositional factors in controlling behaviour. This may be particularly true of events on which attention is focused and which are personally significant or threatening. Hence patients who are able to exercise little control over their behaviour are viewed as willfully manipulative. The consequences of the brain injury are minimized in contrast to stable pre-morbid dispositions ('they were always nasty'). Based on these assessments of cause staff may withdraw from the patient, become punitive and refuse to follow behavioural programmes that are seen as unjustly rewarding to the patient.

To counteract these attributional processes it is important that staff have a clear understanding of brain damage and its consequences. They can be taught how patients are likely to respond in different circumstances and how to intervene as part of a team. Staff must also be taught if necessary how to physically intervene with patients (manual containments). A comprehensive staff inservice programme should include all staff who regularly contact patients (including janitorial staff). A pre-employment orientation period can train staff in the general principles of treatment utilized in the programme with specific inservicing on any special intervention programmes used. Having a defined target population allows for the development of expertise in a range of applicable treatment options.

Treatment planning

Behavioural targets often stand out from potentially competing targets for patient treatment because, until the behaviour disorder is brought under control, it will not be possible to work on other goals. Only a clear understanding of the nature of the behaviour disorder will allow the development of an adequate treatment plan. Behaviour can be defined as the activity of another person which can be directly observed. Observations need to be described carefully and accurately to avoid unwarranted inferences and subjective biases. Behaviour therapy emphasizes specific evaluation of objectively defined target behaviours and the situational, interactive, cognitive and behavioural factors which control them. Here we use the term functional/behavioural analysis. Data derived from the assessment are used to design the intervention programme. The assessment is designed to identify controlling variables so that modification of these variables will effect the production of the behaviour. Intervention may involve modification of the original variables presumed to control the target behaviour (e.g. extinction procedures described below), or may introduce new controlling variables as in antecedent control procedures (see also Chapter 6). An erroneous functional behavioural analysis can lead to ineffective interventions.

The process of observing and recording behaviour is referred to as behavioural baselining. Certain classes of behaviours are only exhibited infrequently or in defined situations (e.g. aggression during personal care) other behaviours occur at various times throughout the day. In a large facility with many staff it can be difficult to know how often a patient engages in a behaviour. Behavioural baselining records the type, frequency and duration of specific behaviours. An adjunctive data collection method attempts to capture more information about a specific behaviour antecedent–behaviour–consequence (A–B–C) recording.

Following the introduction of a treatment recording must continue to establish the patient's reaction to the intervention.

In behavioural baselining the individual is the typical locus of analysis, however observations across a patient population may be helpful in programme design. Because brain-injured people often respond impulsively to minor environmental stimuli there may be a tendency for incidents to occur in corridors, doorways, in cafeteria lines or at specific times of day that are either low or high demand in terms of rehabilitative programming. Analysis of group data may contribute to improved programme design.

Standardized assessments

Despite the frequency of agitated or aggressive behaviour following brain injury few standardized measures are available. The absence of formal measures makes it difficult to know if behaviours seen at different sites are truly comparable and therefore makes it difficult to compare interventions. In addition, in the absence of an accepted standard, comparisons through time and between patients are difficult. Many of the general rating scales available for use with the brain injured have no obvious method to include behavioural data (e.g. the DRS). Adaptive behaviour rating scales, developed primarily for the mentally retarded population have increasingly been used with the person with brain injury (Benton, 1979). Most of these scales allow ratings of a wide range of maladaptive behaviours and are intended to be completed by staff with varying degrees of training and family members (see, for example, Nihira *et al.*, 1993).

Corrigan (1989) has described the development of the Agitated Behaviour Scale (ABS). The scale allows 14 types of agitated behaviour to be rated on a four-point scale from absent, to present to an extreme degree. The scale appears to be reliable and valid (Corrigan, 1989).

The Overt Aggression Scale (OAS) of Yudofsky *et al.* (1986) was developed as an observational report of aggression primarily for the psychiatric population. Aggressive behaviour is divided into four classes, verbal aggression, physical aggression against objects, physical aggression against self and physical aggression against others. Each category is divided into four subtypes of increasing severity. The OAS includes a recording of staff response to the aggression ranging from none to seclusion. The scale has good reliability and validity and can be completed rapidly by staff. Alderman *et al.* (1997) have produced an adaptation of the OAS (modified for neurorehabilitation) (OAS-MNR). The OAS-MNR extends the data captured by the original scale by including a section on antecedents to the aggressive behaviour, and by altering the possible responses to aggression so that they are consistent with best practices in brain-injury rehabilitation. Unfortunately the reliability study only included the authors of the scale and it is not clear that the more complex version of the scale would have adequate reliability when used routinely by staff. However the OAS-MNR is superior to other available scales and warrants further investigation.

APPLICATIONS OF LEARNING PRINCIPLES TO BEHAVIOURAL CHANGE

Reinforcement

A reinforcer is any event following a behavioural response which increases the likelihood of that response being repeated. Positive reinforcers can be divided into two categories primary and secondary. Primary reinforcers are inherently rewarding and are usually attention, praise or consumables such as chocolate, soft drinks and cigarettes. Secondary reinforcers, for example, money, tokens or stars, have no inherent reinforcing characteristics and rely for their value on the meaning attached to them. The selection of primary or secondary reinforcers should be based on the cognitive and behavioural characteristics of the patient. In developing intervention programmes the most valid method of determining what is reinforcing for an individual is to offer a range of options and observe the rate and duration of responding. This procedure is time-consuming and it is usually possible to ask the individual what they would work for. It is important to remember that what is reinforcing for a patient is what has a reinforcing effect on the patient and not what the staff think should be reinforcing. Sometimes patients really want sweets or cigarettes. It is also possible for patients to become satiated on a reinforcer – one can only eat a certain amount of chocolate – having a range of reinforcements may be helpful. When high levels of reinforcement are required the use of secondary reinforcers may be indicated.

The reinforcement of every instance of the desired behaviour is the most efficient way of establishing a preferred response pattern (continuous schedule). The most powerful form of reinforcement occurs when it takes place immediately following a behaviour. The more impaired an individual is the more difficult it is for them to map environmental regularities and the more important it is to have reinforcement immediately following a to-be-reinforced behaviour. In order to increase the endurance of the behavioural change an intermittent schedule of reinforcement may be most successful. Training schedules which include instances of both reinforcement and non-reinforcement of a desired behaviour produce greater resistance to extinction than 100% (continuous) reinforcement schedules. If a subject has no experience of non-reinforcement of a behaviour, the behaviour is likely to be rapidly extinguished in the natural environment when continuous reinforcement is no longer available (Nation and Woods, 1980).

In designing programmes to reduce inappropriate behaviour, it is important to 'start where the patient is' and not to set unrealistic goals. Small reinforcement frequently applied, but for goals which the patient can achieve (with some effort) are preferable to large rewards which the patient is unable to earn because the earning requirements vastly outreach their abilities. The difficulty in generating immediate rewards can be minimized in higher functioning patients by the use of secondary reinforcement. The reasons for using rewards in assisting patients to develop behavioural control include: rewards assist the patient focus on the to-be-eliminated behaviours; rewards increase compliance; rewards assist the patient retain a positive attitude towards the behavioural intervention programme; rewards help staff maintain a positive (non-punitive) attitude towards some difficult-to-like patients. It is not inconsistent for a programme to have positive reinforcement and an extinction component which operate in tandem.

Differential reinforcement (DR)
There are a number of variants of DR procedures. An important advantage of DR procedures is that they provide a positive approach to seriously disturbed behaviour.

Differential reinforcement of other behaviours (DRO)
Where a patient displays inappropriate behaviours with very high frequency and appropriate behaviour with very low frequency, a DRO procedure may be indicated. Here any instance of any type of appropriate behaviour is reinforced.

Differential reinforcement of an alternative behaviour (DRA)
In most cases DRA is preferable to the shotgun approach of a DRO. DRA is the reinforcement of a specified behaviour different from the targeted inappropriate

behaviour(s). The behaviour targeted need not be important from a rehabilitation perspective. DRA is easier to define and therefore to operationalize than DRO procedures.

Differential reinforcement of an incompatible behaviour (DRI)

This approach reinforces behaviour which is incompatible with those which are to be extinguished (i.e. the behaviour selected for reinforcement excludes the possibility of the patient engaging in the target behaviour). This intervention is especially helpful in self-injurious or aggressive behaviour. For example, one patient was taught to lock the brakes on his wheelchair as a DRI to his wheeling after people and hitting them. The patient was taught to respond to a verbal prompt and a mime of putting the brakes on and given social reinforcement for the behaviour.

Differential reinforcement of low rates of responding (DRL)

Also useful when a patient engages in a target behaviour with very high frequency, DRL procedures may at first sight appear paradoxical. Baseline recordings of the frequency of the target behaviour in a specified period are made. Following a period in which the patient becomes accustomed to the reinforcement the criteria for reinforcement are changed so that reinforcement is only available when the rate of the target behaviour is below the initial baseline level. As in other reinforcement programmes changes in earning criteria should occur gradually as the patient demonstrates competence. For example one patient would scream during therapy sessions. Initial baseline frequency recordings were made. The programme was then introduced to the patient and she was reinforced at baseline levels for 1 week. In the following week earning criteria were set at 10% below the baseline rate. As the frequency of screaming decreased the earning criteria were incrementally lowered.

An advantage of DRL procedures is that they can be used in tandem with skill-building approaches. Alderman and Knight (1997) have reported on the successful use of DRL procedures to reduce severely disruptive behaviours in three severely brain-injured adults. Multiple baseline design was used and in each case the DRL programme was carried out in tandem with use of the standard morning hygiene procedures which has been reported elsewhere (Giles and Clark-Wilson, 1988a; Giles et al., 1997). Initially patients were unable to develop independent hygiene behaviours due to their behavioural dysregulation. Reductions in the patient's negative behaviours allowed progress to be made in personal hygiene. Alderman and Knight (1997) report follow-up data up to 18 months post-injury suggesting that the effect of these interventions can be extremely robust.

Token economies

A token system is a way to systematically deliver reinforcement to a group of people and attempts to structure the environment to promote adaptive social behaviour. It allows a variety of individual behavioural programmes to be implemented in a controlled way and, with adequate measurement and recording, can be used to evaluate a response to therapy over time. There are three essential components in setting up a token system: the medium of exchange, the back-up reinforcers and the rules which describe the inter-relationship between the token and back-up reinforcers. A general token economy can be structured to reflect the highly individualized need of brain-injured patients if the targeted behaviours, token exchange and the individual's methods of learning can be reflected in the overall programme design. Additional behavioural interventions may occur in tandem with the token system.

The advantages of token systems are the established expectations of patients and staff based on the concrete and explicit rules which define appropriate and inappropriate behaviour. Established token systems have different time-based reinforcement schedules (15, 30, 60 min); many kinds of back-up reinforcers (attention, food, activities) and different types of currency such as money, tokens or stamps. A variety of rules may govern the earning of the tokens, and means of application of these rules (for example, staff- or patient-governed system). Self-administration must be carefully monitored as individuals tend to become too lenient or too stringent in the delivery of their own reinforcement. Careful evaluation of the system is required to ensure that it fulfils the criteria for helping individuals extinguish inappropriate behaviours and learn adaptive skills.

Extinction

Extinction procedures are customarily used to decrease severe behaviour disorders and are a set of highly effective clinical procedures, the theoretical underpinnings of which are rather obscure. The term extinction refers to the process which occurs when a behaviour is not being reinforced. Typically the reinforcers are naturally occurring and are produced spontaneously by people in the individual's environment (for example, attention for swearing loudly in public). The process of extinction is the weakening of the previously established associations between a behaviour and its (reinforcing) consequences. Exactly how this process occurs, however, is unclear, four of the major theories as they relate to work with the brain-injured are reviewed by Wood and Burgess (1988).

Time-out

Time-out is often considered an extinction procedure and is designed to remove the individual from reinforcement which might occur as the result of inappropriate behaviour (Ullman and Krasner, 1969). Time-out as it is currently used has a number of different forms.

Room time-out

In specialist behavioural units this may involve taking the patient to a bare room where they may remain for a period of between 2 and 5 min. It is most frequently used following episodes of physical aggression. At a practical level this technique gives all staff a response to situations that could be threatening and escalate to situations which could be dangerous to both staff and patients. As noted by Wood and Burgess (1988) it is agreed by many that time-out in the time-out room relies for its effectiveness on its aversive qualities. Therapists should note the patient response to time-out as a small number of patients will seek room time-out as an avoidance behaviour (e.g. the patient may prefer to be in time-out than participate in physical therapy).

Situational time-out

Situational time-out has the same rational as that of room time-out. The goal of situational time-out is to remove the individuals from positive reinforcement. When a special room is not available, staff can place patients in a corridor or at the other end of the room if it is safe to do so.

Time-out-on-the-spot

Time-out-on-the-spot (TOOTS) also involves not reinforcing an individual for inappropriate behaviour. The method is similar to time-out in a time-out room except that the programme is carried out *in situ* (Wood and Burgess, 1988). One method is to not pay attention to the individual (for about 20 s) contingent on the production of inappropriate behaviour (this can be done by moving away or talking to someone else). This time-out to person is most effective when the patient is attempting to engage in interpersonal interaction. A second method is to continue to pay attention to the patient but to ignore the inappropriate behaviour. This latter method is most suitable when therapy is underway and should not be interrupted. After the initiation of an extinction procedures the rate of the inappropriate behaviour may show a transient increase, this 'extinction burst' phenomena, may be unacceptable in the treatment of certain behaviours, e.g. severe head banging, lip biting, such that an alternative type of intervention is indicated.

Response costs

Response-cost approaches are designed to approximate the deterrents which occur in everyday life for inappropriate behaviours, e.g. a parking ticket is a response cost for parking in a no-parking zone. Response-cost programmes are valuable for interrupting continual behaviours, which are potentially dangerous, self-reinforcing, or disruptive of the therapy process. Since the response-cost system allows reinforcement and punishment to be administered along the same dimensions, it can be combined with a token economy. Tangible or secondary reinforcers, for example tokens, may be lost as well as gained.

Control of a behaviour by antecedents

For many clinicians, applied behavioural analysis when applied to brain-injured patients has been synonymous with an operant conditioning model. Antecedents, the 'A' in the ABC chain, may be altered in an attempt to change behaviour. This is a method of setting the environmental conditions – the stimulus events – so as to increase the possibility that the patient will emit the desired behaviour.

Burke *et al.* (1988) have reported a positive approach to the treatment of aggressive brain-injured patients incorporating antecedent control. The following techniques were used:

- Increased density of reinforcement – reinforcement was provided for all pro-social patient behaviours, patients were paid special attention, provided with special dinners or dessert, etc.
- Reinforcement sampling – a special menu of reinforcement was determined for each patient for use in future programmes.
- Antecedent control – a generally low level of stimulation with few demands was provided. The patient was fully oriented to their new surroundings. Patients were frequently reinforced for being calm, speaking in a low tone of voice and generally demonstrating behavioural control. No negative consequences were applied for aggressive behaviour. If patients appeared to be becoming agitated an attempt was made to redirect them to a task at hand. If a patient did become aggressive, punches were blocked and the patient was redirected. Continuous reinforcement was available for appropriate behaviours.
- Appropriate response selection – during the first 24 h in the programme ten things which the patient did well were identified. This was done to reinforce activities incompatible with aggressive behaviour. In addition it was thought that if patients maintained positive self-statements this would be inconsistent with aggressive behaviour.
- Inconvenience review – after the first 48 h patients were taught how aggressive behaviour was inconvenient for them. This inconvenience review was repeated following any act of aggression.
- Self-control training – an attempt was made to teach problem-solving techniques. Patients were trained in overt self-relaxation.
- Self-monitoring – patients were taught to record their daily programmes.

Prior to treatment the average number of aggressive behaviours (sexual assaults, physical assaults and damage to property) was 20.2 per week. During the first week of treatment the number of such incidents was reported to have fallen to an average of less than one per patient and to have subsequently fallen further. The precipitous change does indicate that change in environment (setting events, environmental conditions) may in some patients result in significant alteration in behaviour. Similar reduction in aggression as a response to being placed in a highly reinforcing environment has been reported in other populations (Mace *et al.*, 1983).

Stimulus control

The aim of stimulus control is to interrupt the progression from frustration to physical aggression. Many aggressive behaviours occur 'impulsively' because patients fail to recognize the increase in tension/arousal that would otherwise signal a behavioural predisposition to act aggressively. Patients can be taught to discriminate states of tension or heightened arousal and use this state of arousal as a cue to initiate behavioural alternatives to aggression. Intervention therefore involves the administration of a discriminatory stimulus, i.e. a verbal instruction or physical prompt (e.g. making a stop sign with the hand) when the individual is becoming angry. Once the individual is capable of recognizing an increase in arousal they need to invoke a strategy to manage that arousal. Training in the stimulus control procedure begins on a sessional basis. The patient is taught how the aggressive behaviour is dysfunctional for them. The patient is also taught appropriate verbalizations (which may parallel the cue) and which will later be internalized such as 'I am getting angry – I need to take a time-out'. The patient is then taught by multiple overlearning 'dry runs' how to respond to the verbal and or physical cues. The patient is then cued in all situations in which they become angry or over-aroused. This will help consolidate the verbal strategy, making it easier to evoke in times of stress and high arousal when initiating novel or low frequency behaviours becomes difficult. Whenever the patient engages in the alternative behaviour he or she should be provided with social and or concrete reinforcement.

An example of a verbal mediational strategy:

1 'I feel angry' – the stimulus recognition phase.
2 'When angry I usually hit people' – the response recognition phase.
3 'When I hit people I do not get to go out on the weekend, and people that I like are disappointed in me' – the consequence recognition phase.
4 'I should tell somebody how I feel' – the acknowledgement phase.
5 'It would be better for me to walk away and cool off (or go and tell someone about what has happened)' – the alternative action phase.

Variants of this procedure have proved successfully with numerous patients particularly those whose behavioural control difficulties involved over-responsiveness to normal frustration (affective aggression). Crane and Joyce (1991) have reported the successful application of a modified version of these procedures which they call 'cool down' to two post-acute patients with brain injury. The two patients had relatively preserved cognitive functioning and significant verbal and physical abuse. Initially a sessional training approach involving biofeedback, so that the patient could monitor their own tension level, was used followed by a general unit approach.

Behavioural momentum

Behavioural momentum (Mace *et al.*, 1988) may be considered a special aspect of the antecedent effect on behaviour. It refers to the tendency for low probability behaviours to be more readily performed to request when embedded in a series of high probability of compliance behaviours. The greater the rate of reinforcement available the greater the momentum. Interventions based on this notion can address non-compliance or delayed compliance. By preceding a low probability of compliance request (i.e. an activity which the subject does not normally perform) with high probability of compliance requests the likelihood of compliance is considerably increased. The research of Mace and co-workers (1988) with a mentally handicapped population demonstrates that antecedent high probability of compliance commands increase compliance and decrease compliance latency and task duration, and that these effects are independent of experimenter attention. Behavioural momentum is however only effective when the high probability commands occur immediately prior to the low probability commands (Mace *et al.*, 1988). Treadwell and Page (1996) report the successful use of behavioural momentum in conjunction with an extinction procedure in reducing non-compliance in a patient who was 13 years post-severe brain injury.

Errorless learning

Used primarily to increase compliance with children with developmental disabilities and behaviour disorder (Ducharme and Popynick, 1993; Ducharme *et al.*, 1994) the approach is easily adapted to meet the needs of the brain-injured population. The approach can be thought of as a variant of antecendent control or systematic desensitization and attempts to teach compliance. Initially the individual is exposed to a range of demand situations to which there is a high probability of compliance. The individual can be reinforced for compliance in these situations and then requests that are only slightly more likely to lead to maladaptive responses can be interspersed with the high probability of compliance requests. Over a course of training lower and lower probability of compliance requests can be introduced until the patient is responding appropriately to all requests even those where the initial likelihood of appropriate response was very low. The treatment effects have been shown to be durable on follow-up (Ducharme and Popynick, 1993; Ducharme *et al.*, 1994). Like antecendent approaches the errorless learning approach minimizes the exposure of the patient to high demand situations likely to provoke significantly maladaptive behaviour. Slifer *et al.* (1997) report the use of a combined antecedent control and operant approach to increasing task demands on three recently brain-injured adolescents. Ongoing measures of cooperation (responses to requests to attend therapy), agitation and disruptive behaviour were used to titrate the introduction of escalating demands on the patient in therapy. Two conditions were utilized in sequence. As long as disruptive behaviour continued at baseline rates or were increasing, and cooperation with minimal demands were inconsistent, the training focused on differential reinforcement of compliance with simple instructions and activities which were easy for the patient. When the patient's appropriate behaviour stabilized at low levels the difficulty of the rehabilitation activities were gradually increased but only to the extent that low levels of non-compliance were elicited (Slifer *et al.*, 1997). Further experimental designs are necessary to demonstrate the effectiveness of the procedure but the method shows promise and minimizes some of the difficulties encountered by therapy staff by making the initial behavioural goals explicit to all staff.

A criticism which has been levelled at antecedent control approaches generally is that they alter the environment and not the patient so that relapse is likely when the individual is discharged from the treatment setting. The empirical evidence is quite robust that this is not the case and any method that allows the patient to bring their behaviour under control and reinforce them for doing so may be effective.

Non-specific factors

Although careful analysis of patient behaviours and a grasp of theoretical principles is important so is the manner in which the techniques are used. The methods provide a structure or therapeutic environment within which therapy can take place. It is important to the effectiveness of the treatment that patients live in a potentially highly rewarding environment. Therapists must be capable of providing powerful reinforcement to patients so that the therapist can help the patient to change. Factors such as staff stress, staffing problems, staff turnover and fatigue influences the staff's approach to patients, and appropriate reinforcement for staff is a prerequisite for good patient treatment.

In some cases the reinforcement provided by a therapist who is concerned about the patient and committed to the patient's recovery may be the most powerful reinforcer available. Used within the context of careful functional/behavioural analysis and the consistent application of learning principles these 'non-specific' factors may be central in assisting the patient to recover from brain injury.

SUMMARY

Behaviour disorder is a frequent consequence of severe brain injury. Both learning and organic factors may contribute to the disorders. An understanding of the principles of learning theory is essential to an objective functional behavioural analysis. Until recently interventions were primarily operant, however in recent years a wide range of techniques have been described in the literature. Attention should be directed towards appropriate staff training and the environment so as to develop a rehabilitative culture which fosters adaptive behaviour change in patients.

6

FUNCTIONAL SKILLS TRAINING FOLLOWING SEVERE BRAIN INJURY

Gordon Muir Giles & Jo Clark-Wilson

Severe brain injury often results in the loss or disruption of patterns of adaptive behaviour. In addition an individual's ability to re-acquire adaptive behaviour is often impaired. The frequency of disruption of basic self-care skills among individuals with severe brain injury has been estimated at 5–15% (Jennett and Teasdale, 1981; Jacobs, 1988). Disruption of more complex community skills such as managing personal finances and vocational functioning is more common (Jacobs, 1988). This chapter discusses the theoretical background of functional skills training. Retraining methods are described followed by the application of these methods to various types of functional skills deficits. A model is developed which can account for the effects of functional skills retraining programmes. The chapter concludes with a discussion of the evidence relating to improvement in functional skills that can be achieved by post-acute rehabilitation programmes.

Most survivors of acute neurological damage show some degree of recovery. Although the cause of the recovery is unknown (see Chapter 1) therapists have attempted to potentiate the process by stimulating the patient. In the early acute period coma stimulation is viewed as an important component of treatment by many therapists (Giles and Clark-Wilson, 1993). In later stages of recovery therapists have attempted to stimulate patients by the use of tasks of graded difficulty. Hierarchies in various cognitive, behavioural and physical domains have been constructed and therapists attempt to facilitate patients' progress through these (Soderback and Normell, 1986a, b). It has been suggested that the earlier patients can be exposed to rehabilitation the greater the recovery (Cope and Hall, 1982; Mackay *et al.*, 1992). Rehabilitation during the acute stage of recovery could influence the rapidity of progress and the eventual functional outcome. Alternatively rehabilitation might only affect the initial stages of the recovery process without altering the ultimate level of outcome (Giles and Clark-Wilson, 1993). Improvements might also be due to natural recovery. Accelerated improvement – whether or not it has durable effects – could result in a shorter hospital stay with considerable cost savings. Animal models of recovery from neurological trauma suggest that early physical intervention may be more effective than delayed intervention. In a comparison of early and late motor 'rehabilitation' in Rhesus monkeys, delayed intervention resulted in more rapid improvement but the ultimate level of recovery of the early rehabilitation group was never achieved (Black *et al.*, 1975). There have been no animal studies directly supporting a comparable effect for cognitive functions. Attempts to study the benefits of early intervention on human subjects (Cope and Hall, 1982; Mackay *et al.*, 1992) have been so complicated by methodological difficulties that results have been difficult to interpret (Giles and Clark-Wilson, 1993). There are, however, reports of patients removed from nursing homes and admitted to rehabilitation facilities whose rapid improvement suggests that some stimulation is necessary to ensure that patients function up to the level permitted by their neurological recovery (Shaw *et al.*, 1985; Bell and Tallman, 1995). There is no evidence that one specific form of intervention has a greater effect at this early stage on potentiating recovery than another (Chapters 4 and 9 focus on this early recovery period).

In the post-acute recovery period therapists attempt to directly address the cognitive substrata of perception, attention, memory, judgement, problem-solving reasoning, and so on. The advantage of these basic cognitive interventions, were they to be effective, would be the 'trickle down' effect that improvement in basic cognitive skills would have on all aspects of the patient's functioning. So, for example, improved attention would improve the ability to acquire new information, keep track of ongoing events and increase work performance efficiency. The disadvantage of attempting to remediate basic cognitive functioning is that this type of intervention is of unproved efficacy so that time and effort may result in no functional improvement.

Instead of addressing basic cognitive deficits some therapists have attempted to train brain-injured patients in compensatory approaches to specific deficits. Unfortunately patients are often taught techniques without adequate consideration being given to whether the likely improvement in quality of life warrants the effort required to learn them. To be effective a compensatory strategy must be used by patients confronted by novel situations encountered in the real world. Brain-injured individuals can often learn strategies but be unable to apply them even with training in everyday situations. Compensatory behaviours which are most successful are those which the individual may overlearn to the point of automaticity. Compensatory techniques which despite overlearning remain effortful (such as visualization strategies in memory retraining) are usually too demanding to be used outside the training sessions.

As an alternative to the above techniques specific task approaches train people to perform a specific functional behaviour. In specific task training the therapist attempts to teach an actual functional task. The intervention may or may not involve task specific compensatory training. For example a patient with hemianopia who is being taught to cross the street may be trained to overcompensate by turning their head to the left (a strategy that can also be used in many other situations). Using the terminology of the World Health Organization (WHO, 1997) the intention is to improve abilities and participation. The intervention must address a behaviour of clinical importance and to an extent which makes a real difference. In most cases training must be complete enough to be self-sustaining (i.e. used spontaneously and habitually) by the time the patient is discharged from the treatment setting. Wherever possible the same basic strategy should be applied to multiple areas of dysfunction (e.g. head turning in a patient with hemianopia). The execution of the skill should be taught in multiple real-world settings. Patients should be taught task-organizational skills which can be applied across domains. By focusing on the organization of basic skills (e.g. a methodical approach to the use of a memory aid or using cueing or a check list in vocational settings) it may also be possible to improve patient insight and mental efficiency resulting in continued cognitive improvements. This type of gene-ralization of response set has been described in a number of multiple baselines across behaviours case studies (Burke *et al.*, 1991). Although the effect is probably not a result of improved executive function but rather a reduction in the need for executive control of more basic functions, it is an important technique to encourage generalization within treatment domains (Giles and Clark-Wilson, 1993). Evidence reviewed below suggests that functional improvements may continue in patients provided with functional retraining following the cessation of the training itself.

ASSESSMENT

Functional/behavioural assessment may make use of a range of evaluation techniques. Methods include standardized assessments, questionnaires, checklist and rating scales, and observation. The most important of these is observation. Occupational therapists typically assess patients over a wide range of basic areas of functioning which may be divided into sensory, perceptual, motor, cognitive and affective. Observation of real-life functioning is the primary mode of assessment because there is almost never a one-to-one correspondence between observed cognitive deficits and impaired performance of functional skills. Observational techniques can be described as falling into two categories; naturalistic and struc-tured. In naturalistic observation environmental demands are not specifically manipulated allowing the therapist to develop an understanding of the patient's overall behavioural repertoire. It is important to establish what the patient does unconstrained by external cues or demands. Structured observations fall into two categories. First, specific areas of functioning can be cued and observed, for example, washing and dressing behaviour, street crossing, transfers. Secondly specific behaviours can be evaluated for frequency of occurrence and eliciting factors; frequency baselining or antecedent–behaviour–consequence (ABC) recordings. This second type of recording is often used to describe behavioural disregulation or social-skills deficits. Despite careful observation the underlying deficit resulting in functional skills breakdown can remain unclear. The therapist can reason across functional tasks to deduce the underlying deficits or may use standardized testing to elucidate the cause of the problem so that an adequate treatment plan can be developed.

Functional/behavioural assessment determines current level of functioning and assists in the determination of optimal forms of retraining. In addition it is central to the selection of goals and target behaviours required for the rehabilitation team's integrated treatment plan. Assessment should be conducted under conditions as close as possible to those the person will experience following rehabilitation. There are many variables which influence performance in real world situations, for example, the presence of setting events, cues or environmental conditions.

Standardized assessment

In some instances observation alone will not indicate why a person's performance breaks down. Standardized testing may assist in determining the origin of a performance deficit. Recently a number of tests for use by occupational therapists have appeared on the market which are designed to be ecologically valid (described below).

RETRAINING METHODS

Intervention methods may be thought to exist on a behavioural–cognitive behavioural continuum. All treatment involves modifying the patient's previous responses and replacing them with new and more adaptive ones via practice (Giles and Clark-Wilson, 1993). Patients who are able to develop a new and more accurate model of their own basic cognitive functioning can learn new metacognitive control strategies. Metacognitive control involves learning a new language or way to think about the post-injury self. Functional skills which require the patient to cope with novelty require a complex set of cognitive abilities. For example complete functional use of a diary for prospective appointment-keeping always involves decisions about what information to write down. Practice in how to make entries and what information to enter (e.g. both the type of material to enter such as appointments, work-related events, and the parameters which are important, where and when, what to bring, and so on) reduces the difficulty of these tasks but the patient must nevertheless categorize a particular appointment as one of the classes of events which should be recorded and then initiate the recording.

Training programmes which attempt to address a general behaviour (such as the development of social skills or the use of a memory book) should help the patient develop a compatible metacognitive model. Programmes should include the following three stages.

1 A cognitive overlearning element to focus the patient's attention on the behaviour or area of skills deficit. The therapist discusses the implications of the behaviour or skill deficit with the patient in regard to long-term functioning. The therapist's emphasis is the benefits likely to accrue to the patient from changing the behaviour. If the patient has severe deficits this cognitive component may need to be reviewed once or more per day and may continue throughout and/or beyond the other programme elements.

2 Sessional practice of required behaviours. The patient practices the behaviour for a short period of time in an environment controlled by the therapist. The patient must be able to produce the behaviour with only moderate effort in this controlled environment before progressing to stage 3.

3 The 24-h programme approach. In stage 3 there is an attempt to target each instance of the behaviour throughout the day. This type of intervention requires an interdisciplinary team and a high level of staff training. Each time the patient exhibits the target behaviour a staff member responds in a pre-

determined manner so the patient attends to the behaviour and categorizes it as an instance of the target behaviour, and learns to suppress it and replace it with an alternative or incompatible behaviour.

ANTECEDENT CONTROL

Central to the development of an appropriate retraining programme is an understanding of the features of the environment that elicit behaviour in a patient. Ross (1977) describes the fundamental attribution error as the tendency to underestimate the impact of situational factors in preference to the role of dispositional factors in controlling behaviour. In addition behaviours which we find unpleasant in others will tend to become a focus of our attention. Whatever we focus our attention on is apt to be regarded as a causal agent. Health professionals in general are most familiar with thinking about individuals as causal agents not of systems or environmental events. Altering the environment is often sufficient to elicit a needed behaviour which when practised becomes an increasingly available part of the patient's behavioural repertoire. Part of the therapist's overall approach should include 'cue experimentation' where the therapist attempts different methods of cueing in order to elicit the desired behaviour. Zencius *et al.* (1989) systematically studied the effect of altering antecedents in three patients with marked memory disorder following severe brain injury. Posting a sign regarding breaktimes at the work station of the first patient drastically reduced the number of unauthorized breaks. In another patient the most effective way to increase walking stick usage, a goal of the rehabilitation team, was to provide her with a walking stick to use during her morning ADLs. This technique was found to be more effective than social praise, a contract for money or someone to escort her to get her walking stick when she was found without it. In a third patient the authors found that a map and a written daily schedule was more powerful than a contract for money in increasing therapy attendance. The alteration in the antecedence produced behavioural improvement after attempts to alter behaviour by consequences had proved to be, at best, only marginally successful.

Types of antecedent interventions

Staff can become so busy and task oriented that it is hard for them to see alternatives to making a direct request that a patient engage in a specific behaviour (or refrain from a behaviour). The assumption that individuals understand the world in the same way that we do is so strong that it significantly constrains the types of interventions we contemplate. Often this leads to confrontation, psychological reactance and increased confusion, anxiety and intransigence from the patient. Our limited and familiar behavioural routines and ways of thinking lead us to view our own responses as the only ones available. Therapists should make deliberate attempts to manage factors that can precipitate confusion, agitation and non-compliance. These include overstimulation (often caused by trying to rush the patient), and not managing the patient's perplexity. The patient should be provided with an organized, routine and structured environment that is not overstimulating and which includes familiar people (regular staff). The patient should be provided with explicit and consistent external guidance. These types of interventions can be used in patients with both acute and chronic confusion.

Antecedent interventions can be divided into interventions the primary focus of which is to elicit engagement in therapeutic activities and those aimed at reducing unwanted behaviours (Yuen and Benzing, 1996). Often however they may be used interchangeably. Below interventions are discussed under the headings: 'Engaging the patient in therapeutic activities', and 'Elimination of unwanted behaviours' (Yuen and Benzing, 1996). Some interventions will be found to be counter-productive with particular patients but the authors have used all of the interventions below with success with particular patients. Only individuals with experience in managing people who have behaviour disorder should attempt to use these interventions.

ENGAGING THE PATIENT IN THERAPEUTIC ACTIVITIES

Implicit guidance

The patient may be assisted through an activity using verbal and physical guidance. Patients may deteriorate behaviourally if they become too perplexed or if given direct instructions ('Leave me alone!'. 'Don't tell me what to do!'). The therapist can utilize the client's environmental dependency and conformity to implicit instructions ('let me get your clothes for you' – rather than 'I want you to get dressed'). The therapist 'assumes' that the patient will comply. Options are limited so that the patient does not become overwhelmed.

Biasing cognitive set

Many patients are confused and can easily become preoccupied by a particular thought or misinterpretation of their environment. Biasing the patient's cognitive set involves 'priming the pump' by pre-orienting the patient to an activity, what is happening to them, and the how and the why of the task in which they are to engage. Although very difficult to redirect once the patient has misinterpreted the environment, if initially oriented the patient may be able to maintain cognitive set. This intervention is intended for patients who are confused but who can at times comprehend their situation, it is contraindicated in patients who are actively denying there situation, problems, etc. An alternative strategy, suggested by Yuen and Benzing (1996), is to place a request in the context of pre-injury skills or goals, for example by pointing out to a patient that someone in his or her occupation needs to be able to perform a certain task.

Redirection to new controlling variables

A straightforward prompt or situational demand may elicit a set of specific negative behaviours from a client or rigid non-compliance. For example, one client when asked to go to eat lunch in the cafeteria would refuse stating he was not hungry. The patient would however 'go for a walk' ending up in the cafeteria where he would eat. Another client would state that she had showered the night before and would refuse to shower. A calendar check-off sheet was developed and posted by the nurses' station. Every morning she was prompted to 'check the calendar' where the date of the last shower was written, eliminating the showering problem.

Behavioural momentum

In behavioural momentum a low probability of compliance request is embedded in a string of high probability of compliance requests. Staff may become anxious about making requests of patients who display powerfully negative responses. This can lead staff to go directly to a low probability of compliance request (or even to project an expectation of non-compliance). An embedded or graduated introduction of what has previously served as a discriminative stimulus for non-compliance may be more effective. A staff member might, for example, first have a cup of coffee with the patient, then look at the paper and only when engaged with the patient introduce the shower request.

Structuring the situation so that goal achievement leaves the client in the client's preferred situation

This is a very simple idea. If the client likes their room and the goal is for the patient to ambulate, walk them to the room and not away from it. If they like to be in their wheelchair, transfer them to the mat and ask the patient to transfer themselves back to the wheelchair (this can be done over and over again).

Use of specific staff

The stimulus characteristics of specific staff (appearance/behaviour) enable them to get patients to comply with requests that elicit non-compliance or resistance from others. All of the staff resources should be utilized to increase compliance initially, later generalization can be attempted by pairing staff in what were initially low probability of compliance activities.

Errorless compliance training

Discussed in more detail elsewhere, this technique uses a highly structured approach to develop behavioural compliance. A hierarchy of behaviours is developed from very high likelihood of compliance to low likelihood of compliance behaviours. What the patient practises is compliance to requests. Once an acceptable standard is met for compliance with high likelihood of compliance requests, requests that are somewhat less likely to be complied with are introduced. This process continues until the patient is routinely complying with what were initially low probability of compliance requests. Although superficially similar to behavioural momentum its goal is a durable change in responses to compliance requests. Errorless compliance training has been used extensively with children with developmental disabilities and behaviour disorder (Ducharme and Popynick, 1993; Ducharme et al., 1994) and has been used with patients in the acute recovery period after brain injury (Slifer et al., 1997).

ELIMINATION OF UNWANTED BEHAVIOURS

Distraction and derailment to automatic behaviours

Many patients develop overvalued ideas or behaviours. When confused they may engage in these thoughts or behaviours with very high frequency. The automatic response for staff is often to attempt to dissuade the individuals from a particular inappropriate activity (driving, going home, etc.). The individual does not understand why they should not engage in the activity and the patient's sense of certainty and control may be challenged by the therapist's attempt to dissuade. Both staff and patient become more and more stressed and the situation deteriorates. Saying 'no' to a confused client usually agitates them so staff should look for ways to say yes and then to engage the patient in an alternate activity. For example a client who was very confused and agitated was very insistent about going outside – the client was however quite content when taken to a fully enclosed patio area in the hospital.

Overstimulation

Most individuals without brain injury can only focus for brief periods without the need to rest. This phenomenon is also readily observable in patients emerging from coma. Many patients appear unable to focus their attention. Increasing stimulation can provoke increasing levels of arousal that the patient is unable to regulate leading to increased behavioural production, agitation and distress. Patients with impaired attention have little ability to filter stimuli and are prone to overstimulation. When staff see a patient become behaviourally or emotionally disregulated the natural reaction is to approach, but in the case of the patient who is overstimulated this makes the situation worse. Patients should be assisted to titrate the amount of stimulation to which they are exposed; the introduction of frequent rest periods as well as breaks during therapy sessions can be helpful.

Avoidance of triggers

A variant of the above addresses the precipitants of aggressive behaviour so that they can be avoided. A patient may become irate and assaultive if they ask to smoke and are told 'no', but may accept the statement 'Yes, at the next smoke break, and I will make sure that you get there in plenty of time'. Physical proximity or eye contact may trigger aggressive behaviour in some patients. Positioning patient, staff or objects so that direct eye contact is not possible can be effective. Some patients will become preoccupied with a specific staff member and this may last a few minutes or longer. Removing that staff member from the routine care of the patient can be an effective intervention. Rarely, particular staff are incorporated into an elaborate delusion and this may limit the usefulness of the staff member with the patient. Triggers may be a part of the normal institutional environment. An appropriately designed unit protects patients from reasonably foreseeable triggers. One patient with profound frontal lobe impairment, irritability, and utilization behaviour was repeatedly smashing television sets when left unsupervised. Transfer to a unit where the televisions were ceiling mounted and behind Plexiglas eliminated the problem.

Structured routine

In highly structured behaviour programmes or transitional living programmes much of the work of providing structure for the patient is provided by the treatment milieu. However in acute rehabilitation and less specialized settings a consistent structured environment may be much more difficult to achieve. A patient may not remember from one moment to the next but nonetheless respond to routine by increasing compliance with routine behaviours that serve as behavioural anchors for the patient. A routine of bathing, dressing, eating, therapy and resting, with written schedules when appropriate reduces stress on the patient and staff. Initially it can be difficult for staff to modify their behaviour but it is eventually possible for most staff to comply with a schedule. Initially in a long-term behaviour-management unit run by one of the authors (GMG), patients had to be brought to group settings and continually brought back to the group after they wandered out. However in a matter of weeks patients were coming to the door at the correct time without being able to state why and were able to stay throughout the group.

Walking

Many of the most difficult patients to manage are fully ambulatory but acutely confused. Walking can help a patient relax and provide an outlet if the patient seems to feel the need to move. If the physical environment allows having a walking route or loop in the hospital which does not go near exits this is ideal. Patients will often habituate to the route. For obvious reasons patients should not wander in settings that could place them at risk.

Developing an emotional set

Patients who are labile and disinhibited are often highly susceptible to the emotional environment or setting events. Finding a way to relate to patients that is both appropriate and warm can be very effective. For example, a profoundly impaired highly assaultive male patient had been at a state mental hospital for 16 years before admission to a long-term behaviour-management programme run by one of the authors (GMG). When first admitted it was requiring four to six staff to render ADL care due to assaultiveness. Although multiple interventions were attempted concurrently the most important of these was a humorous cajoling approach in which staff described the patient as a 'ring leader' and 'mad, bad and dangerous to know'. When spoken to in this way the patient laughed uproariously and was compliant with staff requests.

Distraction and redirection

Severely impaired and confused clients can be distracted and attempts made to engage them in alternative (preferred) activities. These interventions can be very simple. One patient is extremely labile easily becoming irate and assaultive but can be readily encouraged to 'give the peace sign' which ends the behavioural outburst. This type of intervention runs counter to how people normally behave with others and can be a difficult skill to acquire. It can be thought of as the antecedent equivalent of the operant-conditioning procedure of differential reinforcement of an incompatible behaviour.

SKILL BUILDING

Reinforcement

A reinforcing event is one which increases the likelihood of the behaviour which immediately precedes it being repeated. Reinforcers may be primary or secondary. There is some evidence that reinforcement aids learning (Lashley and Drabman, 1974; Dolan and Norton, 1977). The reason that reinforcement increases learning is unknown but may be related to the ability of reinforcement to direct attention toward the to-be-learned aspects of the practised behaviours. In addition developing positive cognitions about the learning process itself and what is to be learned is probably very helpful in human beings.

Task analysis

Task analysis involves a process of dividing tasks into component parts which can be taught. The analysis provides a method of organizing behaviours to make them easier to learn. The components of a task analysis may be converted to verbal or visual prompts. When using a task analysis to develop a set of visual or verbal cues, the number of cues depends on the patient's ability. For example, in developing a washing and dressing programme some patients require only a few prompts such as 'wash your face' to produce complex behavioural chains. Other patients require several prompts, for example, 'pick up the wash cloth', 'put soap on the wash cloth', 'wash your face', 'rinse the wash cloth' (Giles *et al.*, 1997).

Chaining

Functional tasks can be thought of as complex stimulus–response chains in which the completion of each activity acts as the stimulus for the next step in the chain (Kazdin, 1994). Three chaining options are available for training functional tasks.

1 Backward chaining (BC) in which the last step of the task is trained first, followed by the second to last step and the last step and so on, progressing backwards through the chain.
2 Forward chaining (FC) in which the first step of the chain is trained first, followed by the first and second step and so on, progressing forward through the chain.
3 Whole task method (WTM) in which each step of the chain is trained on each presentation.

Basic operant researchers have preferred BC on theoretical grounds (Skinner, 1938; Martin *et al.*, 1981), while clinicians have focused on the practical advantages of WTM. Contemporary studies have found WTM to be equivalent or superior to BC (Martin *et al.*, 1981; Spooner, 1981, 1984; McDonnell and Laughlin, 1989).

Prompts

Events which facilitate the production of a behaviour are called prompts (or cues). In many instances prompts are available in the environment but they are no longer sufficient to guide behaviour or they have lost their meaning entirely (e.g. arriving at a busy junction no longer cues safe street-crossing routines). The therapist adds additional prompts to those already available in the environment. Therapists can facilitate the learning of skills with a range of differing types of prompts. Two types of prompting systems have been evaluated in teaching chained tasks: the system of least prompts (SLP) and time-delay procedures. The system of least prompts (sometimes referred to as the increasing assistance procedure) involves the presentation of a prompt hierarchy that is arranged from most general to most specific. The individual is cued progressively through the hierarchy of prompts available for each step in the chain until a correct response is produced. The time-delay cueing system typically involves two training stages.

1 A cue designed to elicit the next step in the chain is delivered so as to coincide with the stimulus (i.e. the completion of the previous step in the chain).
2 A defined interval is inserted between the occurrence of the stimulus and the response eliciting cue. Two types of time-delay procedures are described in the literature: progressive time delay (PTD) where longer and longer intervals are inserted between the occurrence of the stimulus and the cue, and constant time delay (CTD) where a fixed response interval is inserted between stimulus and cue (Wolery *et al.*, 1990).

Some therapists may prefer to begin with CTD and utilize PTD as a fading technique. However PTD should only be used when the patient has already developed the skill to the point where they can be 80–90% correct as otherwise they are likely to 'practice' the propagation of incorrect responses – a situation to be avoided. Questions like 'What's next?' or instructions telling the individual to 'go ahead' can also help the individual initiate the activity and decreases dependence on prompts.

Practice and the development of automaticity

Repetition of a behaviour increases the probability of the behaviour being further repeated (Giles and Clark-Wilson, 1993). This is known as response practice and is the most important aspect of successful behavioural training. As practice is continued the behaviours can become automatic. Overlearning refers to the practice of a skill well beyond the point where mastery has been achieved. Overlearning increases the chances that a skill is consolidated in the individual's repertoire of skills and reduces the effort required for performance of the skill (Giles and Clark-Wilson, 1993). For example, a street-crossing programme should not be terminated on meeting the functional criteria for the first time but on meeting criteria plus a certain number of practice sessions designed to make the behaviour automatic. The number of additional sessions required to develop automaticity is unclear. Automaticity is assessed by ongoing monitoring of the patient's behaviour in everyday life with its attendant distractions.

Shiffrin and Schneider (1977) describe attention in terms of attention-dependent controlled processing and attention-independent automatic processing. Controlled processing is capacity limited, slow serial and effortful and is required for new learning to occur. Automatic processing occurs without conscious control, and places only limited demands on the information processing system. Controlled processing and practice is necessary for the development of automaticity. Studies of individuals in the post-acute stage of recovery from severe brain injury suggest that the amount of practice required for automaticity to develop is increased by brain injury (Schmitter-Edgecombe and Rogers, 1997). It is important to note that that consistent practice of the same activity performed in exactly the same way leads to the development of automaticity. Stimuli which have variable task demands attached to them do not result in the development of automaticity. Many subskills in more complex tasks are invariant and can develop automaticity with highly structured practice (Kramer *et al.*, 1991; Giles and Clark-Wilson, 1993).

Encore procedure

When an individual demonstrates an infrequently displayed skill without prompting, he or she can be prompted to produce several more correct responses. For example, a patient was learning to attract attention appropriately before asking questions or making requests in social skills groups. On any occasion when she interacted appropriately such as by saying the persons name, or 'excuse me' (rather than by screaming or banging objects) and asking a question, she was given social, and occasionally tangible reinforcement and she was asked to repeat the sequence of behaviours again whereupon she was reinforced again.

Highlighting

Many individuals after brain injury have problems in distinguishing the central aspects of a task. Highlighting refers to a strategy that promotes the discrimination of the crucial elements of an activity by exaggerating the salience of some stimulus features. Prompts are progressively faded once the patient is consistently making correct discriminations. Highlighting might be achieved by emphasizing phrases, pointing, touching or by providing specific reinforcement.

Metacognitive control and skills training

The term metacognition refers to a person's understanding and regulation of their own basic cognitive processes (see Chapter 1). Metacognition includes awareness of performance and monitoring and control functions. For example metacognitive functions include assessments of task difficulty and the ability to assess the likelihood of problems in carrying out particular activities. They also include the ability to recognize errors and to adjust performance as a consequence. Meta-cognitive control training may therefore involve the individuals in trials of activities where the individual has to predict the likelihood of error and immediately get feedback. There is a sense in which this new terminology is 'old wine in new bottles' but it also gives a new format to think about interventions. If an individual does not think that their underlying capacity has changed then there will be a tendency not to adjust the strategy for problem solving and there will be repeated failure. Chapter 10 emphasizes the conservatism of self-image and that an individual's conceptualizations of their own capacities tend to be stable.

A number of workers have developed approaches with specific focus on helping the patient develop new metacognitive control strategies (Cicerone and Giacino, 1992; Toglia, 1998). Toglia, in her dynamic interactional model of cognitive rehabilitation (1998), emphasizes the following components: metacognitive training, processing strategies, learner characteristics, the environment and the task. Emphasis is placed on the assessment as an active process designed to determine the features that can be altered to potentiate improved performance. Toglia states that the approach attempts an integration of cognitive psychology theories of how non-neurologically impaired individuals learn and generalize information with the rehabilitation of clients with cognitive dysfunction (Toglia, 1998). Unfortunately because the approach is so dependent on the manipulation of conscious cognitive processes it probably has limited application when used in isolation with individuals with severe deficits following brain injury (a problem recognized by Toglia, 1998) (see discussion of this issue Chapter 1). Increasingly it is recognized the extent to which implicit learning and practice of skills provides the structural underpinning of so much of our apparently cognitive processing. However when integrated with a training approach to both object-level tasks and metacognitive control functions the approach can be useful for patients with a wide range of deficits.

Goal statements

The incorporation of goal statements in treatment has a number of advantages. It may increase participation, help the patient attend to the to-be-learned aspect of their activities (this discriminatory aspect may need to be repeated throughout the session), and it can communicate respect from therapist to patient.

For patients with lack of insight it orients them to their deficits and cues them as to how the to-be-undertaken therapeutic activity will help them achieve their own goals. Therapists may wish to present the session as a scientific endeavour, in which either the therapist or the patient is allowed to have incorrect notions, but in which an empirical question is examined. Goal-directing statements, for example, for 5 min at the beginning of each session and interspersed statements throughout, orienting patients to these issues are frequently indicated. For example, 'as you know as a result of your severe brain injury you have needed some help in washing and dressing yourself – we are working with you every morning so that you can develop a system to be independent – yesterday you performed all but three of the activities of washing and dressing completely independently'.

As with most interventions it can work well with some patients and with some it is contraindicated. With some patients active agreement with the therapeutic intervention is not attainable, and the therapist seeking agreement will only derail the therapeutic endeavour. The therapist is not advised to abandon the goal of developing functional skills by waiting until the patient knows that he or she has deficits.

Debriefing

Regular debriefing about performance (knowledge of results) is indicated in producing positive behavioural change. Telling the patient that they have done well is encouraging, but non-specific and damaging if untrue. Feedback about results should be concrete and accurate. Materials that the patient can refer to such as graphs or logs should be used where possible.

ASSESSMENT AND TRAINING IN SPECIFIC AREAS

Attention

Increased understanding of attention as a set of complex inter-related processes may help clarify how voluntary control is exerted over more automatic processes. Posner and Peterson (1990) highlight three principles central to understanding attention.

1 The neuroanatomical system which underlies attention is separate from the more basic systems (sensory motor, etc.) to which attention is allocated.
2 Adequate attentional processing depends on the interaction of different anatomical areas.
3 The areas involved in attention are specific and distinct from one another and the rest of the brain (i.e. that attention is neither the property of a single centre nor a property of the brain as a whole).

Different components of attention can be identified:

- Spatial attention: the ability to allocate attention to different areas of internal and external space.
- Selective attention: the ability to maintain a consistent behavioural set which requires activation and inhibition of responses depending upon the selection of target stimuli from background stimuli.
- Sustained attention: the ability to maintain a consistent response set during continuous or repetitive activity.
- Alternating attention: the ability to switch response sets as a response to environmental cues so that two activities with distinct response requirements can be performed in sequence.
- Divided attention: the capacity to respond simultaneously to multiple tasks.

Each of these aspects of attentional processing can be disrupted after brain injury. Unfortunately adequate measures of attention have until recently not been available for clinical use so the true prevalence of these attentional disorders and their natural history are unknown.

Assessment

Therapists have typically evaluated attention via cancellation tasks and sustained vigilance tasks utilizing computers. Measures of neglect are available (e.g. the behavioural inattention test) but standardized measures of more complex attentional processes have been lacking. The test of everyday attention (TEA) (Robertson *et al.*, 1994) is the first standardized non-computerized test of attention available for use by psychologists, speech therapists and occupational therapists. The TEA was developed to reflect current theories of attentional functioning and measures selective attention, sustained attention, attentional switching and the ability to divide attention. It uses relatively familiar everyday materials and is plausible and acceptable to subjects. Reliability and preliminary validation data are available and the test takes approximately 45–60 min to administer. Normative data are available for ages from 18 to 80 years.

Interventions for deficits in spatial attention

Standard treatment approaches used to address spatial inattention involve structured and repetitive methods of asking individuals to scan into their affected hemispace. Treatment activities include:

- Identifying objects in a picture.
- Pre-made cancellation tasks (with feedback and instruction in strategy use).
- Letter/word cancellation tasks from stimuli selected by the individual, i.e. crossing out all the capital letters in a passage or crossing out all the words beginning with a letter or all the instances of a specific word or words, for example 'of, and, but' (Diller and Weinberg, 1993).
- Reading from a newspaper (attempting to begin at the beginning of the column).
- Reading and summarizing short articles.
- Computerized scanning tasks.
- Verbal regulation strategies used in simplified retraining tasks and functional settings.
- Diller and Weinberg (1993) suggest a number of strategies to use when individuals are failing to recognize their perceptual deficits:
  - Using patient generated materials as a stimulus. The person is asked to write numbers horizontally from one to ten or to write the alphabet and then to point to the first in the series.
  - Using a conventional standard such as a 12-inch ruler for bisection tasks.
  - Counting money, the individual is given an amount of money ($1, $5, $10 and $20 dollar bills) and is asked to count the money, putting it on the table beginning left to right. The individual is then asked to pick it up again and count it.
  - Placing and picking up objects. The person is asked to place objects on the table and to then pick them up.

Diller and Weinberg (1993) suggest that acknowledging and working with the individual's response pattern is central to effective retaining. Diller and Weinberg (1993) advocate using dramatic examples to increase the credibility to the person of the problem, e.g. placing money in both the attended and unattended field and asking the person to pick up the money.

Robertson *et al.* (1988) describe the use of microcomputer-based cognitive rehabilitation of visual (left) neglect. The authors utilized a multiple baseline across cognitive functions approach and present three single case studies (one person with head trauma and two with CVA). The aim of the training programme was to establish a verbally regulated motor habit for orienting leftward. Utilizing commercially available computer-scanning training the participants were initially loudly instructed to look left just prior to the scanning trial. In the next phase participants were instructed to look left in a quiet tone. This was followed by requiring the participants to say look left and finally to give themselves subvocal commands. Non-treated cognitive functions remained at baseline levels while each participant showed significant improvement in the visual scanning tasks. The authors note that the improvement was extremely rapid and hypothesize that the results might be accounted for by the participants developing a verbal regulation strategy.

Niemeier (1998) has reported the effective use of the Lighthouse Strategy with individuals with hemispatial neglect following CVA. Patients were given a visual cancellation task and provided with feedback about their errors. In this context the visual imagery of a lighthouse was introduced to them as a way for them to conceptualize scanning left and right in functional tasks. Patients were then exposed to simple table-top, computer-assisted and paper-and-pencil tests requiring visual scanning. Any failure led to returning to the lighthouse imagery. Posters of the lighthouse were distributed around the facility and given to family members or caregivers to display at home. The Lighthouse Strategy was then incorporated into other therapeutic tasks. Comparisons of a repeat administration of the cancellation task indicated that the patients exposed to the lighthouse strategy improved significantly and that overall improvement on a measure of attention was greater for the experimental than for the control group.

Conventional approaches to neglect are implicitly or explicitly based on learning theory. Learning-based approaches are atheoretical regarding the cause of neglect and attempt to help the patient develop new overlearned habits to compensate for the deficit. Theory-based approaches suggest that interhemispheric imbalance in orientation tendencies underlies unilateral neglect. The imbalance, it is proposed, can be removed by increasing right brain activation. Three types of strategies that attempt to increase activity in the right hemisphere have been identified: the lateralized task approach, the controlled sensory stimulation approach and the limb activation approach (Lin, 1996).

In the lateralized task approach hemispheric-specific activities are used to modify hemisphere specific activation on perceptual/cognitive tasks, for example spatial stimuli. For example in a comparison of letter (left hemisphere predominant) versus line cancellation tasks (right hemisphere predominant) patients performed better on the line cancellation task (Heilman and Watson, 1978), however this and other studies showing the effect have been difficult to replicate (Lin, 1996). In the controlled sensory stimulation approach specific stimuli and activities are used in an attempt to activate brain-stem attentional mechanisms. The superior colliculus on the side ipsilateral to the lesion controls contralateral space.

Presenting static and dynamic stimuli to the neglected side improves line bisection (Butter *et al.*, 1990). An alternative type of intervention depends on the fact that retinal inflow to the superior colliculi arises predominantly from the contralateral eye. Patching the right eye (the eye ipsilateral to lesion in left neglect) reduces input to the left superior colliculus. Since the right superior colliculus is hyporeactive in comparison with the left, reducing the amount of stimulation reaching the left superior colliculus may have the effect of levelling out the activation and it does improve line bisection (Butter and Kirsch, 1992).

A third set of techniques can be described as limb activation approaches. Enabling individuals to neglect using their left hand has been found to improve spatial attention-dependent task performance (Halligan and Marshall, 1989; Halligan *et al.*, 1991). Left-hand movements are important even when the subject cannot see the hand (Robertson and North, 1992).

Other approaches that simply make the patient allocate attention to the affected hemispace by, for example, tracing the extent of a line or performing an activity in the left hemispace prior to performing a line bisection task all have an effect possibly by enabling the patient to form an intention to act in the habitually non-attended-to hemispace (Lin, 1996). Although many of these interventions show promise as yet there are no published reports of functional generalization so the interventions must be considered experimental.

Attention retraining

Sohlberg and Mateer (1987) have described an Attention Process Training (APT) method for individuals with attentional problems. The authors view attention as a multidimensional cognitive function with the subcomponents of sustained attention, selective attention, alternating attention, and divided attention. The model suggests that placing each subcomponent under stress facilitates improved functioning in that system. The authors developed hierarchies of treatment tasks for each of the four components of attention. Sohlberg and Mateer (1987) describe six basic tenets of the process-specific approach to cognitive remediation: the theoretical model, comprehensive assessment, process approach, repetition, knowledge of results and use of probes to evaluate generalization. The authors used a multiple baseline across cognitive dimensions in four single case studies which provided support for the APT approach (Sohlberg and Mateer, 1987). The mechanism by which the treatment has an effect is unclear. It is possible that new ways of processing material are being developed in conjunction with developing increased automaticity in cognitive subroutines, a process analogous to the improvement of executive functions resulting from practice of strategies for handling real-world functions described earlier, however these ideas are speculative.

Gray and Robertson (1989) describe three single case studies employing multiple baselines across cognitive dimensions design. Three brain-injured men were provided with microcomputer-based training in an attempt to remediate attentional problems. A range of different computer attentional retraining programmes were used. Each of the patients improved in their attentional functions as measured by improvements on the training task while the baseline cognitive function remained stable. In two instances the control measures were memory tests and in one a discrimination-reaction time test. The authors suggest that the development of new verbal behaviours in combination with processes rather like motor learning may have accounted for the improvement (Gray and Robertson, 1989). Because the training task and the outcome measure are identical it is unclear that there is any generalization of effect, however the findings do suggest that real-world tasks which have high loading on an attentional factor can usefully be the target of practise and possibly develop increased automaticity.

Memory

In order to understand the type of memory deficits that can follow brain injury a conceptualization of the different systems of human memory is needed. There has been rapid change in our understanding of human memory since the 1970s largely as a result of studying patients with amnesia following brain injury. It is now widely accepted that there are multiple overlapping memory systems in humans which may be differentially affected in brain injury and which are affected by damage to different brain areas. Some memory systems are available to introspection and some are not (implicit versus explicit learning). The detailed structure of these memory systems remains a subject of debate (Fuster, 1995). Before discussing the assessment and treatment of memory a typology of memory in functional retraining which may be useful in clinical practice is presented.

Retrograde and anteriograde amnesia

The terms retrograde and anteriograde define the period of memory impairment in terms of whether it is for material which preceded or followed the injury. Retrograde amnesia refers to loss of memory for events occurring prior to the injury and anteriograde amnesia refers to loss of the ability to remember (loss of memory) events that follow the injury. Most people do not remember being injured and for some people the period of retrograde amnesia may extend back in time for months or years. As the patient recovers, the period of retrograde amnesia shrinks, so that a person who initially could not remember what happened to them 3 months before the injury might eventually be able to recall all but a few hours or even minutes before the injury. The longer and more overlearned the memories the more resistant they are to loss. This shortening of the period of retrograde amnesia as times goes on suggests that much of the difficulty is due to problems in accessing or recreating memories. It may be that retrieving relatively recent memories involves a different set of mechanisms possibly involving the hippocampus (see below). The process of recording memories itself is disrupted by the injury so that memory for the injury itself (and a least a few minutes prior to the injury) almost never returns.

The patient and the family may be most concerned with retrograde amnesia (because it is the most apparent in the hospital when the patient does not actually have to do anything) however disruption of the patient's ability to consolidate new memories (anteriograde memory) is far more important for the patient's day-to-day life.

Post-traumatic amnesia

A period during which the patient is unable to remember new information is normal after injury. This inability to lay down new memories spans the period of coma and continues into the post-coma period. The name given to this period is post-traumatic amnesia (PTA). The duration of PTA is related to severity of injury. Because of the significance of PTA in predicting recovery it is important to monitor the patient's ability to remember new information on an ongoing basis. As an approximate rule of thumb PTA may be expected to last approximately four times the duration of coma. Initial emergence from PTA is usually inconsistent, i.e. it is not an all-or-none phenomenon. In cases where the injury was very severe the patient may have lasting severe memory impairment and it is not known when the patient really emerges from PTA. Patients can learn during PTA but retention is very severely impaired relative to those who are not in PTA.

Short-term memory

Short-term memory is the ability to remember items for brief periods (from 30 s to a few minutes). It is capacity limited and information in it decays rapidly if not rehearsed. It is this type of memory that allows us to look up a number in the telephone book and remember it long enough to place the call (those of us who often have to look the number up a couple of times will be keenly aware of how rapidly the information decays). The capacity limit has been expressed as seven items plus or minus two. It is possible to hold more information by chunking information together but the limit of seven discrete items is robust. The requirement of conscious attention to be directed towards the material in short-term memory has led to some to conceptualize a short-term memory store as 'working memory'.

Short-term memory may be disrupted by brain injury. Deficits in short-term memory often coexist with distractibility and pervasive attention deficit. Central to the function of short-term memory is its role in facilitating long-term retention. Rehearsal of information (going over it in one's mind) is clearly central in some attempts to place information in long-term storage.

Long-term memory

Failures in long-term memory are the most common forms of memory disturbance following brain injury and have the most functional importance. Long-term memory describes the ability to remember material for longer than a few minutes up to months, years or decades. When individuals are unable to form new memory traces they are described as amnestic. Long-term memory can be usefully divided into declarative (episodic and semantic) and non-declarative memory. These categories of memory are differentially susceptible to central nervous system damage.

Declarative memory concerns memories which are available to introspection – we know that we know them. Declarative memory can be further subdivided into episodic and semantic memory. Episodic memory is memory for personal historical events, for instance facts about the individual's thoughts, feelings and experiences which are often associated with specific times and places. Episodic memory permits the recollection of events as they occur in a continuous stream though time.

Episodic memory is the type of memory most frequently damaged by brain injury. This is why patients loose their sense of time, forget where they are or what they are doing and fail to understand their current circumstances. Episodic memory allows us to carry on our normal daily lives, develop interpersonal relationships, follow the plot of a soap opera on TV and so on.

Semantic memory is knowledge about the world which is not usually temporally or spatially located (for example, most of us know December 25th is Christmas day but very few of us remember when or where we first learned that information).

Non-declarative memory unlike declarative memory is not available to introspection. Usually an action or set of actions which were at one time available to introspection have become overlearned to the point at which they become a procedure. The examples of this type of behaviour with which we are most familiar are riding a bicycle or driving a car. Current evidence suggests that extremely complex forms of learning may be subserved by non-declarative memory. The distinction between implicit and explicit knowledge is increasingly recognized as important. Many individuals following brain injury deny explicit knowledge, but changes in behaviour demonstrate that learning has taken place despite that lack of conscious awareness. A number of sophisticated experimental procedures have demonstrated the wide applicability of the implicit versus explicit dichotomy (see Chapter 10).

Assessment
Orientation
One of the most fundamental tests of ability to remember is orientation. Although there are some exceptions return of orientation usually occurs in the following order: person, place, time.

To person:

- What is your name?

The therapist will also be interested in whether the patient can recall other personally relevant information such as date of birth, names of family members, home address, and so on. (If the individual is unable to speak due to intubation they can be provided with a list of names and asked to indicate which one is correct).

To place:

- Where are you?
- What town are we in?
- What kind of place is this? What is its purpose?

(If the individual is unable to speak they can be provided with a list of alternatives for each question, e.g. is this an airport, a hospital or a bus station? Are we in

Manchester, Birmingham, Leeds, New Orleans, St. Louis or Chicago? Is the purpose of this place to prepare food, repair cars or to care for people who are sick.)

A person is oriented to place if they can tell you exactly where they are. However a person may also be oriented if they can tell you what town they are in and that they are in a hospital. When the person gives a non-specific response they can be told the correct information to determine whether they can retain it.

To time:

- What year is it?
- What month is it?
- What day of the week is it?
- What is the date? Many non-neurologically impaired people cannot answer this question with any precision (plus or minus 2 days is normal).
- About what time is it? Is it before or after breakfast/lunch? (If the individual is unable to speak the therapist can provide the patient with alternatives for each question, e.g. is it 1957, 1982 or 1993? Is it October, February or July? Is it Monday, Thursday or Sunday? or present them with a calendar.)

A person is oriented to time if they know the year, month, date, day of the week and approximate time of day. A person is at least partially oriented if they can state the year, month, whether it is early or late in the month and the approximate time of day.

It is being recognized that remembering is in many instances a reconstructive process in which the individual marshals many sources of information to constrain their responses. Damage to frontal lobe functions may disrupt this ability. Individuals may at times be oriented, and be able to generate information about their actual circumstances, while at other times they may not.

GOAT

The Galveston Orientation and Amnesia Test (GOAT) (Levin *et al.*, 1979a) is designed to chart changes in cognition and orientation during the subacute stage of recovery from brain injury. The GOAT provides a practical and reliable scale designed to evaluate the major spheres of orientation, i.e. time, place and person and may be used by various health-care workers. The GOAT also allows for estimation of the period following injury for which the person is unable to recall events and for the period pre-dating the injury for which recall is absent (retrograde amnesia). All items are presented orally. The GOAT can be used at the patient's bedside and daily administration is recommended. The recording form and detailed scoring instructions are provided in the original report (Levin *et al.*, 1979a).

Assessing other aspects of memory

An individual can be fully oriented but nonetheless have memory impairment significant enough to interfere with everyday functioning. Adequate assessment of memory functioning includes structured interviews of the individual and their family, standardized testing, and observation of the individual in their daily routines (e.g. how long does it take for the individual to learn the location of their room?). A combination of methods will allow the therapist to evaluate where real-world performance breaks down. Memory assessment should routinely include the patient's recall of written, visual and verbal information immediately, i.e. at 30 s and after a delay (after 20–30 min). The therapist can manipulate the task demands to evaluate if the patient is having difficulty encoding the information in the first place (immediate recall) or retrieving the information (by free recall followed by increasingly cued recall). A standardized test of memory, the Rivermead Behavioural Memory Test, is available for use by therapists to evaluate the types of problems a patient may have in everyday life. There are 11 subtests in the RBMT and four parallel versions so that practise effects that might occur with repeated testing can be avoided. There are two scoring methods, a screening score and a standardized profile score. Both are straightforward and are categorized on a four-point scale from normal to severely impaired. The RBMT should be used in combination with other methods of assessment such as the Everyday Memory Questionnaire (Sunderland *et al.*, 1983) and observation of real-world memory performance.

Memory retraining
Therapy for memory dysfunction can be directed at correcting the defective process or function (restitution) or reducing the effect of the deficit by utilizing intact alternative strategies (substitution) (Miller, 1985).

Internal strategies
Everyone uses internal strategies to help store and access information, although these methods are not always recognized, even by those who use them. It has been suggested that the application of some types of internal strategies could assist individuals with neurological damage and resulting memory dysfunction (Pattern, 1972; Harris, 1980; Wilson and Moffat, 1984).

Visual imagery
Visual imagery techniques have been found to assist the non-neurologically impaired in learning novel material. The place method (or method of loci) involves the individual imagining a familiar or schematized area (such as a town or an office) and 'placing' the to-be-remembered information in a specific location. The peg method helps the patient learn to associate a visual image with each of a series of numbers (e.g. one is a bun, two is a shoe). In order to remember a list of novel items (such as a shopping list) the individual imagines the items in combination with the already learned peg images. Often bizarre visual images are used to associate the material. In order to remember the list the individual thinks first of the number and of the peg image associated with it and as a result the item which was remembered in conjunction with it is recalled (Pattern, 1972). Individuals after brain injury are often inflexible in thought and have difficulty in generating images alien to their

immediate situation. Therefore individuals with deficits severe enough to warrant introduction of these types of procedures often have such severe deficits that they cannot use them. However stable associations such as face/name association can be formed using visualization techniques and could be helpful for some individuals.

Verbal elaboration

Some verbal elaboration methods are similar to the visual methods described above except that they use words to form associations. Other methods such as PQRST encourages the individual to process the material more fully. There are a number of well-known variants of the word association technique. A chaining-mnemonic format can be used to sequence information together in the form of a story to aid recall of the material, for example, the airplane list (Crovitz, 1979). However the application of this type of procedure to novel information is even more cognitively demanding than the visualization techniques described above and is therefore not usually recommended.

External strategies

The non-neurologically impaired use external strategies to recall information more often than internal strategies (Harris, 1980). External strategies include asking someone to remind you to do the task, or leaving objects in relevant places so they will be encountered when needed. For example, placing important work papers by the front door, so they will be picked up the following morning before going to work. Although many different types of external aids can be of used by persons with memory disorders here the use of calendars, clocks, posters and timetables, diaries, memory books and electronic memory aids and checklists will be discussed.

Calendars, clocks, posters and timetables

Immediately following brain injury most patients have some degree of disorientation and post-traumatic amnesia (PTA). The period of early confusion is associated with problematic behaviour and decreased functional independence. Duration of PTA is a marker of injury severity and outcome status. Clinicians have used various strategies to address the disorientation associated with PTA. One approach has been to provide multiple sources of orienting information to the patient who is in PTA including in-room clocks and calendars, posters and the use of a memory book. Reorientation groups have also been advocated (Corrigan et al., 1985). There is no evidence that these types of interventions accelerate recovery from PTA (Wanatanabe et al., 1998). They are probably important in helping patients with memory disorders who are post-PTA when used as part of an integrated approach and they do provide staff with a range of 'in the moment' management strategies. Sometimes multiple approaches, used in combination, are effective when the strategies used individually are not. For example, the use of flashcards and questioning or the use of questions in a group context and peer reinforcement (Zencius et al., 1998). Prominently displayed posters can assist patients to learn needed information. The poster should be large and eye-catching so that the patient will read it every time they see it. It may be helpful to have the person sign it to establish that they have registered agreement. Changing the look of the poster and altering its position will prevent habituation. Niemeier (1998) describes the use of posters as part of the programme of training patients in the Lighthouse Strategy to address visual inattention. Niemeier describes use of the posters to help promote the use of the technique throughout the interdisciplinary team and in an outpatient setting by giving copies of the posters to caregivers, family and the patient to take home with instructions to place them in prominent locations such as on the refrigerator door and bedroom mirror.

A timetable can be a simplified version of a diary. People at home, in rehabilitation settings or in long-term care settings have routines which can be presented in the form of a timetable. The timetable can include wake-up time, times to wash and dress, eat, do laundry or household chores and regularly scheduled individual and group therapy times or appointments. A version of this timetable needs to be posted in a prominent place for the individual such as the bedroom as well as in the memory book.

Diaries and memory books

A diary or memory book may be used at many stages of recovery from brain injury (but see the caveat above). A diary or daily planner is most applicable to prospective memory (remembering to do things in the future) while a memory book is best used as an aid to remembering the past. The memory book can include some or all of the following sections. An orientation section including the person's name, where they are and what happened to them. In this section it can also be helpful to include a list of areas in which the individual is currently having difficulty (e.g. remembering new information). This section would also include a calendar with days marked off to assist the patient in locating the correct date and a schedule of events at the hospital or rehabilitation facility to aid orientation to time and place. A section for therapy could be included for the individual to write down what they have done in therapy and record their progress. Visitors can write down when they come to the hospital and record events that occurred with family members and friends. As the patient progresses prospective memory sections can be included; for example there can be a section for questions (subheadings may include 'Questions for my husband', 'Questions for the doctor') and activities to remember. Each section in the memory book should be clearly divided and marked. The daily routine should include the time the patient needs to review their memory book and staff should encourage the patient to have the book at all times to record relevant information (initially as determined by the therapist). The memory book is most useful in encouraging staff to interact with the person and to orient them to their activities. For instance, rather than answer repetitive questions the staff should cue the patient to look at their memory log as that is where the information they need will be. As the person recovers they begin to review the book spontaneously and make entries about events in their day. Effective use of the prospective sections of the memory book usually occurs at a later stage of recovery when the patient is taking initiative and planning and organizing their activities. At this time it needs to be determined whether the patient will need an external memory aid to function in their daily life. This depends on the severity of the person's memory deficits and their vocational and living environment. Since training in the use of a memory aid is usually effortful and time-consuming, it is important that it actually addresses the patient's real-world requirements. For instance many people use the day-at-a-glance diary or other commercially available systems, such as electronic memory aids. In order to use a diary efficiently an individual must be able to read and write and extract the essential components of a plan of action in order to write them down. The individual must also be able to initiate the use of the diary at the appropriate times both for entry and retrieval of information (Giles and Shore, 1989b).

The three-stage behavioural approach (described above) has been effective in training patients in the use of external memory aids. On a sessional basis, the therapist and memory-impaired person review the individual's deficits, the reasons for using the memory aid and the specific techniques and procedures being taught. The second step involves specific practice sessions in the use of the memory aid with appropriate supervision of its use in everyday tasks. The third step involves establishing a system to ensure that the person uses the memory aid on a 24-h basis.

Jennett and Lincoln (1991) found that group therapy for memory problems was effective in increasing use of memory aids and that patients reported a decreased number of troublesome memory problems following the group. Wilson (1991) in a long-term follow-up study of memory functioning 5–10 years post-brain injury or CVA found that the majority of patients used external strategies such as notebooks (65%), lists (50%) and wall charts (50%). Interestingly individuals tended to increase their use of memory aids following discharge from the hospital. In line with our own findings (Giles and Haussman, 1997), once use of a memory aid is acquired it tends to be used consistently.

Check lists
Many patients with memory disorders do not remember whether they have performed a task. This results in them either becoming confused while performing an activity, repeating the activity or refusing to engage in the activity on the grounds that it has already been performed. Individuals can be taught to mark off each instruction/activity on a checklist as it is performed. As a more general strategy, a person with memory deficits can be taught to follow checklists as a 'meta' procedure so that whatever they need to learn can be designed as a checklist. Some patients will be non-compliant when instructed by a therapist but will follow a printed checklist. A prominently placed checklist that the person marks off or signs can be invaluable in increasing attention to task and can reduce non-compliance.

Functional skills

The term functional skills is used to describe the abilities required of an individual to function in their everyday life context. As used here the term functional skills encompasses both basic activities of daily living (e.g. washing and dressing) and complex social behaviours and work skills. Although related to physical, cognitive and behavioural performance, there is no one-to-one correspondence between the constructs we use to understand cognitive functioning and functional performance. Functional skills are therefore an area of analysis and target of intervention in their own right. The skills required of an individual to function depend to a large degree on environmental context. Different contexts exert different task demands and individual performance is often context dependent. In this chapter a small number of specific functional skills are reviewed in detail. As every person is unique (both before and after injury) the methods each individual uses to accomplish functional tasks are highly variable. The various retraining options must be selected and individualized for each person. Only a small number of functional behaviours can be considered in this chapter, however the general principles apply to many of the other domains that therapists are called on to remediate.

A retraining model

While there has been increasing interest regarding the memory deficits that may follow traumatic brain injury there has been very little effort devoted to applied studies of learning. Memory research has been of little practical assistance to those involved in training the neurologically impaired. Putting together the theories and evidence in attention and memory outlined here it is possible to suggest a retraining model with practical implications for occupational therapists and others. We rely particularly on the procedural declarative (episodic/semantic) typology, the work of Shiffrin and Schnieder (1977) on automatic and control processing and the increasing evidence that learning requires attention but does not require understanding of what is to be learned.

Let us take as an example how we might train an individual to cross the street. Crossing the street safely consists of stopping at the curbside, looking in both directions and then walking directly across the street, when there are no motor vehicles within a certain distance (depending on the patients speed of ambulation and so forth). The first time this retraining occurs is an 'episode'. It is processed and the specific to-be-learned activity is associated with the specific street intersection, the traffic which was passing and other incidental information. This episode may not be available later for introspection but a certain priming effect will have occurred. In amnestic individuals, this information will undoubtedly be subthreshold for explicit recall. On the second occasion, retraining occurs, only certain aspects of the situation will have been held constant, for instance, the specific instructions given. As this street-crossing routine is repeated, in very similar ways, the street crossing 'episodes' are not retained (or at least are not recallable). The street-crossing memory becomes an abstraction of many specific experiences, all inevitably slightly different, that eventually produces the generalized memory structure of 'crossing streets'. This experience becomes prototypical and part of the individual's behavioural repertoire and store of knowledge. In optimum cases the patient no longer chooses to cross the street in a certain manner, the patients just 'knows' that this is how they cross the street (Giles and Clark-Wilson, 1993). As we have pointed out elsewhere (Giles and Morgan, 1989; Giles and Haussman, 1997) it is not clear that either procedural or semantic memory fully describes the process taking place and the information may or may not be available to introspection. Even where there are profound deficits in episodic memory functioning, semantic learning may occur (Vargha-Khadem *et al.*, 1997). Whether this is due to retained hippocampal functioning, an ability to encode information in semantic memory that is independent of episodic memory or access to semantic memory from other memory systems is unclear.

The more severely memory impaired the individual the more important it is to limit the opportunity the individual has to propagate errors. In the presence of intact priming and severely impaired episodic memory individuals have little ability to suppress errorful performance. The absence of episodic memory prevents them from recognizing the behaviour as a failed strategy and the priming effect makes the last action the most available action and therefore increases the likelihood that it will be performed wrong again. In these circumstances errorless learning interventions are preferred to trial-and-error learning. In errorless learning sufficient cues are given to ensure adequate performance. As the behavioural response becomes more and more likely the number and depth of the cues needed to elicit the behaviour can be reduced.

Continence

Incontinence is a common consequence of severe brain injury. If unconsciousness is prolonged patients are usually catheterized. Once the catheter is removed the patient needs to be kept dry and clean in order to avoid infection and decrease the risk of skin breakdown. Some patients will emerge from coma and almost immediately be continent. However the greater the length of coma the more profound the ADL impairment and the more marked the frontal lobe injury the more likely the person is to have continuing incontinence (Oostra *et al.*, 1995). When daytime incontinence continues despite regular toileting of the patients it is appropriate to perform a medical and behavioural analysis to determine the cause of the problem. The types of incontinence most commonly seen after brain injury include reflex incontinence (detruser hyper-reflexia), urinary retention (and overflow), functional incontinence and behavioural incontinence.

General

Bladder deconditioning may have occurred due to prolonged unconsciousness with consequent diminished bladder capacity, poor bladder control and detrusor weakness. A regular toileting programme with gradual lengthening of the periods between voids may be sufficient for bladder re-education. Starting frequency for a toileting programme should be every 2 h and twice at night (but toileting may be more frequent) with the aim to achieve a schedule of between every 3 and 6 h (Hartman, 1987). Medical and cognitive factors should be considered, which may include the effects of sedation, decreased attention to bladder cues, depression and inability to communicate needs. In planning the diet it should be remembered that alcohol, coffee and tea, and some soft drinks, have a natural diuretic effect and are bladder irritants. The therapist should establish expectations that the patient should be continent and street clothes worn and clothes changed promptly after a period of wetness to avoid sanctioning incontinence (Hartman, 1987). Adequate nutrition and bulk should be maintained so as to ensure that bowel voiding occurs at least every 3 days. Where a patient is making gains in other ADLs but is not responding to a toilet training schedule a urology evaluation is recommended.

Functional incontinence
Patients may be physically incapable of getting on or off the toilet or adjusting their clothes, have difficulty in asking for help, or be unable to judge the time required to reach the toilet. The physical effort involved may be so great, or take so long, that patients prefer to wet or soil themselves. In these circumstances an alteration in the environment can help the patient achieve continence, for example ensuring the patient's bedroom is near the toilet, that the door is clearly labelled, or that the patient has a urine bottle or commode available. Patients with cognitive deficits require prompting to help them learn how to manage their personal needs; patients should be taught to communicate their wishes, e.g. their need to go to the toilet, and to ask for physical help if this is required.

Behavioural incontinence
There are occasions when patients can be punitively incontinent as a method of showing objections to their treatment. Staff should be hesitant to adopt this formulation since the problems of coming to an accurate assessment are multiple, i.e. determining whether the problem is due to attentional deficits, memory problems, physical limitations or dyspraxia. Once an accurate conceptualization of the behaviour has been established a behavioural programme aimed at increasing the benefits of continence and increasing the costs of incontinence may be useful in treating the functionally as well as the punitively incontinent patient. Behavioural intervention has been demonstrated to be effective with even the profoundly impaired patient. Cohen (1985) described the treatment of incontinence in a 27-year-old woman with encephalitis, basal ganglia damage and profound cognitive and motor involvement secondary to carbon monoxide poisoning sustained in a suicide attempt. Techniques used in treatment included *in vivo* exposure (practice), contingent reinforcement and shaping to reduce urinary and faecal incontinence, to increase toilet usage and to decrease screaming and aggression when undressed or accompanied to the toilet. Results showed a reduced rate of incontinence after the introduction of the programme, with improvements maintained at discharge (Cohen, 1985).

Night-time incontinence
It is important to determine whether the patient is actually asleep when incontinent at night. If asleep, waking the patient during the night may help him become aware of the need to urinate. Alternatively, behavioural programmes similar to those used with children and described by Azrin *et al.* (1974) may be effective. When the patient is not actually asleep, simple expedients such as ensuring a urine bottle is clearly visible or placing a commode by the bed may be effective. Alternatively a programme of reinforcement for a certain number of 'dry' nights may be effective.

Feeding

Patients may have difficulty in the motor control of eating and drinking or in regulating their food and fluid consumption. Inadequate eating and drinking may result from oral motor disorders, decreased arousal, akasthisia, ataxia, apraxia or other motor disorders. Motor control deficits may be complicated by lowered frustration tolerance and behaviour disorder.

Assessment or oral motor functioning may be performed by the occupational therapist or the speech therapist. Assessment and treatment of oral motor dysfunction is an area of specialized practice (Logemann, 1983; Lazarus and Logemann, 1987). Adaptive equipment may be useful in the acute stages of recovery improving the patient's functioning and make eating considerably less stressful. Training the patient in appropriate positioning to maximize stability and control and to decrease the effects of abnormal tone can have a significant effect on eating. Hooper-Roe (Chapter 8) describes a successful self-feeding programme with a profoundly impaired and uncooperative patient who had previously been fed by naso-gastric tube for 2.5 years. The management of swallowing disorders are reviewed in Chapter 9.

Patients with damage to the hypothalamus may attempt to overfeed or hydrate themselves. A condition similar to the hyperorality which may follow herpes simplex encephalitis can also follow brain trauma. Initially this deficit may seem similar to patients who repetitively ask to eat because they have profound memory impairment and have no memory of having eaten. However patients without hyperorality can usually be engaged in other tasks and do not have the constant and repetitive foraging behaviour associated with constant hunger. Patients whose constant requests to eat usually respond to a schedule of meal times and memory strategy training about meals. Patients with hyperorality are notoriously difficult to treat and limiting the patient's access to food may be warranted.

Transfers

Transferring is an important component of independent functioning. Failure to transfer independently can result from combination of poor motor control, inadequate physical position and transfer planning. Therefore a transfer-training programme should consider both the quality of motor control and the organization of the activity.

Assessment involves observing the patient in order to establish how performance breaks down. A training programme should be designed to act as a functional subcomponent of other training programmes (e.g. dressing). The tripartite functional/behavioural approach to therapy should be used during the implementation of a transfer-training programme. Sessional practice can be used to perfect the patient's positioning to non-verbal and verbal cues. The programme can also be rehearsed verbally with the patient to accelerate the patient's acquisition of the organization of the movement. The programme can be used on a 24-h basis when all staff have been trained to carry it out.

Washing and dressing

Washing and dressing difficulties can occur as a result of cognitive dysfunction, limited motor control or behavioural disregulation and a detailed assessment is essential to arrive at an adequate formulation of the patient's problems. Observing the patient's behaviour on three mornings to the prompt 'Do what you would normally do to get washed and dressed in the morning' (Giles *et al.*, 1997) can assist the therapist to develop an adequate conceptualization of the patient's problems. The patient can be reprompted if not engaged in any washing and dressing related activities after a short period of time. If the patient is not performing adequately, more specific cues should be provided. The therapist looks for why performance breaks down, the complexity of behaviour a patient can perform to a cue, and functional behaviours the patient displays spontaneously. By embedding retained skills in the retraining programme the amount of new learning required of the patient is reduced. Wherever possible a whole task approach should be used with verbal cues derived from a task analysis. Central to the success of a washing and dressing programme is that the method used allows the patient to become physically independent as rapidly as possible while remaining consistent with the patient's other rehabilitation goals. Physical routines such as transferring or standing may require multiple cues and physical assistance initially as they are usually difficult new sequences for the patient to learn. Learning is facilitated by sequencing the separate activities of washing and dressing in a fixed and organized pattern. The order of washing and physical routines can be rehearsed with the patient verbally throughout the day. The patient can be verbally and or tangibly reinforced for correct answers. JCW has reported the successful use of a computer program as an adjunctive training device in this procedure (Clark-Wilson, 1988).

Community mobility

Road safety

Inadequate road safety skills are common following brain injury. Deficits underlying problems in crossing the street include visual deficits (hemianopia, neglect), perceptual disorders, disorders of attention and impulsivity. Safe street-crossing is usually automatic prior to injury but often requires conscious attention following injury.

Assessment should include the therapist accompanying the patient on short trips in the community. The therapist can establish a route which includes a number of different types of streets to cross, both with and without pedestrian lights. The therapist should explain to the patient the purpose of the session and then walk a foot or so behind the patient to stop them if necessary from walking into traffic. If the patient crosses the street safely during the early part of the assessment the therapist should engage the patient in unrelated conversation to see if the patient can maintain safe behaviour when distracted. Patients should be encouraged to think about where they cross the street and to use pedestrian crossings. Patients with relatively mild deficits may only require a small number of sessions designed to concentrate their attention on the skills in order for them to achieve an acceptable standard. More handicapped patients and those with specific deficits (e.g. left neglect) require a specific road safety programme. Starting with one or two intersections may assist in the development of an initial schema before introducing more variations (e.g. different intersections).

Topographical orientation

Navigating new environments may be problematic for many patients. Memory impairment as well as deficits in topographical orientation may severely impair the patient's independence in the community. Some patients have difficulty in learning to find their way in new environments whereas others can no longer find their way around what should be familiar environments. Although topographical disorientation occurs frequently in patients with visual neglect there are patients without marked perceptual or attentional deficits who have lost previous geographic schema or have a specific deficit for route finding. An unimpaired person can be shown an unfamiliar route taking 5 min on foot with two to three turns and have no difficulty in finding their way back. If the patient performs adequately on this test and is otherwise safe the therapist can proceed to teach the patient to follow increasingly complex routes. When the patient has difficulty the therapist can establish how many times the patient needs to travel a route to learn it and which type of cues aid learning. The therapist should investigate whether the patient can successfully read a map or follow printed directions on a checkoff board. Some patients will only be able to learn a few routes but being able to do so independently can considerably increase quality of life (e.g. from home to grocery store, library, coffee shop).

Physical deficits and mobility

Many physically disabled patients have difficulty travelling independently in the community even if they are independently walking indoors (with or without an assistive device). Some patients are able to develop this ability if they are provided with sufficient mobility training or if they choose to reside in an area where amenities are close by. Some patients can be taught to maximize their mobility using local transport (buses, taxis) whereas others will require some form of outdoor mobility aid (such as a powered wheelchair). The patient (and staff) sometimes have difficulty in accepting the need for outdoor mobility aids and the timing and methods of introducing the assistive device should be carefully considered.

Driving

Patients are frequently very eager to resume, or if adolescents begin, driving. Jacobs (1988) found that between 1 and 6 years post-injury 37% of severely brain-injured patients were driving as compared with 93.7% who were driving pre-injury. Neither physicians' nor therapists' clinical judgements nor objective (paper and pencil) tests have been shown to predict on-the-road driving skill (Galski *et al.*, 1990). Van Zomeren *et al.* (1988) examined fitness to drive after severe brain injury. Day-time driving was studied in (1) a car that recorded lateral position control and (2) in driving the subject's own car with a professional observer. The brain-injured subjects were all at least 3 years post-injury (mean 6.5) and all were driving. The brain-injured subjects performed significantly worse than a control group with five out of nine patients classified as incompetent, suggesting that there are many brain-injured individuals on the road who should not be driving. Of particular interest is the suggestion by Van Zomeren *et al.* (1988) that sensory motor deficits may not compromise an individual's ability to drive provided that the individual is able to compensate for them. Hence insight and self-criticism may be a more important determinant for a patient's fitness to drive than degree of cognitive deficits. Kewman and co-workers (1985) attempted to improve the performance of post-acute traumatically brain-injured patients on behavioural aspects of driving by providing specific training using a small electrically powered vehicle. The authors' primary interest was whether improvement on these tasks would translate to the functional (and more complex) task of on-the-road auto-mobile driving. Experimental subjects showed improvements both on the specific exercises and in performance on a structured test of on-the-road automobile driving. Matched untrained brain-injured control subjects who only received unstructured experience with the electrically powered vehicle did not show improvement. Results suggest a significant therapeutic affect of the specific training programme and that training in specific tasks is more effective than exposure and unstructured experience. The medical branch of the Department of Motor Vehicles (Drivers Vehicle Licensing Agency) can determine whether a brain-injured indi-vidual can return to driving and there are many specialized centres offering driving assessment, instruction and recommendations for adaptations to handicapped people.

Shopping and meal preparation

Personal circumstances dictate the training needs of each patient in the area of shopping and meal preparation. Some patients receive almost total care and never need to make themselves anything to eat or drink whereas others are primarily responsible for organizing the shopping and meal preparation for themselves. Many patients will be able to redevelop independence in these activities. To shop and cook independently the individual needs to ensure that they have money, decide on a meal, make a shopping list and determine how to get to the grocery store and back with the groceries. Assessment consists of setting tasks of graded difficulty, for example, by beginning with preparing a cold snack (avoiding safety issues around hot surfaces). Planning and shopping for breakfast or a sandwich: progressing to hot meal preparation for instance heating a can of soup or a microwave meal, and finally coordinating many items involving organization and timing of the cooking of different foods using the stove top and oven simul-taneously. Many patients need to practise shopping for and cooking the same or similar menus repeatedly in order to become proficient.

Patient 1 was preoccupied with the idea that staff were attempting to starve him and kept him on 'a pointless pill diet'. Staff hypothesized that if Patient 1 could be taught to prepare a meal for himself he would be less likely to believe that he was being starved. Teaching Patient 1 to prepare a meal was complicated by a number of factors including his profound amnesia, paranoia and by a category specific loss of information for food and objects in the kitchen. Patient 1 could not distinguish food from non-food items; did not know what colour toast should be or what 'boiling' meant; and could not recognize an oven, grill or basic kitchen implements. Patient 1 was observed for 1 week attempting to make a breakfast consisting of two slices of toast with a can of baked beans and sausages (his selection). A programme of written instructions was developed and modified in response to difficulties Patient 1 experienced in carrying them out. Patient 1 was prompted with 'check instructions' on entering the kitchen. All the food items to make breakfast were set out on the counter with a copy of the instructions and a pen for Patient 1 to check off each task as it was completed. For the first two weeks Patient 1 continued to require verbal instructions as well as the written instructions, but by the end of the third week he was independent with the instruction sheet and supervision was withdrawn. After performing the programme every morning for 6 weeks the instruction sheet was removed, food was left in the cupboard and Patient 1 continued to make his breakfast independently. Nonetheless for a further 6 weeks Patient 1 had to be escorted to the kitchen each morning despite his protests that he could not cook. One day approximately 14 weeks after the beginning of the

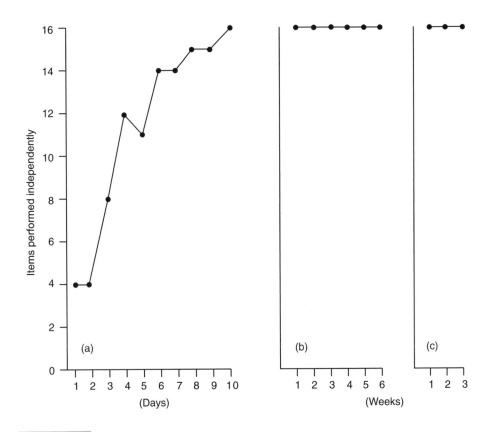

Figure 6.1

The response of Patient 1 to a cooking programme. (a) = Food and instruction sheet on counter and with additional verbal prompts when necessary (primarily 'check instruction'). (b) = Food and instruction sheet on the counter. (c) = Food left in cupboards, no instruction sheet.

programme, Patient 1 greeted every person who entered the unit with a broad smile of excitement and the statement 'I can make my own breakfast!'. Patient 1's protests that he was being starved ceased.

Social skills

Social isolation is recognized as a common long-term consequence of severe brain injury (Thomsen, 1974, 1984). Social-skills training has been used in an attempt to ameliorate some of the patient's difficulties in meeting friends and sustaining established relationships. Socially-skilled behaviours incorporate all *verbal* behaviour, including all aspects of speech, e.g. tone of voice, rate of speech, accent, volume and intonation and *non-verbal* skills like facial expressions, gestures and body movements. Social skills also involve interpreting social cues in order to develop appropriate responses. The aim of social-skills training in a rehabilitation setting is to alter social behaviours in ways which increase opportunities and acceptance in social environments. Research suggests that social-skills training can be effective with brain-injured people if the to-be-learned behaviour is specifically defined rather than an abstract cognitive process. The needs of individual patients are highly variable so accurate assessment is essential to ensure a realistic retraining programme. Assessment of the patient's behaviour and the demands placed on the patient by the environment will suggest the most important goals of intervention. Patient 2 was referred by a group home for treatment. During the assessment process it was determined that the patient could return there if he could learn to stop screaming and not sit so close to the television as he blocked the view for other residents of the home. Another patient could return to live with his wife and family if he stopped shouting at and criticizing his children. Assessment methods include: informal observation data, behavioural observation and role play tests, interviews, self, peer and family ratings and check lists. Any social situation can be a source of informal observational data, and may be used to assess the brain-injured persons non-verbal and verbal skills. Observational assessment of the brain-injured person in their home environment or in functional social settings, e.g. shops and restaurants, can provide the therapist with invaluable data on the individual's social behaviour.

Behavioural observation employs a structured approach to data collection both of the person in natural setting and in structured interactions (role plays). A variety of recording methods can be used, e.g. antecedent–behaviour–consequence (ABC) recordings, frequency ratings and behavioural sampling techniques. Although naturalistic observation is the assessment method most advocated by behaviour therapists (Bellack *et al.*, 1979) role-play situations are frequently used as they are less time-consuming. Representative of role-play tests is the Behavioural Assertiveness Test-Revised (BAT-R) of Eisler *et al.* (1975).

Interviews provide information about the brain-injured person's interpersonal history and provide a setting for informal observation. Interviews can explore the patient's views of their background, family history, social contacts, understanding of social norms; their own evaluation of their behaviour in social interactions, and their perspectives of their present social situation.

Ratings and check-list data can be used to categorize or grade patients' social skills and their problem areas. To assess the brain-injured individual's level of social contact, patients and/or their relatives/friends can be asked to record specific social activities or interactions in a diary, for example, the number of friends that visit or the number of times the patient went out socially during a specified period.

Training procedures

The general model described for social-skills training is that of Trower *et al.* (1978). Social skills are analysed, broken down to component elements and practised. Three types of intervention are described for patients of different degrees of disability. The first type of training described is used with the very severely handicapped and concentrates on teaching non-verbal skills. The second type of training concentrates on teaching basic verbal and non-verbal skills used in social routines, and then generalizing these to realistic social settings. The third type of training aims to help the less impaired patient learn appropriate methods of dealing with social situations that occur in the community. These types of training programmes will be discussed with examples below.

Level 1

The severely handicapped include those with major physical impairments who have little or no usable speech. These patients can have problems in understanding non-verbal cues – such as facial expression, tone of voice and gesture – and have similar difficulties in communicating their wishes. Patients can often be taught the importance of non-verbal forms of communication and how to incorporate them in their normal behaviour. Non-verbal skills include facial expression (smiling is especially important), posture, gesture, eye-contact, proximity to others and body orientation. Many patients are able to make sounds (voice) without being able to produce language (words) and training involves the non-verbal aspects of communication such as volume, tone, pitch and rhythm.

Patient 2, an 18-year-old male, was admitted for rehabilitation 4 years after his severe brain injury. Patient 2 produced no recognizable speech, sat slumped in a chair, and drooled constantly. When he was not given what he wanted he would scream. Many of those around him found it difficult to interact with him because of their feelings of disgust. A potential long-term placement had been found for Patient 2 but he could only go if there were a number of changes in his behaviour. Social-skills training was started in a group of three other patients with similar problems. Appearance, facial expression, posture and lip closure were stressed, the importance of good social presentation explained, and practice in basic non-verbal routines begun. Patients were encouraged to 'sit well' (feet flat on the floor and apart, back straight, head in the midline), with lips closed, and to voice briefly using appropriate volume and pitch, in order to attract attention. They were requested to maintain eye-contact while asking a question (by use of gesture). On all these points Patient 2 needed instruction, but he learned quickly and prompts were gradually phased out as he improved.

The group were trained using the social routines, 'Good morning', 'Please' and 'Thank you'. Patient 2 was taught to sit well, look and orient himself towards the

Table 6.1	Non-verbal	Verbal
Level 1	1. Facial expression	1. Volume
	2. Posture	2. Tone
	3. Gesture	3. Pitch
	4. Gaze	4. Clarity
	5. Personal space	5. Pace
	6. Appearance	6. Speech disturbances
	7. Orientation	

person, voice and smile for 'Good morning'. A similar procedure was used for 'Please' and 'Thank you'. When these were reliably and appropriately being said in the group setting, Patient 2 was asked to use the procedure in the ward setting. For a week Patient 2 was prompted in the use of the routines and praised whenever he used them. After the first week, Patient 2 was no longer prompted, praise and intermittent tangible reinforcement were provided contingent on performance. Requests which were accompanied by screaming, or were in some other way inappropriate, were not acknowledged. Patient 2 was able to maintain his improved performance, and became socially acceptable to such a degree that patients and staff who previously avoided him began to actively seek his company, visiting him in his room and talking with him about their day.

Level 2

The second type of training can be used with slightly less impaired individuals. The organization of the social-skills sessions needs to take into account the patient's physical and cognitive problems and provide structure and consistency to assist learning. Individuals need to have the relevant social skills taught and repeated frequently within short sessions which should be dynamic to maintain the patients' attention and motivation. Social-skills training can sometimes be incorporated into social games to make the sessions more enjoyable.

Patients often require training in how to approach people, and how to converse in social situations. Patients may be taught how to attract attention, ask simple questions, listen to people, take turns in conversation and to initiate and maintain conversation. These tasks can be analysed into verbal and non-verbal components and practised. For example the elements of attracting attention can be divided into:

1 Saying a person's name, saying 'Excuse me', 'Hello there' or whatever is culturally appropriate for the person to attract the attention of the person they are talking to.
2 Once the person's attention is gained, the patient is taught to face the conversation partner, look at him or her (i.e. gain eye-contact), and smile.

These elements of attracting attention can be extended to include conversation management, for instance, initiating communication, asking questions, taking turns

Table 6.2	1. Introduction and exit skills
Level 2	2. Initiating social interactions
	3. Apologizing
	4. Situation-specific routines (e.g. shopping, telephone)
	5. Accepting criticism
	6. Asking for information and requests
	7. Content of speech

in conversation, maintaining conversation and finding appropriate ways to end conversations. To generalize skills it is necessary to gain mastery in sessions, in role-play situations, and then in the real situation.

Level 3

Patients with less severe impairments need to learn methods of adjusting to their changed lifestyle and learn to socially interact with people in the community. Patients frequently have an unusually egocentric frame of reference, rigidity of thinking and lack of sensitivity to, or interest in, the needs and feelings of others. Subjects discussed include skills required for independent community living including; listening and conversational skills, giving and receiving compliments and criticisms, and assertiveness training. Patients at this level can learn through trial-and-error, in role-plays in functional settings, with subsequent discussion and evaluations of their performance. Patient 3 responded to any direction or criticism by moaning and justifying his actions and failed to acknowledge his problems. Patient 3 took instructions literally, got very anxious, and his constant moaning made him very unpopular with other patients. In social skills the fact that Patient 3 moaned was discussed; he apologized for moaning and agreed to work on it as a problem. Patient 3 was asked if he felt the staff could help him remember this and after discussion he asked if everyone would say 'Moaning' to him thereby giving him feedback when this was a problem. This programme was followed, and after 2 weeks staff were finding him more pleasant company and more responsive in other areas of treatment.

Table 6.3	**Conversational management**
Level 3	1. Content of speech
	2. Listening (observing)
	3. Accepting criticism
	4. Assertion skills
	5. Awareness and responsiveness to needs of others
	6. Turn-taking
	7. Giving instructions
	8. Initiating social interactions
	9. Apologizing
	10. Self-disclosure (expression of emotion)

133

A range of problems can manifest themselves as social-skills deficits, e.g. lack of insight, poor anger management, sexual disinhibition or an inability to understand social norms. Patients are often unable to set themselves goals, or may set themselves unrealistic and poorly developed goals. Intervention can be effective with specific behaviourally defined goals and focused training.

OUTCOME STUDIES

Single case or small group studies have demonstrated the efficacy of functional task training with brain-injured adults in the areas of continence (Cohen, 1986), self-feeding (Hooper-Roe, 1988), transfers (Goodman-Smith and Turnball, 1983), personal hygiene (Giles and Clark-Wilson, 1988a, b; Giles and Shore, 1989a; Giles et al., 1997), mobility and community skills (Giles and Clark-Wilson, 1993) and social skills (Gajar et al., 1984; Brotherton et al., 1988; Giles et al., 1988). Single case and small group designs allow treatment to be specifically tailored to the patient's needs while maintaining the controls necessary for determining the effects of treatment (Giles, 1989, 1994a). Lloyd and Cuvo (1994) reviewed results of behavioural interventions concluding that treatment effects are robust and enduring. A number of follow-up studies have examined the effectiveness of post-acute brain-injury programmes. Even when cognitive skills are directly addressed it is often functional skills which improve (Mills et al., 1992). Follow-up of 42 patients treated at an outpatient post-acute cognitive rehabilitation facility found that cognitive measures were not significantly affected by treatment but that there was significant improvement in patient's functional performance and that this was maintained at 18-month follow-up (Mills et al., 1992). Johnston and Lewis (1991) assessed 1-year outcome of 82 patients treated at post-acute community re-entry programmes and found that there were enduring improvements in independent living and productive activities with patients requirements for supervision showing substantial decline. Although improved independent living and household skills were the most frequent dimension of actual benefit they were seldom documented as goals (Johnston, 1991). An outcome study of 21 persons treated at a transitional living programme found that improvements in independence documented at 1 year had remained stable or had improved at 3-year follow-up (Harrick et al., 1994). Other workers have found that functional performance may continue to improve following the end of a programme of functional retraining even in patients who are significantly post-injury (Fryer and Haffey, 1987). Individuals after brain injury can be assisted to redevelop independent living skills which significantly reduce their need for supervision and institutional care. Successful interventions involve carefully designed treatment programmes, manipulation of the environment, the facilitation of success and the development of creative ways to help the patient learn needed skills and graded reintegration into the community.

7 MOTOR LEARNING FOLLOWING BRAIN INJURY

Mary Beth Badke, Gordon Muir Giles, Jill Kerry

MOTOR CONTROL

Therapeutic approaches to rehabilitation of the brain-injured adult are based on implicit assumptions about motor control and motor learning (Gordon, 1987). Traditional facilitation approaches have assumed that nervous system lesions result in a lack of higher level control over movements and a release of lower level primitive and abnormal reflexes. In general, therapeutic intervention starts at the lowest level by stimulating reflex responses and then progresses to automatic responses and then to selective voluntary movements. These theoretically based intervention strategies are often described as 'neurodevelopmental' because progression in rehabilitation involves reintegration of basic reflex patterns into purposeful behaviour which is thought to be a recapitulation/mirror of the development of motor skills in the child. The initial optimism generated by the neurodevelopmental approaches has gradually given way to frustration over the lack of carryover into functional ability. As summarized by Horak (1991), other dissatisfying features of the facilitation models are:

- Lack of incorporation of new developments in the neurosciences and disregard of ideas from such fields as motor behaviour, kinesiology, biomechanics and cognitive psychology.
- No scientific evidence that the nervous system can be modified to control movements more effectively if it experiences normal movement patterns guided by skilled therapists.
- No evidence that inhibition of abnormal tone and primitive reflex patterns promote motor recovery.
- Little direct consideration of the practice conditions and tasks that maximally facilitate long-term functional changes.

In addition, comparisons of neurodevelopmental approaches to other intervention methods have failed to find a consistent superiority for the neurodevelopmental approaches (Logigan *et al.*, 1983; Lord and Hall, 1986).

A new task-oriented model of neurological rehabilitation is emerging, based on new ideas about how the brain controls movement. According to these ideas, movements are not peripherally or centrally driven but emerge as a result of an interaction among many systems, each contributing to different aspects of movement control.

The principle assumptions and features of the task-oriented model are according to Carr and Sheperd (1980):

> the control of movement is organized around goal-directed, functional behaviours. In treatment of the brain-damaged adult the major factor in this learning process is identification of the goal by the patient and therapist.

Consider two cases: both require ankle dorsiflexion as the therapeutic goal. In one, the movement is practised on the mat using positioning and handling to reduce abnormal tone. The other involves stimulation of dorsiflexors during ambulation, stair and hill climbing, with no prominent focus on reducing the level of spasticity. The functional context described in the second case provides a more meaningful perspective compared with the first. There could be many ways in which a particular goal is accomplished, and skill lies in the ability to perform in the most efficient manner.

Movement patterns emerge as a result of appropriate interaction with central, musculoskeletal and environmental constraints. Therapists attempt to assess and improve the patient's ability to adapt to those constraints, by practising tasks in a variety of postures and under varying visual, surface, and biomechanical conditions. In addition therapists alter task demands to elicit specific patient movements.

The same task may be accomplished with a wide variety of movement patterns. Intervention is focused on learning strategies to coordinate efficient, effective behaviours rather than training to one 'normal' movement pattern. An individual with a damaged nervous system will attempt to accomplish important functional goals with whatever systems remain. Gordon (1987) states this is looking at the deficit or abnormal synergies as learned patterns of movement. These compensatory strategies also encompass Taub's (1976) concept of 'learned non-use'. Therapists must determine if the patient has developed useful, compensatory strategies and help him or her eliminate less efficient strategies (including refusal to engage in the activity). For example a patient in the early recovery period may have learned not to perform a task or may have learned to perform it in a way which is unnecessarily limiting. One patient learned a wide-based staggering gait early in recovery. Later he found this very difficult to unlearn even though his neurological recovery had progressed to the point where he was capable of an unimpaired gait.

On occasion the therapist may teach the patient unhelpful compensatory strategies. For example, allowing the patient to extend at the hips in order to scoot forward in a chair (i.e. extending the hips against resistance in sitting) may increase tone causing the patient to lose his or her balance backwards when attempting to stand.

In summary, the contemporary task-oriented model attempts to incorporate accepted concepts of motor control that have not yet been included in traditional neurological rehabilitation approaches. Based on systems theory, the task-oriented model assumes that control of movement is organized around functional goals rather than on muscles or movement patterns. Thus, it is a model of neurological rehabilitation that allows therapists to ask better questions of their patients' motor control problems and to define success of intervention by accomplishing specific functional goals (Horak, 1991).

COMPONENTS OF A MOTOR CONTROL MODEL AND RELATED DYSFUNCTIONS

Normal movement strategies

All movements consist of functionally related patterns of muscle contractions (synergies), which have fixed spatial–temporal relationships. These normal synergies simplify the control of movement for the central nervous system (Bernstein,

1967; Duncan and Badke, 1987). In patients with brain injury, the organization of movement may be disturbed in several ways (Duncan, 1990). With severe injury, the patient's movement may be limited to primitive reflexes (asymmetrical tonic neck, symmetrical tonic neck, tonic labyrinthine reflexes, and positive support). Milani-Comparetti reports on the basis of human fetal movement observations, that many of our 'primitive movements are primary motor programmes: genetic modules which are genetic endowments of the species and are available for motor programming' (1980). The problem in patients with brain injury is that the stereotypic movements are not modified and elaborated upon in the same way as the primary motor programmes are in the course of normal human development and in normal human movement control. In central nervous system (CNS) damage the abnormality is not due to acquisition of abnormal reflexes but to loss of a variety of movement patterns. Well-controlled intralimb and interlimb coordination may be replaced by mass limb movement patterns and difficulty in coordinating movement among the limbs. Often the brain-injured patient's movements are limited to stereotyped patterns of flexion (flexion, abduction, external rotation) and extension (extension, adduction, internal rotation).

Gross movement patterns in the lower extremity may be sufficient for a functional, yet abnormal, gait. These gross movement patterns are less likely to be functional in the upper extremity (Duncan, 1990). A lack of selective motor control may be due to factors that originate centrally, peripherally, or both (Giuliani, 1991). Central factors may include malfunction of the upper motor neuron centres which participate in the programming and execution of movement or abnormal motor neuron recruitment. Peripheral factors may include changes in muscle stiffness or length and muscle fibre atrophy.

Patients with brain injury often have difficulty producing and controlling the muscle forces necessary for generating normal patterns of movement. Weakness or paresis is frequently a primary motor deficit following brain injury. Patients are unable to generate normal muscle tension and often experience a tremendous sense of effort when they produce minimal muscular force (Duncan and Badke, 1987). Alterations in motor unit recruitment and timing may also be factors that affect movement patterns. Abnormal regulation of the motor neuron pool causes prolonged recruitment of motor units and delays cessation of antagonistic contractions at the end of the movement (Sahrmann and Norton, 1977). Disorders of reciprocal inhibition may also contribute to increase the resistance to active movement (Miller and Hammond, 1981). The paresis associated with brain injury is not due solely to an overactive antagonistic muscle, but may be caused by alterations in motor unit discharge patterns and reduced firing rate caused by damage to supraspinal descending systems.

In summary, patients with brain trauma may have the synergistic organization of movement disturbed in the following ways:

1 Movement may be limited to primitive reflexes.
2 Movements may be limited to stereotyped patterns of flexion and extension (dysfunctional synergies).
3 The timing of muscular contractions are abnormal during posture and movement. These timing deficits produce the symptoms of ataxia and tremor.

Musculoskeletal factors

Normal movement strategies depend not only on neuromuscular control but on musculoskeletal factors which both limit and enable movement within certain defined parameters. Factors include planes of joint movement, range of motion and length and tension of muscles and associated structures. The paralysis and immobilization associated with brain injury predisposes many patients to contractures and subsequent loss of range of motion. Pain and heterotopic ossification are additional factors affecting range of motion (ROM). Loss of joint motion limits the functional range of movement, alters the normal muscle length–tension relationship, as well as impairing normal biomechanical alignment. The patient's alignment over his base of support will influence which movement strategies he will use for mobility and stability. Poor biomechanical alignment can therefore contribute to some of the observed motor control deficits. A careful analysis of joint motion is necessary to identify factors which may be contributing to excessive effort in movement, faulty postures, and gait deviations.

Some patient compensatory strategies involve a subtle interaction of their own deficits or musculoskeletal limitations. For instance one patient with bilateral tendo-achiles shortening was able to maintain an upright standing position without difficulty. However following surgical lengthening of the tendons he was constantly involuntarily crouching. The problem did not appear to be one of strength *per se* but of maintaining a chronic level of muscle contraction. The contracture appeared to have functioned as bilateral ankle foot orthosis. At 5-year follow-up his gait had not returned to its pre-lengthening level of function.

Central set

Central set is the ability of the nervous system to prepare the motor system for upcoming sensory information and to prepare the sensory system for upcoming movements (Evarts *et al.*, 1984). For example, if a standing person voluntarily lifts his or her arm, muscular activity in the trunk and contralateral lower extremity precedes the muscle activity in the upper extremity (Lee, 1980). This sequence of muscle activity provides the postural support for the movements. Patients with neurological damage have been shown to have delayed or absent preparatory responses which may result in inadequate proximal stabilization required to perform smooth selective distal movements.

Movement strategies

Everybody uses movement strategies in order to achieve specific goals. For example, there are numerous possible strategies to achieve the functional goal of putting on a sock; some individuals stand on one leg, others sit and cross one leg over the other leg while other individuals bend down to floor level and so on. Some individuals following brain injury may be unable to identify a range of movement strategies to achieve a goal or may adopt strategies which have negative consequences for the patient's overall rehabilitation goals. However, some patients are able to use compensatory strategies to maintain function despite their muscle weakness and/or musculoskeletal problems. If this is true, attempting to eliminate these 'abnormal movements' may decrease the patient's utilization of efficient, effective strategies for day-to-day functions. For example, it is common for people to stand all the way up during a transfer but this may not be efficient or safe if the patient has balance deficits. Learning to reach for/push off from surfaces during a squat pivot may be safer and more independent.

Environmental adaptation

Adaptability is the flexibility in the CNS that allows an individual to programme and execute movement patterns under a variety of conditions and environments. Patients with neurological damage may have lost the ability to adapt quickly to changes in environmental conditions (Horak, 1991). For example, patients with brain injury may require more time to adapt their postural responses to new surface and visual conditions, e.g. carpet, grass, stairs, reduced lighting. The following motor task illustrates the concept of context-dependent movement:

> While practising the progression of sit to stand in the clinic, there is no change in the environment, since the patient is the only thing moving. However, the patient also needs to be able to perform during the rest of the day when the environment changes. The therapist might practise the task with the patient using different chairs, soft surfaces, or while compensating for additional challenges to the patient's ability to adjust posture (i.e. performing the sit to stand procedure on a moving bus or train).

Behavioural goals in motor control

There is a fair amount of evidence that the nervous system is organized in order to accomplish goal-directed activities, not to perform specific movements out of the context of a goal (Reed, 1982). Therapeutic goals should concern the completion of a functional task and not the methods or the movements used to accomplish the task. The goal should be specific and at the individual's functional level. For example, rather than just working on locomotion, a specific goal would be to walk from the Occupational Therapy Department to lunch. For patients in the early stages of recovery, a goal may need to be the completion of an 'automatic' behaviour (for some cognitively impaired patients engaging in overlearned automatic movements appears to be reinforcing, i.e. if allowed to engage the behaviour it will occur with high probability). For some patients finding the right automatic movement can be very helpful in that it acts as a starting point for the development of other behaviours; for example the goal of climbing stairs may improve foot clearance, reciprocal movement and weight shifting necessary in gait. The specific task (stair climbing) elicits these movements without conscious effort to complete each component of the task.

Initiation and termination of movement

Difficulties with the timing of muscle activation produce the symptoms of ataxia and tremor and are common for patients with damage to the cerebellum or basal ganglia. If the patient is unable to produce adequate antagonist force at the appropriate time, he or she may have difficulty terminating movement. Patients with brain injury may also have difficulty controlling appropriate forces of the agonist at the end of a movement. Goal attainment, accuracy and changing directions of movement during a task may be affected if the patient has difficulty with movement termination. Sensory deficits may contribute to these difficulties so, for example, if the patient does not perceive distance or location correctly, he or she may produce inaccuracies at movement termination. Initiation problems may be due to weakness, paresis and poor stabilization and/or cognitive impairments.

Postural adjustments

Abnormalities within postural muscle activation have been reported to cause instability in patients with brain trauma. Examples of abnormal postural adjustments include: significantly delayed onset of postural responses (Shumway-Cook and Olmscheid, 1990), abnormal sequencing of synergistic muscles within a movement strategy and delayed postural adjustments prior to voluntary arm movements (Horak *et al.*, 1984). In addition, abnormal muscle tone may limit a patient's ability to recruit muscles necessary for balance (Shumway-Cook and McCollum, 1991). The extent to which abnormal muscle tone interferes with postural movement control remains controversial (Sahrmann and Norton, 1977; Duncan, 1990).

Sensory, perceptual and cognitive problems

Perceptual and cognitive damage may cause motor control impairments and may significantly affect the individual's ability to relearn motor skills. The impact of perceptual and cognitive impairment on motor-retraining programmes is considered later in this chapter.

The ability to attend to stimuli (both internal and external) and the ability to act in space can be disrupted by brain injury (Giles and Clark-Wilson, 1993). There is evidence that individuals may develop visual neglect disorders related to lateral hemispace, vertical hemispace and peripersonal space, and somatesthetic hemi-inattentions. Hemianopsia may lead individuals to walk into walls or doorways. Individuals may be unable to make successful adjustments to movements based on impaired perception of task demands. Perceptual deficits in patients with brain trauma lead to misinterpretation of the environment and inappropriate movement performances. The inability to attend to information present in the environment prevents the individual from guiding their movements. Cognitive processing deficits may affect both the initiation and termination of movement. The patient may not recognize the need to move or may have difficulty recalling and selecting the movement plan.

Some of the motor control problems described in earlier sections, such as inappropriate co-contraction, timing deficits, slow velocity of movement, inability to combine limb synergies, and decreased coordination, may be attributed to disorders of sensory perception as well as to involvement of the motor system itself (Duncan and Badke, 1987).

ASSESSMENT

Due to the complexity and variability in motor control problems in patients with brain injury, there is no one form of assessment that is sufficient and appropriate for all patients. The most important evaluation that can be performed with brain-injured adults is a clinical evaluation to determine which of the manifestations of CNS damage are contributing to the patient's difficulty in performing functional tasks. Testing can pinpoint the specific deficits associated with the functional impairment.

Below we consider some of the domains of functioning which require assessment and factors which affect the timing of assessment.

Observational assessment of the minimally responsive patient

Following chart review, we recommend a period of observing the patient in their usual movement patterns. The therapist can see the patient at different times of day to determine if the patient's behaviour shows significant variability. Can a particular response be produced once in a half-hour or more than once? In looking at the patient's response to stimuli it is important that the stimuli is closely defined. So, for example, is the patient really following a command or is actually engaging in a stereotyped reaction to noise? The therapist should have the following questions in mind:

- is the skin intact, are fractures present, or are there signs of nerve damage or swelling?
- does the patient move spontaneously?
- are there stereotyped movement patterns? Are the limbs held in characteristic positions?
- is there restlessness or constant movement?
- does the patient have localized or generalized responses, massed movement patterns or locating responses?
- is the patient awake observing the environment?
- is the patient arousable to sound (a startle response to a loud noise, response to any noise, a specific response to their name) or tactile stimulation?
- can the patient respond to one-, two- or three-step commands?
- is the patient able to communicate non-verbally, verbally?

Affect and attitude
Is the patient:

- agitated?
- irritable?
- labile?
- apathetic?
- impulsive?
- depressed?
- unmotivated?

- perseverative?
- euphoric/excited?
- negativistic/oppositional?
- denying disability?

Sensation and perception

When watching people move, assess for deficits in the following areas:

- vision
- hearing
- tactile
- postural position sense
- joint position sense
- neglect
- body schema disorders
- apraxias
- left-right discrimination.

Range of motion

Range of motion (ROM) testing should be performed slowly and passively. Active range of motion is captured under muscle strength. If ROM is less than within normal limits the available range should be recorded. State the possible causes for decreased ROM. Does decreased ROM affect function, hygiene, positioning? Does it pose a risk to skin integrity?

ROM may be limited by

- pain
- soft tissue limitation (i.e. muscular, capsular, ligamentous)
- bony block
- tone
- heterotopic ossification.

Biomechanical alignment

Accurately identify pre-existing musculoskeletal alignment dysfunction. With the patient both sitting and standing observe for postural deviation from midline, differential weight bearing, trunk shortening or elongation, retracted or protracted pelvis or scapula, head and shoulder position, leg length.

Strength

Evaluation should include the following key muscle groups:

- lower extremity: hip flexors, extensors and abductors; knee extensors and flexors; ankle dorsiflexors
- upper extremity: scapular protractors; shoulder flexors and abductors; elbow extensors and flexors; wrist extensors
- neck and trunk: flexors and extensors.

A six- or eight-point scale is widely accepted for the assessment of muscle strength.

0 – no contraction (visible or palpable)
1 – flicker or trace of contraction (but no movement observed)
2 – active movement with gravity eliminated
3 – active movement against gravity (must be able to move fully within own range)
4 – active movement against gravity and resistance (4– slight, 4 moderate, 4+ strong resistance)
5 – normal power.*

Flaccidity, muscle tone (resistance to slow passive ROM), spasticity (resistance to quick stretch)
Scoring:

0 – flaccid
1 – moderate to minimal hypotonia
2 – normal tone
3 – moderately increased resistance to PROM
4 – severely increased resistance to PROM.

Tone must be evaluated passively and during patient-initiated movement (functional activities).

Synergistic organization

Volitional movement

Observe the patient's volitional movements in supine, sitting and standing and make the following qualitative assessments of the available motor patterns of the extremities and trunk:

- no movement
- movements are performed only in stereotypical flexion and extension synergies
- there is an ability to combine components of the stereotypical synergies
- movements are selective without synergy dependence (isolated movement outside of the flexor/extensor patterns of movement)
- movements are influenced by primitive reflexes (asymmetrical tonic neck, tonic labyrinthine, positive support) or associated reactions
- movements are ataxic
- there is resting or intention tremor
- movements are normal in speed and coordination.

*After Medical Research Council (1976) *Aids to the Examination of the Peripheral Nervous System*. Her Majesty's Stationery Office, London.

What alters the patient's muscle tone and quality of movement?

- position
- effort
- fatigue
- emotional stress/anger
- temperature
- pain.

Ask the patient to slowly and then quickly reciprocally flex and extend the elbow and knee.

Ask the patient to move unidirectionally (i.e. flex the knee only). Then compare the force produced and the range of motion during unidirectional movement with that produced during reciprocal movement (i.e. extension of the knee and then flexion).

Scoring:

0 – patient is unable to reverse the direction of movement
1 – impaired: patient is able to reverse, but reversal is slow and jerky
2 – normal: quick reversal of direction of movement is possible.

Functional mobility assistance levels

Assess the spontaneous automatic use of head, neck, trunk and extremities during functional activities of bed mobility (rolling, scooting, bridging), supine to sit, sit to stand, simple transfers, wheelchair mobility ambulation, stairs.

Scoring relates to the amount of assistance required for the patient to perform a specific activity:

I – independent
SBA – standby assistance
VC – verbal cues
CG – contact guard
Min – minimum assistance
Mod – moderate assistance
Max – maximum assistance
Dep – dependent.

Balance activities

Balance activities can be assessed with eyes open and closed. The patient's balance can be assessed in sitting, standing, unilateral stance on the right leg and unilateral stance on the left leg (static and dynamic).

Adaptability of motor patterns

If the patient has volitional and spontaneous movement patterns, qualitatively assess motor patterns as the speed, force, amplitude, postural base and sensory conditions are altered. For example, many patients can meet the basic requirements of ambulation but have great difficulty with running, transfers onto or off a moving surface, e.g. escalators, moving walkways or conditions with rapidly changing motor control requirements.

For example, if the patient is ambulatory you may assess adaptability of gait pattern by altering:

- speed
- sensory conditions lighting, uneven surfaces
- pattern requirements toe walking heel walking
- balance on balance beam
- accuracy following a defined motor pattern (dancing)
- adjustment to environmental conditions
- following changing movement requirements and rapid postural adjustments to command.

MOTOR LEARNING PRINCIPLES

The principles of motor learning discussed below are derived from physical education research with normal subjects. The principles describe the processes involved in teaching relatively contrived motor tasks, sometimes sports, to normally functioning young adults. Currently there is very little evidence regarding how specific motor learning principles apply to patients with abnormal neuromotor systems. There is however considerable evidence regarding more general aspects of learning following neurological insult. Particularly, evidence suggests that the type and frequency of feedback and conditions of practice will impact learning in brain-injured individuals. Below we discuss principles of motor learning and consider how best to modify learning parameters in the light of neurological impairment.

Performance vs learning

One of the most fundamental ideas in motor learning is the distinction between performance during the acquisition phase and learning. Performance refers to the carrying out of a motor act on a given occasion. 'Learning' however is defined as a relatively permanent change in behaviour. Motor learning consists of an ability to generate an appropriate motor pattern in a particular context and environment. Improved performance within a given practice session is not the important outcome, but rather what the patient does at the beginning of the following session (i.e. what the person has learned).

Stages of motor learning

Fitts and Posner (1967) have identified three stages of motor learning: cognitive, associative and autonomous. In the cognitive stage the learner is focusing primarily on developing an execution programme of the skill. In order to do this the learner must understand clearly what is expected and must attend closely to the task. During this initial phase, the learner may be dependent upon environmental cues especially visual and verbal cues to organize information. Frequent errors and variable performance are expected and allowed in this stage. The learner needs to recognize how a performance differs from the goal and actively correct a movement on the next attempt. Thus, errors are considered critical to the learning process.

The associative stage begins when the learner has developed a successful basic strategy and begins to refine its performance. The emphasis shifts from 'what to do' to 'how to do it'. During this stage, the learner relies less on visual and verbal cues and more on kinesthetic or proprioceptive feedback. It is hypothesized that the learner develops an internal reference for correctness which allows for self-correction of error rather than reliance on the external model. The individual can perform relatively well with less error and more consistent performance.

In the autonomous stage, the learner can carry out the task with good quality and with minimal cognitive attention during skill execution. After a great deal of practice, the performance has become largely automatic. Minimal error and little effort are noted in this phase.

FACTORS AFFECTING PERFORMANCE AND LEARNING

Cognitive deficits

Cognitive set

The initial stages of recovery from brain injury are probably a complex interaction of spontaneous recovery, avoiding complications that would mask the spontaneous recovery, and learning. A patient will be in the cognitive stage of learning during the early recovery period of rehabilitation following a neurological insult, therefore the issues of goal development, information processing and memory systems are critical to early intervention (Duncan and Badke, 1987). Evaluating the patient with brain injury for selective attention and attention switching ability, and the ability to concentrate or practice for adequate time periods will offer valuable direction to the physical and occupational therapist. In addition the patient's sensory system must be operating adequately for learning to take place. If the patient is not getting adequate feedback about performance this will impede learning. Multiple memory systems participate in motor relearning. Memory can be defined as the ability to recall information whereas learning can be defined as a change in behaviour based on experience. Response acquisition (motor learning) may take place in even profoundly memory-impaired individuals providing they attend to the task. In many ways the ability to attend to the task appears more central to motor skills learning than remembering the task. The brain-injured individual need not remember ever having practised the task for their performance to improve (Giles and Clark-Wilson, 1993):

1 a certain level of arousal is necessary in order to participate in the activity
2 the learner must have motivation to obtain the goal
3 the learner must be able to pay attention to the task
4 some memory framework is necessary to allow signals to be recognized and movement plans developed and recalled.

These conditions are met only to a limited degree or under very circumscribed conditions in patients in the initial stages of recovery from severe brain injury. It is the goal of the therapist to maximize the patient's chances for learning by manipulating the stimulus conditions and performance parameters.

The patient may not recognize or understand movement commands or instructions. The patients may have difficulty sequencing actions or being impulsive. Participation may be limited by behavioural disregulation, psychiatric disorders or anxiety or failure to recognize why the patients should engage in often very uncomfortable procedures. The patient may have a limited ability to decide to engage in the task due to executive control deficits.

The therapist can assist the patient by:

- finding the time of day when the patient is most able to sustain attention
- providing frequent rest breaks throughout the day
- limiting distractions (i.e. working in a quiet treatment room)
- helping the patient compensate for sensory or perceptual deficits by augmentive feedback (tactile, visual, verbal cues)
- making the activity functional
- making the activity motivating (i.e. walking to the patient's room)
- using stimulus demands to constrain the patient into producing the required behaviour (e.g. the patient may not know how to use a walker but may understand how to use a shopping cart as a training tool for ambulation; a patient with hemineglect pulled up her pants bilaterally without much impairment of motor control).

Verbal instruction/demonstrations

Once the patient has chosen the goal and is able to recognize environmental conditions which regulate the movement, he or she begins to formulate a motor plan to accomplish the task. At this point, it is appropriate for the therapist to provide fairly global verbal instructions. For example, if the patient is working on transferring from a wheelchair to a bed, information about positioning the wheelchair, and how to start out the movement may be useful. The goal is for the patient to be responsible for recognizing his or her own errors. Brain-injured people however often have difficulty with using naturally occurring environmental feedback and it may be necessary to highlight the error verbally or in some other way so that the individual can acquire knowledge, i.e. let the patient start to lose his balance in order to give him the opportunity to get intrinsic feedback about performance errors and to to elicit balance reactions.

Demonstrations may be provided before each attempt at accomplishing the task. There is some evidence that watching a peer learning or performing the skill enhances the performer's ability to learn the skill (Carroll and Bandura, 1982). Demonstrations can be provided in person, or using photographic media.

Feedback

Once the patient has completed his or her first attempt at performing the task, the therapist can provide feedback about the performance. Feedback refers to information received by the learner regarding the degree of success of a movement in attaining a particular goal. Intrinsic feedback can be defined as the sensations associated with the movement. This includes cutaneous, vestibular, kinesthetic, auditory and visual information. Extrinsic feedback is information about the achievement of the goal obtained by the learner from an outside source. This information provides an 'augmentation' of intrinsic feedback by, for example, the therapist telling the learner something about the performance which they had not perceived. Extrinsic feedback can be further classified as knowledge of results (KR) or knowledge of performance (KP). KR refers to information about task outcome provided to the performer after a practice trial has been completed. It is generally verbal (or verbalizable), post-response information about the movement outcome (in terms of the environmental goal rather than about the movement *per se*). This kind of feedback serves as a basis for error corrections on the next trial and therefore can lead to more effective performance as practice continues.

According to Bernstein (1967) what is important is not repetition in and of itself but the repetition of problem solving through the act of generating a solution to the motor problem. In addition to information about the outcome of a movement, feedback can also be provided to learners concerning the movement execution. KP, which refers to information about the movement itself, was viewed as the most effective form of information for the acquisition of motor skills (Gentile, 1972). Two methods of KP are kinematic and kinetic feedback. Kinematics provides information about movement positions, times, velocities and patterns of coordination. When therapists give information about movement patterning (e.g. 'You bent your knee that time'), they are really providing a (loosely measured) form of kinematic information. While kinematics refers to measures of 'pure motion', kinetic measures refer to the forces that produced them. The few empirical studies conducted in this area suggest the relative effectiveness of these measurement categories as information feedback will depend upon the criterion of the skill being learned (Newell and Walter, 1981).

In addition, a number of interesting parallels to the work on KR can be found in other learning paradigms. For example, artificial sensory feedback (EMG biofeedback) has been shown to facilitate the learning of a novel motor task (Mulder and Hulstijn, 1985). Visual feedback including movements of the body via videotape replays appears to be effective for learning skilled movements (Del Rey, 1971) and unskilled movements if verbal cueing or modelling is also provided (Rothstein and Arnold, 1976).

Regardless of the type of feedback, in order for motor learning to occur, the learner must receive information regarding the correctness of a given attempt. In patients with brain injury, we can not assume their intrinsic feedback systems are operating correctly. One hypothesis might be that external or augmented feedback in the form of KP may substitute for the damaged intrinsic sensation, to produce improved motor output.

Structure of the practice session

Assuming the learner has been successful at accomplishing the task a few times, he or she is now ready to move into the later stages of learning. Although few performers would deny the necessity of practice for the learning and performance of motor skills, practice is not a sufficient condition in itself. According to Bernstein (1967):

> The process of practice towards achievement of new motor habits essentially consists in the gradual success of a search for optimal motor solutions to the appropriate problems. Because of this, practice, when properly undertaken, does not consist in repeating the means of solution of a motor problem time after time, but in the process of solving this problem again and again by techniques we have changed and perfected from repetition to repetition. It is already apparent here that, in many cases, practice is a particular type of repetition without repetition and motor training, if this position is ignored, is merely mechanical repetition by rote, a method which has been discredited in pedagogy for some time. (p. 134)

How practice is structured appears to be an important contribution to the effectiveness of motor learning. A number of studies have found that practice sequences in which the task conditions are varied from trial to trial are more effective than constant practice conditions, especially in children (McCracken and Stelmach, 1977). It has been suggested that variability with practice is allowing the learner to practise problem solving. In therapy, one might ask for slightly different forms of a movement in adjacent trials as well as practising the skill under different environmental conditions.

Some environmental factors which could be altered in a treatment session could be biomechanical constraints, visual surround, or support surface. Manipulation of the treatment situation can emphasize a problem/deficit so as to maximize the patient's intrinsic feedback and stimulate error correction and problem solving.

Random vs blocked practice refers to the type of variability in a practice session (Winstein, 1987). If, for example, you want the learner to be able to perform three different variants (A, B, C) of the same task you can present this variety in a blocked or random fashion. In a blocked mode the pattern of practice would be AAAABBBBCCCC or the schedule could be randomized by interspersing practice on all task variations (ACBCBACAB). Blocked practice does appear to enhance the initial stages of acquisition, however, random practice appears to be more effective for learning (Shea and Morgan, 1979). For this reason we provide blocked practice in the early stages of skill development. At this point the patient is still having to devote maximum effort to produce an acceptable response. As the process of skill acquisition continues we recommend increasing the task variability and randomizing practice. However if the patient is repeatedly propagating errors or is perseverating on an inadequate performance of the task we interrupt this and move to an alternative task (see the discussion of errorless learning in Chapters 6 and 15).

Part/whole transfer of training

Therapists have traditionally divided skills into their component parts and often have the patient practise isolated pieces of the task. However, the subtask, when practised separately, may not be the same when performed as an integrated portion of the entire skill. While it is intuitively appealing to assume that working on one part of a complex movement by giving KR for that part over a series of attempts will ultimately enhance performance of that skill, research has found little support for this approach (Schmidt and Young, 1987). In addition dividing tasks in this way may ignore the functional dimension of the task. It appears that the effectiveness of part/whole training depends upon the nature of the task. For tasks which are serial in nature (no overlapping parts) practice of a difficult segment followed by practice of the whole task may be helpful. Such training could be applied when teaching a sliding board wheelchair transfer to a patient with paraplegia. If the task were continuous, meaning that all the parts intermingle and overlap, then part/whole training is much less effective than actually practising the whole task for the same period of time. For example, Winstein *et al.* (1989) have shown procedures which enhance interlimb weight-transfer capability do not necessarily provide for a more symmetrical and effective walking pattern. Our clinical experience suggests that pre-gait weight-shifting and swing phase part-training may be beneficial if the patient can utilize the cues, otherwise whole training is more effective.

Feedback schedule

In addition to structuring the environmental conditions of practice, the feedback schedule needs to be determined. Two descriptors related to the scheduling of feedback are absolute and relative frequency. Absolute frequency is the total number of KR presentations in a given practice session. Relative frequency is the proportion of practice trials during which feedback is given. Although contrary to traditional motor learning views, more recent studies suggest that fewer KR presentations lead to increased learning (Schmidt *et al.*, 1989; Winstein and Schmidt, 1990). These results suggest that the learner can become overly dependent on feedback. Thus, if the therapist is giving too much information, the performer never learns to detect his or her errors and then resolve the problem. Reduced KR frequency appears to enhance the ability to process information and actively correct errors.

On clinical grounds we provide more feedback early in the process of skill acquisition and then decrease relative frequency of KR to trials as the patient develops increasing mastery.

Summary of applications of motor learning principles to rehabilitation following brain injury

Physical and occupational therapists must learn to assess the functional impact of diminished, inappropriate, or untimely sensorimotor behaviour so that a process of building or rebuilding body–brain interactions can be incorporated into appropriate therapeutic interventions. The use of external feedback in the reha-bilitation process is an empirically sound approach. If movement, even if incorrect, can be initiated by a patient, perhaps the motor pattern can be shaped through feedback to produce a functional outcome. In therapy, visual, vestibular, auditory and/or somatosensory input may be provided to guide a movement to an appro-priate outcome. For example, relearning a symmetrical gait pattern may require verbal cues or some visual monitoring of the extent of weight bearing on the more involved side. During ambulation there is a continuous intrinsic sensory feedback concerning performance of the gait pattern. In cases where patients with brain injury have isolated sensory deficits, such as loss of position sense, other sensory modalities can be substituted to develop an appropriate motor response (e.g. visual).

During the initial phases of learning, the performer needs an external model to guide his movements (Mulder and Hulstijn, 1984). In early stages of treatment, patient-generated movement may be dependent predominantly on peripheral feedback. When sensory feedback is absent or distorted, other sources of information, such as EMG biofeedback, videotapes or kinetic feedback, can serve as an external model and inform the patient and therapist about the consequences of a movement. As learning progresses, internal control structures are developed and there is less need for peripheral feedback (Winstein, 1987).

Certain qualitative and quantitative factors that may affect any method of learning or relearning have been previously described and these factors should be considered in the rehabilitation of patients with brain injury. In summary, these principles of motor learning are listed below.

Therapists need to set up environments that challenge the patient to perform functional skills under different conditions. The ability to adjust speed, force and amplitude of movements and to move in different environments should be addressed.

1 Treatment needs to be carried out in the context of goal-directed activities. The nature of the task should be considered in choosing the types of feedback and practice conditions used. The task should be in a realistic environment so that the context is understandable to the patient.
2 The patient must be actively problem solving not just actively moving. When-ever possible rather than trying to elicit movements on a purely automatic basis, the therapist asks the patient to specifically pay attention to what the movement feels and/or looks like. Was the goal accomplished? Was the move-ment the way it was planned? The therapist can then help the patient make decisions about what to try on their next attempt.
3 The goal is not to facilitate 'performance' in practice, but to organize practice in a way that proficiency, retention and generalization is maximized. This means not using neurotreatment techniques that demand performance accuracy, require strong guidance, or do not permit performance of abnormal movements (Winstein, 1991).

4 Select the type of feedback and practice conditions which are appropriate for the task and most likely to facilitate learning. According to Schmidt (1988) these are:

- verbal post-response information from another person, such as a therapist, about task outcome (KR) is the most important variable for motor learning
- both the relative frequency of KR (percentage of attempts on which KR is given) and the absolute frequency (the number of KRs given) are important for learning. Intermittent feedback in therapy may be more beneficial for learning than continuous feedback
- part-to-whole procedures may or may not facilitate transfer of learning to some criterion task. For those tasks which are continuous in nature, part-whole training is much less effective than actually practising the whole task
- variable practice sequences are slightly more effective than constant practice conditions for adults and much more effective in children. Randomly ordered practice is more effective than blocked practice
- knowledge of performance can be given through videotapes, mirrors, kinetic or kinematic feedback. All appear to enhance performance and may have a positive effect on learning
- prior to practice, methods such as motivation for performance, goal setting and modelling/demonstration are all beneficial to learning.

8

REHABILITATION OF PHYSICAL DEFICITS IN THE POST-ACUTE BRAIN-INJURED ADULT: FOUR CASE STUDIES

Jennifer Hooper-Roe

INTRODUCTION

Physiotherapy texts often divide patient's problems into categories such as ataxia, spasticity and flaccidity, which are considered as individual items. This does not take into account how these separate physical disabilities combine and affect the whole person and their real world functioning. The person with severe brain injury can have a multitude of physical problems, but it is the overall functional loss which is the central factor to be considered in designing a programme of rehabilitation.

In addition to the brain-injured person's physical disabilities, other factors such as behaviour disorders, memory deficits and poor drive and motivation may all interfere with function. These problems have often been compounded by months or years of inappropriate placement and rehabilitation.

This situation presents a seemingly impossible task for the therapist. Regular and thorough assessment is vital, both to evaluate the person's disabilities as a whole, and to highlight particular problem areas to be worked on as priorities. Continual re-evaluation of treatment will demonstrate if it is appropriate and achieving its aims.

In dealing with mixed physical and behavioural problems, however important each therapist regards her particular priorities, these must take second place to working with cognitive and behaviour disorders. It is these disorders that have often made previous attempts at physical rehabilitation unsuccessful so that the patient has never reached his or her full potential.

When determining treatment priorities it is essential to consider that the patient may have impaired powers of concentration and attention. The patient may only be able to process one item of information at a time, and may only be able to cope with one area of rehabilitation at a time. For example, if a person's physical priorities are to sit so that the individual can feed him or herself effectively, the initial priority may be to concentrate on sitting well. Likewise, the therapist should take into account the way that instructions are given. Are they presented in such a way that they are easily understood? This can often be achieved by giving a series of one-word prompts rather than full sentences. For the person with severe memory deficits it may be necessary to break an overall treatment programme into very small items and to repeat a few simple tasks over and over again until they become automatic before being able to progress any further with the treatment programme. The physio-therapy assessment may usefully be a combination of a scoreable assessment, and a qualitative assessment looking at posture, balance and gait, fine motor control and any other significant factors. These might include swallowing and feeding difficulties, physical deformities or disorganization of movement. The scoreable assessment deals with locomotor ability, an assessment of abnormalities of muscle tone, joint position sense and superficial and deep sensation as well as some functional indicators.

With behaviourally disturbed patients it is often not possible to gain enough help and participation from them to fully complete the assessment, and it may require long periods of careful observation to reveal the true extent of the physical disabilities and functional deficits.

Only when as much information as possible has been collated can one then decide on which problem is a priority, and set out the aims and goals of the treatment programme. Where behaviour disorder is a factor a behaviour-management system can help with this aspect of treatment (for example, see Eames and Wood, 1985a, b; Giles and Clark-Wilson, 1993; and Chapters 4 and 5). Treatment programmes must be tailored to an individual's needs for them to be of the most advantage, and to make the maximum and most effective use of the treatment time available. Whilst group work has an important part to play in an overall treatment programme, particularly when a number of people need to be taught the same skill, such as sitting posture, it cannot take into account every individual's specific needs and requirements. Nor is it possible within the confines of a group situation to reinforce a desired behaviour from an individual every single time that behaviour occurs, which is essential where an individual has problems in new learning. Also, certain problems do not easily lend themselves to group work, such as walking or standing, when a 'hands-on' approach is often necessary.

In an individual treatment programme the treatment is tailored to the person's unique needs and reinforcement can be provided, contingent on a desired behaviour, every time the behaviour occurs. There is also no opportunity for other patients to give positive reinforcement to any inappropriate behaviour the individual might demonstrate. The benefits of individual treatment programmes will be illustrated in the cases studied later in this chapter.

The treatment programme needs to take into account functional activities used by the person on a day-to-day basis. For example, a person who has been working on gait re-education and fine motor control in physiotherapy sessions might be involved in outings to local shops where the main aspects of his individual therapy sessions can be focused on. The patient will need to be able to walk down a street, or around inside a shop, will also need the fine hand control needed to get money out of his pocket and then select the right amount of money. The patient can also be given the opportunity to practice the skills he is learning in treatment sessions, but more importantly he is taking part in in a normal, everyday activity. It will also be far more rewarding than practising walking in the physiotherapy department and sitting at a table picking up different-sized coins. Other examples of this kind of use of functional activity are gardening – where balance, walking, bending, kneeling and hand control can all be practised, or horse riding – where balance and hand control are vital skills. Hopefully, too, these activities provide pleasure and satisfaction for the patient who may be unaware that he is actually practising what he has been working on in more formal physiotherapy sessions.

Whatever skills a person acquires in an individual treatment programme he or she should be given every opportunity to practise those skills functionally, and to be able to generalize them into different situations.

The following studies exemplify the treatment of patients with physical and behavioural problems. The actual physical treatment programmes illustrated were provided as part of an overall treatment programme, and should therefore not be considered in isolation. They show how particular functional problems can be dealt with despite their association with behaviour disorders.

CASE STUDIES

CASE STUDY 8.1

Patient 1, a 27-year-old female, was involved in a road traffic accident in which she sustained a severe brain injury predominantly affecting the brain stem (coma duration unknown but at least 3 months). In addition to left temporoparietal damage she sustained a fractured left femur and a partial dislocation of the left side of the pelvis and fractured vertebra. Residual impairments included severe left-sided hemiplegia, and loss of speech. Heterotopic ossification occurred surrounding the left hip which became fixed.

One year after injury Patient 1 was described as being totally dependent on 24-h nursing care. She was still being fed 6 hourly by nasogastric tube, and was unable to stand or walk but could propel herself in a wheelchair. She was very poorly motivated and she sat with her head hanging forwards, tongue protruding with saliva constantly flowing from her mouth. Any attempt at having her engage in activity was met with furious outbursts of screaming.

It was decided that the first priority would be to tackle the problems she had with swallowing and feeding and therefore a feeding programme was designed, using contingent reinforcement. This programme was performed by a speech therapist and a physiotherapist, concentrating on lip closure and movements and positioning of the tongue, and also correct posture, and efforts to initiate the swallowing reflex.

Initially Patient 1 was maintained in a semi-reclining position with her head supported by pillows in mid-line. At this stage the mouth was hypersensitive and work was begun on desensitizing the lip and mouth area. Desensitization was achieved by introducing various tastes, textures and touch using glycerine swabs, wooden spatulas, small quantities of sweet sauce, and ice. This procedure was necessary first to enable attempts to feed her and to complete her oral hygiene. In addition to this desensitizing programme Patient 1 was given combined speech therapy and physiotherapy sessions working on posture, and movement of the lips and tongue.

In the feeding programme every attempt at swallowing was reinforced with attention and social praise, whether the swallow was purposeful or just a reflex. Swallowing rapidly improved, and small quantities of soft food were introduced. At this stage advice from the dietician was vital on which foods should be offered, taking into account the ease with which they could be swallowed, and to offer as much taste and variety as possible so that feeding could be a pleasurable experience.

As purposeful swallowing improved therapists only gave reinforcement to this and ignored any pure reflex swallowing. As the programme continued, reinforcement became dependent on Patient I making an attempt at chewing the food in her mouth, moving it to the back of her mouth and swallowing it. Whilst this programme continued, the nasogastric tube feeding was reduced by an amount equivalent to the measure of pureed food that Patient I was consuming at each feeding session. Again, the help of the dietician was invaluable in calculating the amount and variety of food that was offered.

Patient I gained a great deal of reinforcement from all the attention she received when being fed by nasogastric tube. Therefore when the feeding programme was started, being fed by nasogastric tube was done in silence, giving her as little attention as possible to decrease the reinforcement attendant upon it.

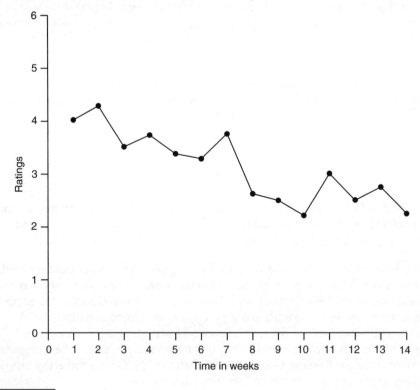

Figure 8.1

Improved swallowing in a patient who had been maintained on nasogastric tube feeding for 2 years and who refused to attempt to swallow. Progress rated on a 1–6 scale where 6 = no effort and 1 = purposeful swallow.

Careful documentation was used throughout the feeding programme so that it could be continuously evaluated. This was based on the following scoring system:

1 = chewing and purposeful swallowing
2 = purposeful swallowing only
3 = reflex swallowing with minimal food loss
4 = reflex swallowing with substantial food loss
5 = no swallow – food lost out of sides of mouth
6 = purposefully spitting food out.

Entries in the clinical notes during this period included the following:

June   During tea-time Patient 1 picked up a jam sandwich, bit a piece of it, moved it around her mouth then spat it out. She repeated this until the sandwich was 'finished'.

July   Feeding programme going well. She now assists by putting the fork into her mouth. She is only having one nasogastric feed a day and the rest of the time is being fed a softened diet in the dining room.

August   Patient 1 is now feeding herself with a minimum of prompts. She holds her head up and swallows effectively.

In just over 3 months Patient 1 was feeding herself satisfactorily after being fed by nasogastric tube for 2.5 years.

CASE STUDY 8.2

Patient 2 had been involved in a head-on collision in May 1983 and suffered a severe brain injury. He was unconscious for 7 weeks, and had a residual left-sided hemiplegia.

Initially he made good progress despite his excitable behaviour, and as the weeks progressed the residual hemiparesis became quite mild. However, Patient 2 became increasingly more aggressive and began to assault staff and then patients. This behaviour escalated to such a degree that it could only be controlled by large doses of sedative drugs, which the made Patient 2 unable to cooperate with any kind of rehabilitation procedures.

On admission to a rehabilitation unit 10 months after injury, Patient 2 was unable to walk but could propel himself in a wheelchair. He was extremely demanding, very noisy and disruptive. He kept up a more or less constant barrage of repetitive questions and comments, which seemed to be his way of keeping others at a distance and making it almost impossible to do anything with him. He responded very well to a time-out programme for his aggression, but any meaningful therapy was severely disrupted by his demanding behaviour and the constant flow of verbal abuse and repetitive conversation.

Physically, Patient 2's main problems were those associated with his hemiparesis. He had great difficulty taking any weight through his left side, there was increased muscle tone in both the left arm and leg, and there was no voluntary movement in his left ankle and toes. Coordination was also impaired on the left side. He also had problems with functional use of his left hand. It was decided that the main priority physically was to try and get him walking, and a walking programme was started.

Patient 2 could stand unaided, but his balance was precarious and his agitated behaviour was enough to cause him to fall easily. Initially physiotherapy was aimed at increasing his ability to balance in all positions, to take weight through his left side and to increase his awareness and use of his left side. He had a below-knee leg cast to allow him to take weight through the foot in a corrected position. This was not very successful and so was followed some weeks later, more successfully, by a below-knee calliper. Despite his constantly noisy, uncooperative behaviour, particularly in group sessions, he made significant progress in all his major physical problem areas.

For his walking programme Patient 2 was given a rollator frame (a four-wheeled walker) to assist him. In an attempt to minimize the constant tumult of chatter and abuse, verbal regulation of his actions was used very loudly and firmly by the physiotherapist. The instructions given were: 'push, step, stretch', to which he pushed the frame forwards, took one step and then straightened up. After each correct sequence he was praised profusely and given lots of attention. He responded well to this, and after a few days Patient 2 was encouraged to use the verbal regulation himself, which he did, however he interjected a great deal of repetitive chatter and verbal abuse. After a few days of performing the walking programme twice daily the prompt words were changed to 'one, two, three', in an effort to promote more rhythm in his gait. Within 2 weeks of starting this programme this patient was walking a distance of 100 yards using the rollator frame and prompting himself with 'one, two, three'. He was also inhibiting all other language whilst he was walking.

As a progression in the programme Patient 2 was encouraged to think of the prompts, but not to say them aloud. Within another week he was walking the same distance in total silence. Three weeks after this the patient was walking independently around the unit with the rollator, and only using his wheelchair for outdoor mobility.

Then, in physiotherapy sessions, Patient 2 was given a short wooden baton to hold horizontally in his hands with his arms stretched forwards fixing his shoulder girdle. The rollator was discarded for the walking programme, but in the meantime the patient started walking outside the unit with the rollator. In the walking programme verbal regulation was used again, this time the prompt being 'step, stretch' as he took one step and straightened up. The same sequence as before was used, 'step, stretch' became 'one, two', and this in turn was internalized. Because Patient 2 sometimes used the baton as a weapon it was taken away, and he repeated this part of the programme using clasped hands. At this point the patient was using the rollator to walk at all times other than during the physiotherapy programme when he was walking with his hands clasped.

Coinciding with Patient 2's ability to walk in this way, an event occurred which precipitated the decision to take the rollator away from him for walking in the unit. During one particular walking session the patient became upset with the therapist and just walked off with his hands clasped, so it was felt he was quite able to walk without the rollator, and it was taken away except for walking outside.

As Patient 2 continued to improve, the programme was generalized into other situations. Trips to the local town were made first using the rollator, then without. Patient 2 was encouraged to join in a gardening project where he was expected to manage all the necessary walking without any assistance. He was very motivated by his own success and his increased mobility spurred him on to try activities that he had previously refused to do. However, this generalization procedure was not without its problems. With the introduction of each new situation the patient became very excitable and noisy and it was often necessary to use prompting again, and go through the sequences used at the start of the walking programme to help him overcome his agitation.

Physiotherapy continued in many other settings, for example in the kitchen where he not only had to walk unaided but also carry and move items around. The walking programme also included increasing his range of walking in that he was able to walk through the grounds of the hospital to the industrial therapy unit, and so that he could eventually walk to the nearby shops, half-a-mile away, do his shopping and walk back. In total the walking programme lasted for 14 months.

CASE STUDY 8.3

Patient 3 fell off his bicycle and sustained a severe brain injury at the age of 13. He was unconscious for several months following the accident but actual coma duration is unknown. There was a previous history of behavioural problems, including being uncooperative and disruptive, and he was in a remedial group at school. Two years after his accident this patient was both blind and aphonic (Patient 3 is referred to as Patient 2 in Chapter 6).

In 1982 he returned home in a wheelchair; he was able to dress himself, transfer from his wheelchair and crawl. Over the following 2 years the home situation broke down completely.

Following admission and during assessment Patient 3 was found to have increased muscle tone in all four limbs. He was unable to isolate movements in his right wrist, hand, foot and ankle. All four limbs were poorly coordinated, particularly the right arm. Joint position sense was impaired in the toes. He could move fairly well from one position to another in lying, sitting, and kneeling and was able to achieve a high kneeling position. He was unable to stand up unaided or walk. Sitting was also a problem in that the patient usually flexed at the waist, and because of a flexion deformity at the junction of the cervical and thoracic spines he had to rotate his head to the side in order to see anything. This poor posture had many further implications. Breathing and swallowing were both difficult. The patient's poor posture and his visual problems compounded one another and he also found non-verbal communication difficult due to limited eye-contact.

Walking was just possible using a ladder-back frame and two people supporting him. Trunk control was poor and Patient 3 flexed to the left side. His head and neck were flexed and his head rotated to the left.

Patient 3 had no heel-strike on either side and ankle stability was extremely poor on both sides, and both feet were everted. He had very little hip extension past neutral whilst walking. Physiotherapy sessions were initially aimed at improving the patients posture in sitting and standing, and in joint speech/physiotherapy sessions work was done on the control of breathing and swallowing. Head control, balance and gait were also areas worked on with the patient who made good progress in all of these areas, particularly balance and gait. His sitting and standing balance improved with better head control than he had shown previously.

Patient 3 started a walking programme. The patient was able to walk short distances using just a rollator for support and a series of prompts designed to encourage a more functional and rhythmic walking pattern. The prompts consisted of:

1 'push' – prompting him to push his frame a short distance forward
2 'step' – to take one step
3 'stretch' – this prompted him to stand up straight, and hold his head up with his mouth closed.

This programme worked well, but it was noticed that the patient only ever stood up correctly following a prompt of 'stretch', so therefore collaboration with the psychology department led to the development of a programme to overcome the problem. Utilizing the patient's love of music a procedure was instituted to help the patient increase his ability to stand up straight. The patient wore a headband fitted with a mercury switch such that when the patient's head was correctly positioned the switch completed a circuit. When the patient's head was in the correct position the switch operated a portable cassette player containing a tape of the patient's favourite music. Thus, the correct positioning of the head produced immediate reinforcement of the desired behaviour.

Figure 8.2 demonstrates the effectiveness of this procedure. Following the completion of the programme Patient 3 demonstrated appropriate head posture well above the baseline level, possibly because the patient gained the reinforcement of attention and eye-contact.

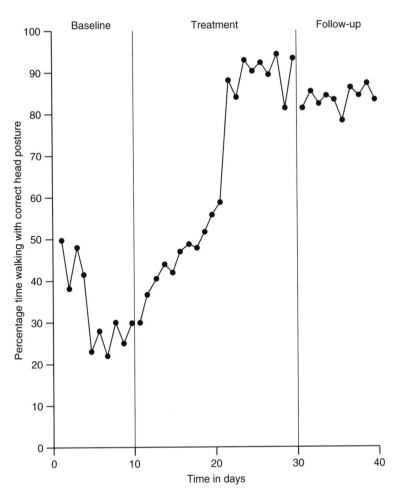

Figure 8.2

Improvement in the percentage of walking with correct head posture using a mercury switch headband to provide contingent music reinforcement.

CASE STUDY 8.4

Patient 4 sustained a severe brain injury at the age of 28 when involved in a road traffic accident. Following the accident he was unconscious for 13 days. Previous attempts at rehabilitation had been unsuccessful.

Initial assessment revealed his principal problems as lack of drive and motivation, aggressive outbursts, poor attention to task, incontinence, immobility due to a severe spastic hemiplegia with sensory inattention. He was unable to walk and had poor

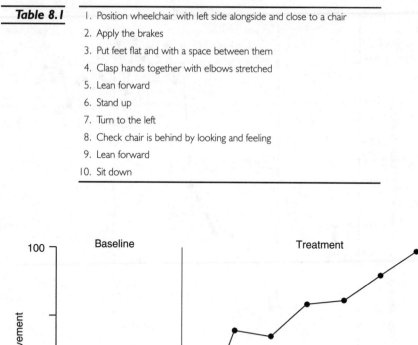

Table 8.1

1. Position wheelchair with left side alongside and close to a chair
2. Apply the brakes
3. Put feet flat and with a space between them
4. Clasp hands together with elbows stretched
5. Lean forward
6. Stand up
7. Turn to the left
8. Check chair is behind by looking and feeling
9. Lean forward
10. Sit down

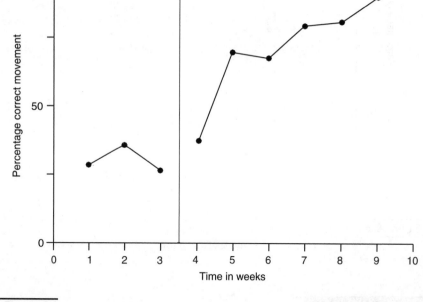

Figure 8.3

Improvement in transferring from wheelchair to chair using a shaping procedure and contingent reinforcement.

and often dangerous wheelchair control. Transferring was also a problem in that he literally threw himself from chair to chair with little regard for his own or anyone else's safety.

Many different aspects of his physical rehabilitation were treated during his stay on the unit, but one particular problem was that of transferring. Baseline measures were completed and a transfer programme implemented, aimed at improving his skill and performance in transferring (Goodman-Smith and Turnbull, 1983). It was hoped that this would increase his awareness and effective use of his left side.

The transfer programme consisted of ten units (see Table 8.1). The number of words used in each instruction were kept to a minimum to aid understanding. For example in prompt 3 the command given was 'Feet flat and apart', and in 4, it was 'Clasp hands, stretch elbows'.

Each element of the programme completed was immediately followed by a small edible reward and plenty of congratulation and praise. The programme was repeated five times each day (see Figure 8.3).

During baseline recordings the proportion of correct movements completed in the transfer programme was 26%. During the course of the programme, which continued for 6 months, this increased to 90%. At this stage the patient was 5 years post-accident. He was eventually able to walk unaided.

Conclusion

The attentional and cognitive problems associated with severe brain injury present a major challenge to physiotherapists. Traditional forms of physiotherapy, it is argued, must give way to techniques that are functionally based. The task of the physiotherapist is to help brain-injured people to relearn skills. However, attentional and cognitive deficits severely decrease learning ability and therefore to set the task in a functional or lifelike setting is to increase the chances of satisfactory outcome.

The need for close interdisciplinary liaison is demonstrated, in order to increase the functional relevance of tasks to be relearned, and of course this requires the physiotherapist to become more aware of learning processes, and how they can be disrupted. This is exemplified by the breaking down of tasks into units that are relevant to the patient. For the brain-injured person, physiotherapy can only produce meaningful change by facilitating the relearning of tasks that are likely to be relevant to the patient in the future.

9 TREATING COGNITIVE/LANGUAGE AND ORAL MOTOR DYSFUNCTION IN THE BRAIN-INJURED ADULT

Ann L. Dill, Gordon Muir Giles

In a study of severely brain-injured residents of Los Angeles, Jacobs (1988) found that 40% of those surveyed had problems in speech and language functioning. The individuals' communication abilities declined as the task demands became more complex, abstract or occurred outside the home. Many of those surveyed had problems in interpersonal relations, assertiveness and social communication. Language impairments following traumatic brain injury often occur as part of a constellation of deficits which compromise the individual's communicative and social competency (Lubinski *et al.*, 1997). The aphasia syndromes typically associated with cerebrovascular accidents are unusual following closed-brain injury but may follow some types of focal injury. Nonetheless, communication disruption is almost universal following severe brain injury (Sarno, 1984). Communication deficits lead to handicaps in community, home and vocational functioning. The therapist should approach communication disorders in the context of the patient's overall functional ability. Language skills cannot be analysed without considering cognitive processes (e.g. attention and memory) and cognitive/behavioural factors (e.g. self-monitoring and impulsivity).

The patient comes to treatment not only with a unique neurological presentation but with a complex psychosocial history, individual preferences and response styles. The patient has an interpersonal, familial and wider cultural context which also has to be considered in treatment. The World Health Organization (WHO) has recommended a distinction between domains of functioning: impairment, disability and handicap (recently redefined as impairment, abilities and participation) (WHO, 1980, 1997). Impairment refers to abnormality of psychological, physiological or anatomical structure or function. Disability (abilities) refers to the functional consequences of impairment defined in terms of cognitive, emotional or physical performance. Handicap (participation) refers to an individual's disadvantage in a society because of an inability to fulfil socially approved roles. Speech and language therapists must work with impairment but more especially at the level of disability and handicap to ensure the relevance of the therapeutic interventions to the patient's everyday life.

A fundamental issue in treatment planning is how to identify and prioritize the problems to be addressed. In the acute stages after trauma, many patients are minimally responsive and the therapist's goal is to encourage responses to environmental stimuli. Other goals emerge as the patient improves. As more complex and goal-directed behaviours are demonstrated by the patient, the selection of individual treatment goals becomes more complex. When prioritizing the goals of treatment, the following principles should be considered:

1 Whatever is important now will be important later. Cognitive/language deficits and behaviours which influence functioning during rehabilitation will usually continue to affect the patient post-discharge. Discussions between the patient, family and therapist identify speech and language problems and highlight the important aspects of communication for therapeutic intervention. For example, one patient in the post-acute stage never said 'hello' or 'good bye' and appeared sullen and uncooperative until engaged in conversation by others. Since the patient was intending to return to his previous employment as a retail sales clerk, this was considered to be significant problem.

   Many patients lack awareness of specific areas of dysfunction and therapists do not feel comfortable informing them, as they are concerned about how the patient may respond. Therapists may ignore the patient's behaviours because they are 'recovering from injury' or because they are 'patients' and so they consider the behaviour normal. Families may not notice because they are so relieved that the patient has survived and they assume that their relative will recover fully.

2 Whatever drives the staff crazy will drive the world crazy. Those cognitive/language deficits and behaviours which cause adverse attention to the patient or which interfere with the individual's ability to perform social roles should be addressed in therapy. The real-life responses that the patient will experience in the world matter. By working with the patient in the everyday environments, it is possible to determine how the patient reacts to others and what upsets the patient in social situations. Therapy should assist the patient develop ways to manage these reactions.

3 The patient and staff should address only a limited number of practical goals so that both the staff and patient can focus and not feel overwhelmed.

4 Functional goals should be selected from the beginning of treatment. A hierarchical, graded approach (i.e. working from easy to more complex) is most likely to motivate the patient. For example, being able to vocalize is a prerequisite for being able to talk.

EVALUATION OF THE MINIMALLY RESPONSIVE PATIENT

Most patients demonstrate rapid improvement in the early stages of recovery following severe brain injury. The rapidity of the recovery process depends on the severity of the injury and the presence of complicating factors. During the early stages of recovery it is the therapist's role to monitor the patient and ensure that appropriate interventions occur at suitable times. Interventions may include family and staff education about how to communicate with the patient. At this stage, it is also important to consider the impact of the environment and to provide appropriate stimulation without increasing the patient's agitation. The following sections will describe the role of the speech and language therapist as the patient emerges from coma.

COMA

Patients in coma do not obey commands, utter words or open their eyes. Patients in vegetative states, like patients in coma, do not obey commands or utter words (although they may vocalize) but unlike patients in coma, patients in a vegetative state resume sleep–wake cycles (with eye opening). Some therapists use coma stimulation in an attempt to accelerate recovery/emergence from coma. Stimulation can be provided unimodally or multimodally. An example of unimodal stimulation is music, which has been found to have short-term limited effects (Wilson *et al.*, 1992). Multimodal stimulation involves visual, auditory, tactile, olfactory and gustatory stimulation provided in sequence. Protocols for administration vary from relatively short sessions to many hours per day (Wilson and McMillan, 1993). There is evidence that multimodal stimulation has a short-term limited effect (Wilson, S. *et al.*, 1991). Evidence regarding the effect of multimodal stimulation on arousal from coma and on long-term recovery is mixed (Rader *et al.*, 1989; Wilson and McMillan, 1993) and further research is indicated.

Repeated evaluations of the patient's responsiveness can be performed using the Glasgow Coma Scale (GCS) or the Western Neurosensory Stimulation Profile (see below). With these diagnostic tools, the therapist evaluates the patient's cognitive status by measuring the patient's ability to give systematic responses to stimuli. Patients can demonstrate simple purposive behaviour in coma, however, the simplest communication is to indicate affirmation or rejection in some way to verbal questions or instructions. Approach or rejection to tactile stimuli may simply represent a behavioural response tendency and does not indicate higher cognitive processes. Initially, patients rarely say 'yes' or 'no' but indicate affirmation or rejection in some other way (see 'augmentative communication' below). Patients will often have brief periods of being able to respond to simple yes/no questions such as 'do you have a sister?' but consistent and reliable yes/no responses may be very difficult for the patient. Patients often demonstrate perseverative movements or response sets or may only be able to give one or two purposeful responses before either internal or external 'interference' prevents the patient from responding. Patients will often be able to engage in automatic purposeful behaviours such as turning the pages of a magazine or putting a toothbrush in their mouth before they can give reliable answers. In addition, difficulties in maintaining arousal and attention as well as apraxia and perseveration may make yes/no responding problematic. A small number of patients appear to be in a vegetative state but in fact suffer from 'locked in syndrome'. They have retained cognitive function but have profound motor impairment (see 'augmentative communication' below).

At the next stage the therapist's aim is to determine if the patient is understanding what is said to them. In order to give a yes/no answer, a patient must have the following component skills:

- receptive: arousal, attention, discrimination, auditory sequencing, categorization, processing, auditory memory, problem solving
- expressive: selecting response mode, response selection, initiation, response termination and output monitoring for accuracy.

Therapists attempt first to elicit a response before focusing on accuracy. It is often difficult to determine the patient's receptive ability because it is compounded by difficulties in expression. Consistent shrugging or waving when asked a question may indicate understanding that a question has been asked but show an inability to respond with content. Concrete questions about personally relevant information (e.g. 'Do you have a sister?') are more likely to be answered accurately than abstract yes/no questions (e.g. 'is the sky blue?').

Family members may overstate the patient's functioning, interpreting random or repetitive movements or reflexes as purposive. However, family members, who are often spending the longest sustained periods of time with the patient, may also be the first to appreciate subtle changes in the patient's responses (Freeman, 1993).

FORMAL RATING AND ASSESSMENT SYSTEMS

It is important to monitor patient behaviours in the coma and early post-coma stage with precision. Accurate monitoring of changes in patient behaviours enables the clinician to detect any signs of deterioration, determine the rate of recovery, and may be used for research purposes to determine the effects of coma stimulation or other rehabilitative interventions. Horn *et al.* (1993) have reviewed a wide range of available scales. Scales commonly used in clinical practice are described below.

The Glasgow Coma Scale

The Glasgow Coma Scale (GCS) of Teasdale and Jennett (1974) is a standardized assessment procedure for use with the comatose patient. The GCS uses three independently measured aspects of behaviour; motor responsiveness, verbal performance and eye opening. Patients are rated on their best response. The GCS can be applied rapidly and consistently by any member of the treatment team. Recording of GCS scores can be completed on first admission to the emergency room or neurological trauma unit. A severe injury may be defined as a GCS of 8 or less (the lowest obtained score is 3), a score of 9–12 indicates a moderate brain injury and of 13–15 a mild brain injury (Rimel *et al.*, 1981).

The Western Neurosensory Stimulation Profile (WNSSP)

The Western Neurosensory Stimulation Profile (Ansell *et al.*, 1989) is used with slow to recover (STR) patients (Rancho levels II–V). The WNSSP is a reliable and valid instrument for the assessment of responsiveness to various types of sensory stimuli. The WNSSP consists of 33 items which rate a patient's arousal and attention, expressive communication and response to auditory, visual, tactile and olfactory stimulation. The items were selected to capture the broad range of behaviours exhibited by patients at Rancho levels II–V. For each of the 33 items, responses are rated using a scoring hierarchy which captures both extent of cueing required and response latency (higher scores indicate more impaired functioning).

Table 9.1

Glasgow Coma Scale* with explanations of terms

	Motor response
Obeys commands:	**6** Patient follows simple commands; care must be taken to avoid interpreting a grasp reflex or a postural adjustment as a response to command
Localized pain response:	**5** A stimulus applied at more than one site causes movement in an attempt to escape it
Withdrawal:	**4** A normal flexor response; patient withdraws from painful stimulus applied to nailbed with abduction of the shoulder
Abnormal flexion response:	**3** Patient withdraws from painful stimulus applied to nailbed with stereotyped mass flexor pattern (including adduction at the shoulder)
Abnormal extensor response:	**2** Patient withdraws from painful stimulus applied to nailbed with stereotyped mass extension pattern (including adduction and internal rotation at the shoulder and pronation of the forearm)
No response:	**1** Usually associated with hypotonia (ensure adequate stimuli and absence of spinal cord injury)
	Verbal response
Oriented:	**5** Patient oriented to time, place and person
Confused conversation:	**4** Patient can converse but the content indicates disorientation and confusion
Inappropriate speech:	**3** Patient utters comprehensible words but only in a random way (e.g. purposeless shouting and swearing)
Incomprehensible speech:	**2** Patient utters grunts and groans only (no recognizable words)
No speech:	**1** Self-explanatory
	Eye opening
Spontaneous eye opening:	**4** Does not imply awareness (includes sleep/wake cycles)
In response to speech:	**3** Patient opens eyes in response to some speech (includes shouting) but does not imply that the patient opens eyes to command
In response to pain:	**2** Patient opens eyes in response to painful stimuli applied to the chest or limbs
Eyes do not open:	**1** Self-explanatory

Glasgow Coma Scale Score = sum of motor, verbal and eye opening score (3–15)

*After Teasdale and Jennett (1974).

Assessment in the early post-coma recovery period

After the stage of coma, it is important to be able to track patient progress. A number of more general scales are available and widely used for this purpose. The Disability Rating Scale (DRS) of Rappaport and co-workers (1982), charts the recovery of the severely brain-injured patient beginning with coma. The DRS consists of four categories. The first category measures arousal, awareness and responsivity, and is adapted from the GCS. The second category grades cognitive ability for self-care activities (feeding, toileting and grooming) and relates to the patient's knowledge of how and when to perform such tasks. Ability is rated as complete, partial, or minimal and the rating is dependent on stating or demonstrating how and when to perform, and not on actual performance. The third category measures level of functioning. The patient is rated on actual performance as independent, independent in a special (modified) environment, and mildly, moderately, markedly and totally dependent. The fourth category rates employability. In the original study, no patient was rated as being without disability at discharge. Inter-rater reliability was 0.97–0.98. The scale can be used easily and applied rapidly (usually taking no more than 5–15 min).

Although not an evaluation tool, an overall categorization of purposive behaviour is provided by the Rancho Los Amigos Scale (see Table 9.2). The scale consists of eight categories ranging from no response to purposeful and appropriate behaviour. The scale is a useful shorthand method for describing patient functioning but as a result may obscure subtle but important changes in behaviour. In addition, patients may demonstrate behaviours from two different levels at the same time. It should also be recognized that environmental stimuli can influence behaviour and recovery patterns are not always linear and so a patient may demonstrate behaviours consistent with level IV one day and level III the next.

Table 9.2

Ranchos Los Amigos levels of cognitive functioning* with explanation of terms (not all patients go through all stages nor do all patients progress at the same rate)

1. No response	Patient exhibits complete absence of observable response when presented with any stimuli
2. Generalized response	Patient exhibits generalized responses to painful stimuli; may respond to repeated auditory stimuli with increased or decreased activity; responses are the same irrespective of the type or location of stimuli
3. Localized response	Patient demonstrates withdrawal or vocalization to painful stimuli; may turn towards or away from auditory stimuli; responds to discomfort by pulling tubes or restraints
4. Confused/agitated	Severely impaired processing of environmental information; patient responds primarily to internal state; attention span very limited; profound difficulty in encoding new information; behaviour may be bizarre or aggressive; dependant in all aspects of care
5. Confused/inappropriate non-agitated	Patient is able to respond to simple commands fairly consistently; patient is able to attend to some aspects of the environment but attention span remains limited; memory function severely impaired; patient requires assistance or close supervision for functional tasks; performance deteriorates when structure decreases or complexity increases
6. Confused/appropriate	Patient follows simple directions consistently; patient inconsistently oriented to time and place; completes overlearned tasks with supervision
7. Automatic/appropriate	Orientated consistently; may retain significant memory disfunction; initiates and carries out basic routines completely independently; displays some insight into disability but may be unable to realistically plan for own future
8. Purposeful/appropriate	Patient is alert and oriented consistently; demonstrates more responsibility for self and may be able to plan realistically for own future; able to learn new tasks and can apply learned skills independently in new situations; may be able to work or be a candidate for vocational rehabilitation; may continue to show reduced ability relative to premorbid functioning

*After Hagen et al. (1972).

ACUTE EVALUATION AND TREATMENT

Initial contact with the patient

Care needs to be taken when interacting with the minimally responsive patient (Rancho level III and IV). Repetitive and/or excessive environmental stimuli (visual and auditory) should be minimized. The therapist models for staff and the patient's family and friends how to approach the patient. In the early stages of recovery interactions should focus on basic orientation. Individuals entering the patient's environment should introduce themselves, tell the patient where they are, why they are there, what is going on around them, what day it is and the time of day. The patient should be oriented to where the therapist is (i.e. the side of the bed) and the therapist should speak calmly and softly. Simple concrete statements should be used and abstractions (i.e. conditional clauses or sentences with implicit meaning) avoided. The patient may have attention deficits and be unable to cope with overstimulation so it is important that only one person should speak or give instructions to the patient at a time.

Cognitive/language disturbance

The language/communicative impairments of patients in the early period of recovery from brain injury have been described as cognitive/language disturbances (Hagen, 1982) and cognitive/communicative impairments (Ylvisaker and Urbanczyk, 1994). These terms indicate the close relationship between cognition and language functioning at this early stage of recovery. Cognition and language should be assessed together by the speech and language therapist. During the early post-coma period, the patient may have very poor attention skills and become easily overstimulated and agitated. Disturbed verbal behaviours including coprolalia (repetitive and stereotypic use of profanity), verbal aggression, sexual talk, verbal disinhibition and other socially inappropriate behaviours are often directed towards family members or care staff.

Patients who rapidly emerge from coma may make an almost immediate motor recovery but demonstrate severely impaired cognitive/language functioning. The patient's speech and mental life may be full of fantastic combinations (of what should be separate stimuli or events) and misperceptions. The patient at this stage in recovery does not have the capacity to sort or to categorize information efficiently. Without this ability the patient is unable to self-monitor thoughts for accuracy. The confused patient will misperceive or mislabel current stimuli and may attempt to understand their current circumstances by trying to make it consistent with their previous environment. Since the patient can neither remember nor understand the events which took them from their previous circumstances to the hospital setting, the patient has a view of the world which does not incorporate these changes. The patient may believe that he or she are in their own home or workplace so for example an injured metal worker may mistake the oxygen cylinder in the corner of the room for an acetylene torch familiar to him from his work. The hospital room is the workshop, staff are seen as co-workers or family members, etc.

Patients can become fixated on bizarre ideas and the patient's speech may include high-frequency words or references to the patient's previous environment. Paraphasic errors are common and patients often perseverate on the error becoming agitated when they are not understood. At this stage, both non-verbal behaviours such as physical proximity and eye-contact as well as verbal behaviours such as conversational management are likely to be impaired. Deficits in receptive and expressive language skills, fluency and self-monitoring are related to the patient's overall cognitive functioning (see Chapter 4). Other errors include echolalia (repetitions of the speech of others) and deficits in both receptive and expressive language skills are evident. In very severely injured patients, both voice and fluency are likely to be impaired.

It is important for the therapist to reorient, reassure and redirect the patient. It is important to keep the patient safe and not to unduly support the patient's fantasies as patients may attempt to act on their confused ideas. The therapist can validate the patient experience and redirect: 'I know that it really feels like you need to leave the hospital but let's call your wife now and she can talk to you about what has happened'. Arguing with a confused patient usually only serves to escalate their anxiety. Prevention is far more effective than cure, frequent short and concrete orientation can prevent the patient from becoming fixated on behaviours which place them at risk. Indirect reassurance and orientation reduces the likelihood of psychological reactance.

The treatment team needs to develop ways to redirect the patient. Developing high-frequency and preferred alternative activities is an important strategy to use in managing the confused patient at this stage in recovery (e.g. playing checkers, card games, going for a walk, or engaging in other non-demanding physical activities). Activities which were enjoyed by the patient pre-morbidly are often the activities the patient will engage in most easily. High-frequency behaviours may be rewarding to the patient and can often be easily developed by staff.

The speech and language therapist should be alert to the following questions: Has communication taken place? Is the patient communicating what they think they are communicating? Can they use the strategies they are attempting to use?

Oral motor

Swallowing

Oral motor functioning requires early and repeated evaluations in the initial stages of recovery from coma. Most patients when first seen are intubated and frequently have total parenteral or enteral nutrition. Early nutritional management involves recognition of hypermetabolic and catabolic condition (Clifton, 1988). Yorkston *et al.* (1989) found that of 151 brain injured patients admitted consecutively to two hospitals, 77.5% had swallowing disorders after emerging from coma. Yorkston *et al.* (1989) used clinical criteria in the absence of videoradiographic studies so may have underestimated the true incidence. Patients may exhibit swallowing disorders including reduced oral motor control, delayed or absent swallow reflex and pharyngeal or laryngeal involvement. Early in recovery, swallowing disorders are common and frequently occur in isolation from motor speech disorders.

The patient's responses should be observed for evidence of awareness of oral stimulation and increasing oral motor functioning. Limited awareness of oral stimuli increases the risk of aspiration and can be due to decreased arousal, attention or an alteration of oral and pharyngeal sensation. Therapists can assess the patient at rest for lip closure and observe the patient's breathing, (nasal versus oral) as well as how the patient manages secretions (swallowing, coughing, wiping of the mouth or apparent unawareness). Visual examination of the oral cavity may indicate injury, asymmetry and the location of dysfunction. Therapists evaluate voluntary oral motor control but must recognize that voluntary oral motor control is not necessarily indicative of motor control in swallowing.

Pre-feeding skills are evaluated by multisensory stimulation, temperatures, smells and tastes (i.e. ice chips, lemon, glycerin swab) (see Logeman, 1989 for a detailed discussion of oral motor, oral sensory and physiological swallowing assessment). Pre-feeding activities may begin at Rancho Los Amigos level III (snacks) but a full oral diet may not be appropriate until Rancho Los Amigos level VI. Complicating the swallowing dysfunction, some patients may have heightened sensation and demonstrate abnormal reflexes such as a hyperactive gag or bite reflex. Desensitization approaches may be used with these patients. An approach which is often effective is to have the patient present the desensitizing stimuli to himself or herself.

In addition to traditional approaches to oral and pharyngeal sensory and motor disorders, the speech and language therapist assesses a range of other factors of particular importance to the management of the brain-injured person (Avery-Smith and Delarosa, 1994). The speech and language therapist assesses how alteration in posture, self-feeding behaviours, as well as cognitive and perceptual disorders affect swallowing. Among dysphagia patients, more severe cognitive impairments are associated with increased severity of dysphagia (Cherney and Halper, 1989). Facilitating hand-to-mouth responses has been shown to increase orientation to eating and swallowing (Groher, 1992). The patient's eating behaviours can interact with the patient's swallowing ability. For example, patients with frontal lobe injuries may eat impulsively and 'stuff' food into their mouths creating a choking risk especially in patients who have reduced oral motor control.

The environment for eating needs to be considered as well. At this stage of recovery, brain-injured patients are distractible and sensitive to stimulation often resulting in behavioural disregulation during eating. Reducing stimulus complexity and attentional demands of the environment can help the patient concentrate on the task. For instance, only one food item and one utensil on an uncluttered surface may increase the patient's independent eating. Inattention may also increase the risk of aspiration of food or liquid. Additionally, patients with impaired initiation may not feed themselves despite being hungry, having food and having the physical capacity to do so. For further descriptions of types of dysphagia which may occur following brain injury, the reader is referred to Logeman (1989). Various rating scales are available to chart the progress of patients with dysphagia (see, for example, Cherney et al., 1986).

Practical problems in dysphagia management

Successful management of the patient with impaired oral motor functioning requires the balancing of various practical considerations. For instance, due to institutional and economic constraints, the speech and language therapist may only have limited time to treat the patient forcing prioritization between swallowing and communication training.

The therapist must consider whether the patient can get enough nutrition/ hydration by mouth before having the feeding tube removed. The therapist should consider the technical skill required to feed the patient and the amount of supervision required to ensure that the patient can eat for the length of time required.

Staff and family should be trained in how to use the strategies required for the patient and initially be supervised when feeding the patient. Issues surrounding swallowing are foreign to most staff and family members and these issues may be difficult for them to understand. It is obvious when a person cannot stand or talk but swallowing is usually not observed directly. Some swallowing deficits may be truly invisible. Frequent repetition of the information in a straightforward way with opportunities for discussion are important.

A major challenge can be helping the family understand that giving their relative a type of food that they cannot swallow, can be potentially life threatening. This can be an issue at any stage in recovery but is particularly difficult when the patient is starting to ask for food. Cultural traditions and specific social relationships involving food may complicate the family's ability to respect the restrictions which the speech and language therapist establishes for the patient's diet. Wherever possible the therapist should take the opportunity to work closely with the family. Cultural food preferences may be particularly important in motivating the patient to resume eating and very difficult to accommodate given dietary limitations. Patients who are stimulus bound and unable to understand what is going on around them may be simply unmotivated to eat pureed foods. Showing and discussing with family members the results of the videofluoroscopy is a potentially powerful intervention.

Most patients with severe traumatic brain injury are discharged home to the care of their family. The importance of family dysphagia education cannot be overstated (Hutchins, 1989). Hutchins (1989) describes a 30-min single family approach to dysphagia information for the family which includes a videotape, review of the patient's video study, written materials and an opportunity for discussion.

Dysarthria, dysphonia and apraxia of speech

Severely brain-injured patients should be assessed for dysarthria (i.e. motor speech disorders due to impairment originating in the central or peripheral nervous system), dysphonia (a disorder affecting the patients use of voice) and apraxia (i.e. disruption of voluntary or purposeful programming of muscular movements). In the early stages of recovery, many patients present with severe dysarthria although the actual incidence of the disorder is unknown. For many, this resolves as the patient improves neurologically. Yorkston *et al.* (1989) evaluated speech and swallowing disorders in 151 traumatic brain-injury patients during the patients' acute medical hospitalization, during acute rehabilitation and during outpatient treatment. The percentage of patients who were unable to communicate due to speech disorders showed a steady decline from 25% in the acute stage to 20% during rehabilitation and then to 10% during outpatient treatment. Many patients respond to long-term intensive treatment. Oral motor exercises can be used to improve basic oral motor skills and hence speech intelligibility. Patients who can sustain attention for 10-min intervals up to 30 min can progress using an articulation skills-building approach (i.e. drills involving sound production progressing through the following stages: isolated sounds, single words, short phrases, sentences, structured conversation and spontaneous conversation). Since self-monitoring skills are frequently impaired, the patient needs auditory or visual feedback about their performance. For a small number of patients, post-acute treatment may include prosthetic or surgical interventions (Ylvisaker and Urbanczyk, 1994).

Voice and fluency disorders

Some of the most common communication disorders involve impaired self-monitoring and self-regulation (Giles and Clark-Wilson, 1993). Patients often have limited awareness of their voice or fluency and have difficulties in interrupting their own speech flow.

The speech and language therapist assesses vocal parameters for appropriate quality, pitch and volume. Organic aphonia or dysphonia from intubation typically resolves without therapy. Often behavioural interventions are appropriate and effective techniques to improve voice. The patient, with practice in individual sessions with the speech and language therapist, is able to bring the voice deficit under conscious control. A programme is then developed to assist the patient to generalize the skill. Parameters for designing intervention programmes are described in more detail below. There is considerable evidence that these kinds of problems are amenable to behavioural strategies (see Giles and Clark-Wilson, 1993).

Similarly, the speech and language therapist assesses fluency parameters (i.e. the flow and rate of speech). The patient may present with cluttering, stuttering and other rate disorders. Like interventions for voice, the patient is taught to self-monitor and self-correct. Specific pacing strategies can be applied.

Hearing

Hearing impairment, resulting from damage to the vestibulocochlear (eighth) cranial nerve, often occurs in patients with severe brain injury with associated skull fracture (Giles and Clark-Wilson, 1993). Total or partial hearing loss occurs in 6–8% of patients with severe brain injury. The speech and language therapist needs to assess and rule out the possibility of a hearing loss. Physical trauma may have been noted at the time of the trauma and medical records should be reviewed. Once the patient is medically stable an audiological evaluation can be performed.

Augmentative communication

Simple non-verbal systems such as gestures, eye blinking, switching devices and communication boards may aid communication in the early stages of recovery.

However, patients are unlikely to be able to use anything but the simplest systems and will have to be constantly reoriented to them. It is unfortunate that the easiest movements for the patient to produce, such as hand squeezing and eye blinking, occur as reflexes and are therefore difficult to interpret reliably. Natural systems (i.e. those used in normal social interaction such as head nods and gestures) are preferable to artificial systems such as one eye blink for yes and two for no.

Early post-acute rehabilitation

As the patient improves, the speech and language therapist should move from continuous evaluation to active retraining. Evaluations become more detailed and there is a gradual shift in the patient's treatment programme in both content and method of intervention. Higher level language and communicative functions are more likely to be addressed and specific cognitive retraining strategies incorporated in the programme.

Post-acute evaluation

Evaluation of the language and communication abilities of the traumatic brain-injury patient is complex. Patients often show adequate or only minor impairment in speech and language functioning on formal testing but are nonetheless socially and communicatively ineffective. This may be due to the interplay of impaired self-regulatory mechanisms (executive function deficits) and subtle language disorders. Assessment of the patient's communication skills is made more complex by the wide range of factors which can affect performance, such as environmental context and the stimulus demands of the testing itself. Structured tasks often provoke better performance than spontaneously generated responses. The situation is made more difficult by the relative simplicity of the hospital environment which may not tax patients sufficiently for them to demonstrate functionally relevant disability. This combination of factors requires that the speech and language therapist utilize multiple functional tasks in real-life contexts for assessment. A functional skill assessment is a measurement of how the patient performs daily tasks. Following the informal assessment procedures, formal testing can take place. The evaluation may begin with an informal assessment, this includes both an interview and a functional skills assessment (see Table 9.3).

Informal assessment

The initial interview should be preceded by obtaining background information when possible (i.e. medical history and physical, neuropsychological evaluations and prior speech and language therapist assessment results). Information from family and friends is essential in establishing pre-morbid functioning. The therapist needs to gain an understanding of how the patient was before the injury in order to appreciate the patient in all functional environments. The speech and language therapist should know the patient's previous and current medical status and medication regimen (which may complicate oral motor, language and cognitive functioning). Baseline social and behavioural functioning are established by asking about the patient's ability to live independently, maintain interpersonal relationships, hold a job and lifestyle. The informal assessment should begin by viewing the

---

Table 9.3

A. Pragmatics

1. Proximity: the patient's physical closeness to another in space. For instance whether the patient invades intimate or personal zones or create too much distance between speaker and listener or touches others excessively or not at all

2. Body language: including posture, facial expression, eye-contact and use of gestures. For instance, whether the patient exhibits a flat facial expression or is expressive; moves impulsively or erratically

3. Prosody: whether the patient has a melodic voice or whether it is flat, monotone or characterized by odd or unusual inflections

4. Social rules: for instance whether the patient follows the turn-taking of conversation or uses socially acceptable language and behaviours

B. Speech and language

1. Speech intelligibility: for instance whether the patient can articulate precisely and be understood

2. Receptive and expressive language functioning: for instance whether the patient evidences disruptions in syntax such as telegraphic speech or paraphasias, circumlocutions or perseverations, use both written and verbal forms of communication

3. Fluency: for instance whether the flow, rate and pressure of speech are within normal limits

4. Voice quality: for instance whether the patient has a hypo-/hypernasal quality to their speech, has a disturbance in pitch or speaks too loudly or too softly

5. Hearing

6. Cognition: this includes how the patient uses language to communicate, self-monitors, uses feedback, or demonstrates evidence of impaired memory, problem solving, or judgement

C. Oral motor

1. Breath control

2. Apraxia

3. Dysarthria

4. Dysphagia

D. Affect and mood

E. Other

1. Use of augmentative communication devices?

2. Use of hearing aids?

3. Other assistive devises (memory aids, computers)?

---

patient as a communicating, socially interacting person. Individual deficits can be noted but in an informal assessment the speech and language therapist should focus on overall communicative ability and social presentation. This stance should be adopted intermittently throughout treatment.

Functional assessment

Although functional assessment is initiated early in the assessment process (usually begun immediately following the initial interview) it is also an ongoing process. Functional assessment suggests the areas to be targeted in formal assessment. Tasks used in functional assessment may include a variety of brief functional behaviours which can give the therapist information regarding the patient's cognitive processes and communication competence. The task should be selected according to the patient's physical and cognitive capabilities and should be relevant to the patient's rehabilitation goals. Tasks included in an informal assessment might include making orange juice from concentrate, using a telephone directory to obtain information, telephoning a business to request information, ordering coffee and a doughnut in a restaurant, following instructions to go shopping and make a specific purchase or completing a specific project such as making photocopies which requires following verbal or written instructions.

The therapist needs to observe how the patient approaches the task. For instance the patient's ability to plan the activity and to anticipate what is needed to carry out the task (i.e. money, directions, appropriate clothing for a shopping trip) characterizes planning and problem-solving skills. The patient might have difficulty paying for goods and using strategies to remember information. During observations of functional activities, the therapist takes special note of how the patient's linguistic skills affect their performance during functional activities. From a process oriented approach, it is important not only to note the patient's ability in formal testing but also to observe how the patient's performance breaks down in functional settings and how, if at all, they attempt to compensate for their difficulties.

The therapist should restrict himself or herself to the observation and the recording of behaviours to obtain an actual picture of what the patient would do in the natural environment. It is important for the therapist to be aware of how their own actions may influence the patient's behaviour. Unfortunately, premature intervention often prevents the therapist from seeing how the patient attempts to problem solve. Obviously, the patient's safety and the therapist's professional relationship with the patient are more important in the long term than obtaining accurate information (as there should be additional opportunities for data collection), but help should be restricted to when the patient is ceasing to function effectively and requires help. For example, the therapist should determine what the patient will do when the patient is failing to communicate effectively in the grocery store, i.e. will the patient begin to cry, start shouting, or give up and leave the store?

Formal testing

Formal or standardized tests help pinpoint the precise nature of the patient's speech and language disorder. Formal tests are available for the same areas listed under the heading 'Informal assessment'. Formal tests may be administered in a routine battery approach or individual tests can be used to elucidate deficits identified on informal assessment. Commonly used tools include the Boston Diagnostic Aphasia Examination (Goodglass and Kaplan, 1972), the Western Aphasia Battery (Kertesz, 1982) and the Minnesota Test for Differential Diagnosis of Aphasia (Schuell, 1963). Most speech and language therapists select subtests from these batteries and devise a test battery which specifically addresses the patient's problems. The Communicative Abilities of Daily Living Test (Holland, 1980) and the Ross and Spencer (Ross-Swain, 1996) test of cognitive abilities are more functionally oriented communication assessments. These tests measure communication skills used in daily life and allow the patient's performance to be compared to group norms.

These formal tests assess the process which the patient uses to answer questions. Observing the process is often more helpful than the answer itself as it reveals both the language and communication deficits and the compensatory strategies naturally adopted by the patient. Careful observation of how and why the patient's performance breaks down can be useful in determining therapeutic interventions. This approach is similar to the process approach to neuropsychological testing advocated by Kaplan (1988). For example, a subtest of the Ross and Spencer, the test of Rapid Naming, measures the patient's ability to cluster words into semantic groups to facilitate recall. One question asks the patient to name 'toys'. The patient who answers 'I don't play with toys' demonstrates an attempted rejection of the task and a concrete egocentric response to the question.

TREATMENT PRINCIPLES AND METHODS

Treatment of language and communication dysfunction is best carried out by a team in the patient's own natural environment. The environment initially may be a hospital bed and gradually change to the person's home, school or work settings.

Type of treatment environment: multidisciplinary versus interdisciplinary

The treatment environment influences the type of treatment approaches that can realistically be provided. For example, teaching a patient sign language is not helpful if no one else understands it. Staff organization is an important factor in service provision. Although many treatment facilities claim to be transdisciplinary, many continue to follow the structure of the multidisciplinary team. In a multidisciplinary team, the treatment team in conjunction with the physician determine the goals for the patient in their respective disciplines and report back, usually once per week. Any coordination of treatment is done in an *ad hoc* way. In a transdisciplinary team, the whole team develops a small number of goals without regard to therapy discipline boundaries. Treatment programmes based on these goals are then implemented by the whole team working together. See Case Study 9.1.

CASE STUDY 9.1

Patient 1 exhibited a rapid rate of speech with marked cluttering (a fluency disorder). The team, in consultation with the speech language therapist, decided to have Patient 1 pace his speech by tapping his leg. The therapist trained the staff in the procedure and demonstrated the technique for all staff at a group meeting. All staff were then responsible for cueing the patient in use of the technique.

The benefit of the transdisciplinary team is that the desired behaviour is practised and reinforced consistently and the patient can reach the desired goals more rapidly. However, the transdisciplinary team has disadvantages: it is challenging to staff's professional identities. In the USA, there are documentation and third-party payer constraints. It takes time and effort to coordinate a treatment plan. There may be financial benefits to the institution of multidisciplinary teams so it is often the structure imposed on therapists in a hospital setting. The interdisciplinary or transdisciplinary team is particularly challenging to some because the focus of the individual disciplines is to train all staff to interact with the patient in a therapeutic way. All staff are therefore responsible for, and take credit for, the patient's progress. The more effective the speech and language therapist is in training the staff, the more effective the patient's overall treatment, but there is some loss incurred in the patient–therapist relationship (see also Chapter 12).

The hospital is not the best environment for rehabilitation once the patient is past the acute phase of recovery and progressing towards community integration. The treatment setting should be the community and preferably a 'home-like' environment. The rehabilitation setting should be accessible to transportation, stores, restaurants, schools and other community resources, and it should attempt to replicate the types of demands that are placed on an individual in a community environment.

Individual treatment

Individual treatment is the most appropriate format for assessment, education and skill development. On meeting the patient, the therapist should explain the professional purpose of seeing the patient, as well as the purpose of assessment and treatment. For higher functioning patients, neuroeducation involves describing the type of disorder the patient has and the likely effects of treatment. Some patients can state their problems and the approaches they believe will help them, others will need to have a programme designed for them. A joint understanding of the goals of treatment is a prerequisite for most successful rehabilitation. The patient does not need to completely understand all the nuances of their problems or of the treatment plan, but whenever possible, there should be some agreement as to the goals and methods of treatment.

The speech and language therapist is also involved in helping the patient with the psychosocial aspects of loss of communication. Some patients are reluctant to admit that they have problems and are reluctant to work on them because they are unable to admit that they could have a 'mental' problem. Providing gentle and persistent approaches to overcoming deficits while maintaining the prospect of improvement with treatment is recommended.

Sessional practice

The speech and language therapist and patient develop treatment goals and the initial stages of skill development take place in the context of sessional practice. The individual treatment session allows the therapist to facilitate patient performance by controlling task demands. For example, a patient who has a disruption of fluency can initially be asked to practice short, simple phases ensuring successful performance. A hierarchy of structured tasks could progress from phrases, sentences, brief conversations to long conversation of increasing complexity (see, for example, Giles et al., 1988). Maximal feedback about the patient's performance can be provided initially but later, the speech and language therapist can fade cues and introduce self-rating (excellent/good/average/poor). Finally, the self-rating can be faded and the patient encouraged to attend to spontaneously arising social cues such as facial expression in the natural environment. This type of sessional practice can be applied to articulation, language (structure and content), fluency, voice, use of specific compensatory strategies, cognitive retraining, and social behaviours. The speech and language therapist can use role-play to develop compensatory strategies and work in a hierarchy of systematic desensitization around functional social situations involving communication. Individual sessions with the speech and language therapist provide a secure environment for teaching the patient communication skills which the patient can find extremely frustrating and anxiety provoking.

Group treatment

The use of groups introduces a greater range of stimuli to which the patient has to respond while in a safe and controlled setting. Patients work on individual goals but the unpredictability of multiple individuals is introduced. Patients benefit from group encouragement and support when working on similar goals and may gain greater understanding of their circumstances through shared experiences. The number of participants in a group can vary from two to many. Groups may also play a role in assessment as some subtle deficits may only be apparent to the speech and language therapist when observing the patient in group conversation. Groups may have a single focus (e.g. articulation or dysphagia) or may be parallel where participants are working on a shared project such as a newsletter but each have individualized goals. The parallel group allows full scope for the therapist's creativity. For example, a patient with deficits in executive functions could be the editor of a newsletter; a task which requires the patient to work with all the other patients to put the project together. A patient with mild expressive aphasia can practice written language skills. Lower functioning patients can do page layout, photocopying or distribution.

The therapist designs the framework of the project with the group, but the work is the production of the group. The standard of the work will depend on the level of functioning of the patients in the group and the organization of the group. Groups can be particularly useful for patients who have limited insight as to how their language deficits interfere with their day-to-day functioning. Group processes, for instance, humour, working together and team spirit, allow mutual support between group members. Social-skills training occurs in the naturally occurring social interactions in these sessions. A group project does not have to be based on a speech and language task for the skills of the speech and language therapist to be effective. For example, cooking groups can involve attention, convergent and divergent thinking skills, sequencing and organizational skills, memory, self-monitoring, categorization, problem solving, and the social pragmatic aspects of speech in the functional lunch or dinner environment.

The 24-h programme

Once the patient has been able to learn particular skills in individual sessions and in controlled group settings, a 24-h rehabilitation approach can be used to help the patient generalize the behaviour. All staff can be taught to prompt the use of the skill developed in individual therapy (see Case Study 9.1 where Patient 1 is taught to tap his leg to pace his speech).

Other treatment considerations

Treatment to overcome the language/communication deficits of severely brain-injured patients most commonly focuses on ameliorating the impact of the combination of communicative deficits and frontal insight/control disorders. The aim is to limit the negative impact of these disorders on social and vocational functioning. Specific deficits can be addressed in skills retraining programmes developed according to the parameters described above. Other approaches include environmental modifications and selective use of community resources.

Environmental modification

In the acute stages of rehabilitation, the environment can be modified to assist the patient to become oriented. There is evidence from studies of both traumatically brain-injured and stroke patients that impaired sustained attention ability is associated with poor outcome (Tatemichi et al., 1994). A quiet non-distracting environment should facilitate learning. Prominently displayed clocks and calendars assist the patients to reorient themselves. A memory book divided into different sections and used together by patient and staff provides a focus for repetitive interactions around information the patient needs to learn.

Later in recovery, the patient can be taught to be an active modifier of the environment (see Stimulus control, Chapter 5). As the patient begins to understand what they find difficult, they can be taught metacognitive control strategies. Compensatory metacognitive strategies include internal strategies, for example, word finding strategies, self-pacing, behavioural/social interaction routines, learned problem-solving strategies and frustration management skills. External strategies might include the use of notebooks or electronic memory aids. The patient can be taught to be proactive in modifying their own social environment but with care to ensure that they do not appear strange. One approach is for the patient to help others understand their limitations. However the patient should be discouraged from telling everyone that they meet that they are brain injured as this will not help them further their social goals. A more effective and less stigmatizing strategy to gain understanding might be to ask for help in social situations, for instance to ask others to write down appointments for them in their diary.

Augmentative communication devices

Some patients require equipment to aid speech or communication and the therapist trains the patient both to use, and to become comfortable using, the device. Patients will only use the equipment if it suits the purpose for which it is intended, is effective, easy to use and does not require excessive effort. Some types of equipment can be stigmatizing. Hours of work on using a communication board or other augmentative communication device is irrelevant if the patient refuses to use it.

The patient's motor, cognitive and behavioural skills and their social environment must all be taken into consideration when a communication system is being selected (see DeRuyter and Becker, 1988). Many different types of electronic aids are now available, including hand-held devices and devices designed for use with desktop computers. Although technological progress has increased the capacity and complexity of electronic aids, the majority of severely brain-injured patients use relatively simple augmentative, devices such as word and alphabet communication boards (DeRuyter and Lafontaine, 1987). If sign language is considered, the therapist should establish whether the patient is going to be with individuals who could help them use and maintain their skills with the signing system.

Communication social-skills retraining

A central issue for many patients is pragmatics or the paralinguistic aspects of communication/conversation management. Patients may only choose conversational topics biased towards their own interests. Information required for the listener to make sense of what is being said may be missing from the patient's speech and there may be rapid topic shifts. Information may be imparted very slowly making the individual's conversation seem 'dull' (Ehrlich, 1988; Godfrey et al., 1989). While there is little evidence regarding the efficacy of rehabilitation for these types of communication deficits (Ylvisaker and Urbanczyk, 1994) the limited information available suggests a behavioural learning model may be effective (Giles et al., 1988). Interventions should be within the cognitive capacity of the individual, behaviourally operationalizable, and negotiated with the individual. Non-verbal communication may also be an appropriate target of intervention (see Chapter 6).

Severely impaired brain-injured patients often become socially isolated. Many individuals adapt to having social acquaintances rather than the social intimacy which was enjoyed prior to injury. Patients can be encouraged to actively participate in their community, for instance to go to particular cafes so they become 'regulars', go to a particular church and attend church-related events, join a bowling league, amateur dramatic societies and so on. While initially this may require very consistent encouragement, it can also help many individuals feel that they can maintain social connections and be a part of the life of the community.

CASE STUDY 9.2

Patient 2 sustained a severe brain injury as a pedestrian in a road traffic accident (coma duration 5 weeks) with severe damage to the left frontotemporal region. When first evaluated at a transitional living centre, Patient 2 was found to have moderate memory impairment, moderate to severe receptive and expressive aphasia, and an impaired ability to follow social rules, including verbosity, lack of turn-taking and pausing, and poor self-monitoring. Patient 2 was also paranoid and perseverative leading him to have difficulty depersonalizing feedback regarding his language skills. Instead the patient believed that the therapist was making a personal attack on him rather than attempting to help him develop more effective ways to communicate.

Training in individual therapy included education around his difficulties as well as skills building. The initial focus of sessions included practising conversation where he was cued to pause. The patient practised the give-and-take of conversation with the therapist. At times, the patient interpreted the cues from the therapist to be insults addressing the content of his spoken message, however, with continued practice, the patient began to understand the cue 'clear and concise please'. Patient 2 was unable to fully utilize a memory book, but was capable of handling a less complex approach which was simply to write down as much of what happened during the day as possible.

Following sessional skill acquisition Patient 2's verbosity was treated by using all staff within a transitional living centre. A behavioural programme was devised around Patient 2's most salient social problem, the lack of pausing (note the behavioural specification of this problem). All rehabilitation staff were given a watch with a second hand. As soon as Patient 2 initiated conversation, staff ostentatiously looked at their watches. If Patient 2 had not paused in 30 s, he was cued '30 seconds' and then had 30 s to finish his thought. When Patient 2 engaged in conversation the staff member placed a mark in the patient's memory book. The conversation interaction could be rated as independently stopped, cued stopped, or staff terminated. As the programme progressed, the percentage criteria for acceptable performance went up. A specific reward of a trip out to a favourite pizza restaurant for successful performance was negotiated with the patient prior to initiating the programme 'as a token of our appreciation of all your hard work on your recovery'.

Similar issues were addressed in his writing. A hierarchical approach was taken toward increasing his use of skills with the memory book. Patient 2 was able to make use of sections in his book which included a list of words he commonly used and had difficulty retrieving (dysnomia).

Patient 2 was able to develop a range of effective language routines enabling him to ride buses independently, participate in a volunteer job and finally to live independently managing his own affairs with support of a case manager.

CONCLUSION

The communicatively impaired patient should be considered holistically in their environmental context. Specific intervention techniques for the speech and language therapist are discussed for the patient emerging from coma, in rehabilitation settings or living in the community. Treatment approaches are described for work with patients with acute cognitive/communicative impairment, behaviour disorders, dysphagia, and motor speech disorders. Emphasis has been placed on the interaction of mild communication deficits and frontal insight/control disorders. Effective approaches to treatment include a skills building approach in conjunction with the development and implementation of compensatory strategies which translate into natural and effective communication experiences. The individual needs to practise communicative skills and use them on a daily basis for effective integration of the skill into use following the end of therapy. A unit-based approach can result in rapid generalization of skills.

10 LACK OF INSIGHT FOLLOWING SEVERE BRAIN INJURY

Gordon Muir Giles

My experience is what I agree to attend to.

William James (1890)

Denial (or lack of insight) regarding physical illness is a common phenomenon (Strauss *et al.*, 1990). Lack of insight is associated with illness which is life threatening or other events or circumstances which threaten the individual's self-image in other important ways. Significant rates of denial have been found in patients with cancer (Aitken-Swan and Easson, 1959; Katz, 1982; Zervas *et al.*, 1993), severe coronary artery disease (Froese *et al.*, 1974) and patients recovering from cardiac arrest (Croog *et al.*, 1971). Denial does not always have negative consequences for the individual and has been associated with both increased quality of life (Havik and Maeland, 1988) and longevity (Hackett *et al.*, 1968; Greer *et al.*, 1979). Lack of insight becomes problematic when it leads the affected individual to act dangerously, impedes rehabilitation efforts or prevents the person from making good judgements (Levine *et al.*, 1994). Lack of insight occurs in both neurological and non-neurological conditions but different explanatory models are used with the different populations. Definitions are often imprecise and do not discriminate between different forms of the phenomenon (Ramachandran, 1996; Small and Ellis, 1996; Ellis and Small, 1997).

Patients who deny their deficits and who refuse to accept apparently obvious features of reality can be mystifying to professionals and present intractable management problems. The brain-injured person who does not see their own limitations may become angry with professionals or family members who are trying to help them. Assisting patients in developing insight into their deficits is an important goal of therapy as increased insight among brain-injured people is associated with better participation in rehabilitation (Lam *et al.*, 1988). The understanding of lack of insight has been hampered by the predominance of a medical/neurological framework in which the structure, content, and values in the person's beliefs are viewed as unimportant except as a symptom of the pathology. The approach followed in this chapter, attempts to understand the neurobehavioural symptoms of lack of insight in terms of damage to the normal psychological processes and neurological systems.

Lack of insight may be considered a multidimensional problem. Historically there has been considerable interest in how personality and neurological factors might interact to produce the observable manifestations of lack of insight (Weinstein and Kahn, 1950; Ullman *et al.*, 1960). Workers in the neurological sciences have rejected dynamic explanations of denial (Starkstein *et al.*, 1992) in favour of neurological accounts or have seen them as distinct phenomena (McGlynn and

Schacter, 1989), despite the continued respectability of psychological explanations in other branches of science (Zervas *et al.*, 1993; Ramachandran, 1996). Possibly because patient behaviours are often extremely unusual or bizarre, neurological damage may seem to be the only explanation. The attempt to divide neurologically based lack of insight from non-neurologically based lack of insight suggests a rigid dividing line which is difficult to reconcile with the observed phenomena (Ramachandran, 1996). The assumption seems to be made that people without neurological impairment know why they do things and have direct access via introspection to their true capacities. However there is considerable evidence that the explanatory models that non-neurologically impaired people use to explain their own behaviour are inadequate or erroneous (Hefferline *et al.*, 1958; Nisbett and Wilson, 1977; Svartdal, 1991; Riccio *et al.*, 1994). In addition the view of lack of insight as a straightforward manifestation of neurological illness fails to explain why patients without neurological damage demonstrate lack of insight (e.g. cancer, cardiac disease) and why family members of the neurologically impaired may manifest lack of insight at least as marked as that of their injured relative. There is no reason to believe that individuals with brain injury do not fall prey to the same types of lack of insight which beset the non-neurologically impaired, such as denial of impending loss of employment, loss of a treasured relationship, financial difficulties, or the impact of health compromising behaviours (e.g. smoking) (Schoenbaum, 1997).

No generally accepted theories of lack of insight exist in neuropsychology (Burgess and Shallice, 1996). No single theory explains all of the important insight-related clinical phenomena encountered in the rehabilitation of brain-injured people. Important questions which remain unresolved include: is lack of insight function specific? (Levine *et al.*, 1991); does the same lesion which leads to a motor or cognitive deficit lead to lack of insight? are there as many types of lack of insight as there are functions which can be impaired? (Schacter *et al.*, 1988; Schacter, 1992); where is the lesion which underlies lack of insight and what is the mechanism involved? what is the role of memory impairment in lack of insight? (Ramachandran, 1996).

Recently a number of workers have begun to emphasize detailed analyses of the cognitive content of neuropsychiatric syndromes as a way to understand how a particular symptom comes to be manifested by a particular individual (Halligan and Marshall, 1996). Theories which attempt to bridge the cognitive neurological divide have been described for the Fregoli delusion (Elliss and Szulecka, 1996), Cotard's delusion (Young and Leafhead, 1996) and reduplicative paramnesia for places (Luzzatti and Verga, 1996) among others (Halligan and Marshall, 1996). Much of the symptomatology of neuropsychiatric syndromes can be seen as resulting from:

1 changes in the patient's circumstances, or perceptual experiences as a result of changed neurological processes plus
2 the person's own attempts to account for the changes they are experiencing
3 the patient's account is often affected by the changes in their brain function (for example, depression in Cotard's delusion).

Table 10.1	• Denial that the trauma occurred
Types of unawareness associated with brain injury	• Denial of the trauma's significance
	• Denial of current deficit
	− Sensory
	− Motor
	− Cognitive
	− Personality
	• Denial of current functional implications of a deficit
	• Denial of future implications of a deficit

The current chapter is then a contribution to this trend in neuropsychiatry.

This chapter presents the outline of a theoretical integration of the diverse phenomena described as denial of deficit. It attempts to build a bridge between psychological and neurological levels of explanation but is only an outline because various aspects of the theory have yet to be specified. This chapter draws some distinctions between varieties of lack of insight and discusses theories of how human beings develop understanding of their own behaviour. Clinical manifestations of lack of insight in neurological conditions are reviewed and a multidimensional account of lack of insight is presented which incorporates both neurologically and non-neurologically mediated factors. The chapter concludes with sections on assessment and treatment.

DEFINITION OF TERMS

Initially the term 'anosognosia', meaning lack of knowledge of disease, was primarily associated with unawareness of hemiparesis. The phenomenon was first described by Pick (1898) and the term anosognosia was introduced by Babinski in a 1914 paper describing two patients with left hemiplegia. However, use of the term was quickly expanded to include lack of awareness of blindness, incontinence and other forms of physical disorder. The terms anosognosia, denial of deficit and lack of insight are used interchangeably in clinical settings. Denial of deficit is used to describe disorders ranging from those that are almost only found in people with specific and identifiable neurological damage (i.e. hemiplegia, blindness) to those which are frequently found in those with no known neurological impairment. Although for theoretical reasons the term lack of insight is preferable to denial of deficit, here the current convention of using them interchangeably for convenience of expression is retained.

Insight and denial are terms with multiple meanings. First, knowing about abilities and causes is a social phenomenon and relates, at least in part, to what are customary explanatory models within a community. For example a patient or family member may have a volitional model of behaviour whereas a clinician may have a clinical/neurological model. With different explanatory models it is difficult to come to a consensus on the existence of lack of insight. A clinician may see a patient's failure to recognize repeated memory failures as a lack of insight because the clinician understands memory failures as stemming from the type of neurological impairment the patient has suffered. The patient's family may claim that the patient's memory was never very good basing their claim on an observable consistency in the patient's behaviour and a history of less than perfect memory in the patient. The patient's family and clinician are basing their understanding of observed phenomena on different explanatory frameworks. It is important to note that most lack of insight refers to a capacity that observers would agree was possessed by the individual prior to injury.

Second, denial or lack of insight is applied to failure to appreciate many behavioural changes ranging from the very concrete to the very abstract. These include: denial of the traumatic event (e.g. the belief that the injury or surgery never occurred); unawareness of physical changes or the inability to perform various motor behaviours or to recognize the absence of sensory capacities (e.g. hemiplegia, blindness); denial of cognitive changes; denial of personality changes; and denial of the current or future implications of changes. With such a wide range of phenomena categorized as lack of insight it is not surprising that adequate definitions are lacking.

A third difficulty is that a person can demonstrate insight or lack of insight in different ways. Most discussions of denial focus on what people say of themselves. For example a person who has recently had a severe brain injury and has a concomitant hemiplegia may insist that they can walk but that they choose not to 'just now'. Such a person appears to have learned behaviourally but not cognitively of the impairment (underlining that physical and verbal behaviour are dissociable). Another person may admit to severe amnesia but similarly discuss their plan to return to their occupation as a business executive in a large corporation. Just as there are multiple memory systems which most often work together, there are probably multiple ways of knowing – some of which are available for introspection and others which are not. A distinction into three types of knowing is proposed: behavioural or action knowing, concrete cognitive knowing and implicational knowing. Behavioural and cognitive knowing are doubly dissociable. Implicational knowing requires cognitive knowing and is therefore only singly dissociable.

In *behavioural or action knowing*, which is not available to introspection, the person's actions are consistent with the person's limitations but their verbal behaviour is not consistent with the presence of a deficit (i.e. they lack explicit knowledge). That this type of learning can take place should not be a surprise as acquisition and retention of motor skills and classical conditioning without conscious awareness has been demonstrated in patients with different types of brain damage (Glisky *et al.*, 1986; Giles and Morgan, 1989) and that the learning without awareness can relate to very complex real world tasks (Giles, 1998). Implicit knowledge of consciously unavailable information has been described for memory, vision, facial recognition and motor skills (Weiskrantz, 1997). There are many instances described in the literature describing behavioural 'recognition' of limitations and acquisition of competencies without awareness.

In *concrete cognitive knowing*, the person is able to describe deficits if asked. However in other contexts they may make statements that imply the absence of deficits. The individual has not incorporated the deficits into a consistent view of themselves and their abilities. The person's view of themselves and their life goals have not been revised in light of changed capacities.

In *implicational knowing* the individual behaves and makes statements consistent with their deficits and their likely future implications. The ramifications of the specific physical or cognitive deficits are integrated into a view of the self (alteration has occurred at the level of the self-schema). This level of awareness need not be completely available to conscious awareness (see the section on 'Cognitive behavioural models of self-awareness' below).

These various ways of 'knowing' will be discussed throughout the chapter. In order to place lack of insight associated with neurological disease in context the next section examines awareness in individuals without neurological disease.

THE NATURE OF SELF-AWARENESS

Skinner (1938) pointed out that the assumption that humans behave with the causal mediation of consciousness (i.e. that mental events cause behaviour) is one that is very difficult to challenge because it appears to be substantiated on a daily basis from direct personal experience. Contemporary commentators make a similar point, i.e. that natural theories of consciousness seem to 'stand to reason' (Dennett, 1991). Natural theories of consciousness treat reporting one's mental state as analogous to reporting an event in the external world (Dennett, 1991, p. 306). However the idea that consciousness may not be causal in human behaviour is not new.

People are sometimes unaware of the existence of stimuli that significantly influence their responding (Hefferline *et al.*, 1958; Goldiamond, 1965; Svartdal, 1991). Individuals may be unaware of the existence of a response, or that a stimulus has affected their response. When people report on their cognitive processes they do not do so on the basis of true introspection (Dennett, 1991). Their reports are instead based on *a priori*, implicit causal theories, or judgements about the extent to which a particular stimulus is a plausible cause of a given response (Ross, 1977). Socially accepted explanations are reinforced. Accounts of behaviour are therefore most likely to be consistent with normal language explanatory models (i.e. spontaneous accounts of behaviour in the general population do not make reference to impaired brain functioning, possession by spirits or having ones thoughts and actions controlled by aliens). The individual gives an account of the behaviour which is within the terms of normal social discourse (even if the behaviour and the justification for it are socially unacceptable to most listeners). So, for example, if the individual does not recognize that they are disabled then a socially acceptable account of not walking must be found. In order to account for aberrant behaviour an individual may simply describe the behaviour as motivated, 'I wanted to ...'. These accounts may be *post hoc* rationalizations but the account makes personal sense to the individual. Much of our difficulty in empathizing with the individual with lack of insight is the belief that were we in similar circumstances we would know that we were impaired. However there is considerable evidence that this may not be true.

Individual's erroneous reports about their cognitive processes are not haphazard but regular and systematic (Dennett, 1991). Nisbett and Wilson (1977) describe a series of experiments in which subjects were unaware of influences on their responses. For example, in one experiment prospective shoppers were asked to indicate preferences among purportedly different (but actually identical) stockings. Most shoppers preferred stockings positioned to the right of the display. When asked to account for their selection none of the participants indicated that position had been important but noted differences in the colour and texture of the stockings. When it was later suggested that position may have been a factor in determining choice most shoppers stated that position was irrelevant. Further evidence that individuals' views of their own cognitive processes, although not accurate, are not random either comes from 'observer subjects', individuals who did not participate in experiments but who read verbal descriptions of them. Observer subjects are found to make the same erroneous predictions about the determinants of responses to stimuli as those made by the subjects who had actually been exposed to them. Subjects and observers are drawing on a similar source for verbal descriptions of stimuli effects (i.e. culturally sanctioned rules for determining what are acceptable explanations). A number of recent commentators have argued that human consciousness is profoundly influenced by cultural factors (Dawkins, 1976; Dennett, 1991). In the cultural context of the USA and northern Europe there are advantages to seeing oneself as independent, competent and self-reliant. Introspection, admittedly an unreliable indicator, would suggest that our own natural views of our own mental processes are erroneous. For example, the generally accepted notion that people have continuous conscious mental life when awake will be recognized as flawed by anyone who has been ill or very bored and has 'come to' and realized that they have been thinking nothing.

Lack of insight can be interpreted as maintenance of the customary, socially sanctioned, explanatory frameworks. To avoid 'lack of insight' the brain-injured person would have to demonstrate a radical alteration in their explanatory model. As a result of the natural history of recovery from brain impairment (and the nature of some types of brain impairment) this is exactly what some patients cannot do.

Some work reported by Toglia (1993) can be interpreted as a partial test of this hypothesis. Toglia (1993) in developing a test of contextual memory compared the ability of acutely brain-injured persons ($N = 62$) to control subjects ($N = 310$) to recall 20 line drawings of thematically related objects and to predict how well they would perform. The control subjects predicted that they would recall an average of 13 items while the subjects with brain injury predicted that they would recall an average of 14 items. The actual ability of the subjects with brain injury was considerably worse than that of the non-injured controls, however the prediction of performance was almost identical. Toglia concludes that the patients are basing their predictions on their estimation of their capacity prior to injury (1993).

Most people do not include neurological functioning as an explanation of their own behaviour. Particularly when placed under stress individuals are more likely to use explanations with which they are familiar from their normal life experience. Part of the rehabilitation process may be to develop new explanatory terms or ways of understanding the world (Spencer *et al.*, 1995). It is also true that the contingencies of reinforcement for the 'verbal community' (a group of people who share a common and somewhat deviant set of words and meanings) of the rehabilitation setting are very different to the reinforcement contingencies which exist in the wider community (see, for example, Spencer *et al.*, 1995). Patients are rewarded for statements which are couched in terms of 'deficit', 'recovery', 'limitations' and 'working towards independence'. Explanatory models which assume competency and which account for errors as momentary and normal lapses which are typically rewarded in normal life are not rewarded in the rehabilitation setting. This also partially accounts for the families' denial of deficit, cognitive deficits are not part of the way people explain their own behaviour or that of loved ones.

DYNAMIC THEORIES OF DENIAL

In psychodynamic theory an individual may have thoughts, fears or wishes which are unacceptable to their conscious mind and which are held repressed in an unconscious state. Events in the environment can cause unconscious material to become pre-consciousness. This provokes anxiety and leads to the implementation of defence mechanisms. The individual is unable to accept that the environmental event which triggered the unconscious thought or impulse really occurred. Denial can be defined as a defence mechanism that has the goal of avoiding unpleasant emotional states by disavowing certain aspects of reality (Freud, 1967). The psychodynamic construct of denial depends on the assumption that the person has knowledge of the illness. The person is assumed to have unconscious knowledge, but this knowledge is too anxiety-provoking to be allowed access to consciousness. Self-deception cannot occur without some knowledge of the illness (Levine *et al.*, 1994). Dynamic theories of denial may be adequate when applied to some patient groups but inadequate when applied to the severely neurologically impaired, such as patients with traumatic brain injury, cerebrovascular accident (CVA) or dementia.

Theories of motivated denial of deficit are attractive in that they explain problematic aspects of anosognosic behaviour. Popular dynamic accounts of denial offer plausible accounts of why patients continue to deny deficits when to an outside observer the deficits are clearly apparent. The fact that patients accept hospital routines, take medication and so forth is considered to be evidence that the patient actually knows what is wrong.

Another line of evidence interpreted to support the popular dynamic views of denial is the hypothesized relationship between denial and depression. According to psychodynamic theory there should be an inverse correlation between denial and depression. However, the fact that increased awareness of deficit can lead to increased emotional distress does not necessarily mean that avoidance of the anxiety-producing material prevents depression. Rather than denying in order to avoid depression, individuals with lack of insight may simply not know that they have anything to be depressed about. Recent tests of the depression hypothesis suggest that there is no increased incidence of depression in those with, as opposed to those without, insight, i.e. anosognosia does not protect against depression (Starkstein *et al.*, 1992).

METACOGNITION

The term 'metacognition' describes a person's understanding and manipulation of their own cognitive and perceptual processes. Nelson and Narens (1994) describe a two-level, two-process model of cognitive functioning. The two levels are the object level, which includes basic motor, sensory and cognitive processes, and the meta level which further processes information and controls strategies used at the object level. The two processes are monitoring, in which the flow of information is from the object level to the meta level, and control, in which the flow of information is from the meta level to the object level. Contained within the meta-level is a model of how the object level works (the model is necessarily imperfect). Individuals have beliefs about how their cognitive processes work. The beliefs include judgements of competency and these judgements affect behaviour. For example if a person believes that they can easily remember appointments they are unlikely to write them down. If, following neurological damage, there is no change in the model of object-level functioning then the individual will have no ability to adjust their control functions to compensate for the impairment. A readjustment of the model would however give the patient the opportunity to engage in new regulatory behaviours which could significantly improve functional performance.

COGNITIVE BEHAVIOURAL MODELS OF SELF-AWARENESS

Recent cognitive models view personal identity as being central to an individual's understanding of the world. These models also view resistance to change as natural, and, in some cases, beneficial (Dobson, 1988). Human beings attempt to understand the environment and to predict and reduce the effect of environmental challenges. The way in which we learn about ourselves in the world can be conceptualized as a self-organizing system for knowing. The person establishes and maintains his or her own identity and develops idiosyncratic ways of understanding themselves and the world. These ways of knowing are called schemas or constructs. Self-knowing is intrinsically conservative as it relies primarily on activation of previously existing constructs. New schemata/constructs can be developed, but under conditions of stress people rely on overlearned and automatic modes of thinking. The mechanisms of identity are interwoven with the mechanisms of knowledge so that what an individual knows about the world and the self are intimately connected. Developmentally individuals acquire knowledge about themselves and the world through associative and cognitive processes resulting from continuous interactions with their environment. Development occurs through a process of progressive reorganization of self-knowledge. An important and counter-intuitive implication of this view is that the highest level of self-knowledge is not fully available to introspection.

Information which is consistent with the person's view of the self is easily assimilated while events which do not fit may be rejected or trigger adjustments in self-understanding (assimilation versus accommodation) (Piaget and Inhelder, 1969). Events may be known by their emotional or pre-aware associations. The dimensions 'feels good/feels bad' form an extremely powerful basis for judging whether to accept or reject information (Fulcher and Cocks, 1997). There is now an extensive literature that suggests that evaluative associations utilize a unique associative system, that the learning may take place outside awareness and that it is both automatic and immediate (Levy and Martin, 1975; De Houwer *et al.*, 1994; Martin and Levy, 1994; Fulcher and Cocks, 1997).

Believing that one is in control of events is highly rewarding, as a result people will try to fit new experiences into familiar ways of thinking. In periods of confusion or stress automatic functions are used in preference to cognitive controlled processing. Only frequent repetition of new ways of thinking will increase their availability and the likelihood that they will be used. Most of us will be familiar with this phenomenon where we respond as if a previous, but no longer existing, set of circumstances were present (when this behaviour is brought to our attention the response is often 'yes! of course! I knew that') (Reason, 1984). Insight is influenced by a variety of factors, for instance increased stress on an individual can reduce their ability to process new information and restrict their opportunities to gain knowledge of themselves and the world.

STRESS AND COPING

Another important set of explanatory models are those found in the stress and coping literature (Weitz, 1989; Aldwin, 1994). These concepts have been developed to understand the behaviour of people dealing with life-threatening events and terminal illness. The effect of a stressor on an individual appears to be the result of a complex interaction of a number of factors. Stress arises from an imbalance between the requirements of the situation and the person's appraisal of their ability to cope with it. Individual differences in motivation and cognitive traits (e.g. dispositional optimism) lead to markedly different reactions to potential stressors. Lazarus (1993) uses the term 'relational meaning' to emphasis how personality and environmental variables combine to affect the person's appraisal of the potential effect of life events on their well-being. Coping appears to be highly dependent on the type of stressor, the environmental conditions and the state of the person under stress. Lazarus suggests that the coping methods employed depend on the person's appraisal of whether or not anything can be done to change the situation. He describes two basic types of coping responses: problem-focused coping and emotion-focused coping. The person who believes that the situation can be brought under control will use problem-focused coping. This person is likely to be actively interacting with the environment, attempting to gain mastery and change the situation so that it becomes less stressful. The person who believes that nothing can be done to change the situation is likely to use emotion-focused coping. This can involve changes in the way the stress is attended to or in the way the event is understood and integrated into the person's life. Both types of coping are useful and help people manage stressors. Problems arise if a particular type of coping is misapplied: what is highly adaptive in one context can be counter-productive in another. Weitz (1989) has described two basic strategies used by indi-viduals under stress as vigilance and avoidance. In vigilance the individual becomes hyperaware of indications of illness and tries to gather all pertinent information and to actively manage their circumstances. In avoidance the individual ignores signs of illness, avoids physicians, etc. and denies that the events are happening. Although vigilance and avoidance can appear to be opposites they can be regarded as separate strategies to reach a common goal: the construction of a normative framework that enables an individual to explain their situation to themselves. Although lack of insight presents a major problem to rehabilitationists, hyper-vigilance regarding deficits is not uncommon following neurological impairment (Prigatano and Altman, 1990).

DENIAL IN NEUROLOGICAL ILLNESS

Historical views of denial in neurological illness

The exclusion of motivational factors in discussion of anosognosic phenomena following neurological insult is comparatively recent. Up to the early 1960s the subject of the interplay between neurological (capacity) factors and motivational (dynamic) factors was a subject of debate (Weinstein and Kahn, 1950; Ullman et al., 1960). The attitude of the observers and the patient's relatives were considered important in determining the degree and duration of the denial. Ullman et al. (1960) reviewed both physiological and psychodynamic factors associated with anosognosia. Weinstein and Kahn (1950) in describing a series of patients with denial of various deficits noted the following general patterns of responses; first, the patient stated that he was perfectly well and denied any manifestations of illness. Second, the patient denied the major illness but lay stress on some trivial aspect of his condition (which the authors suggest is a form of displacement). Third, the patient expressed some awareness of his illness but attributed the manifestations to a benign cause. The patient expressed awareness of the deficit but rationalized it or minimized it to the point where it was not regarded as a defect. Varying methods of explaining away the deficit could be used by the same patient at different times.

Weinstein and Cole (1963) in examining possible personality variables which might affect denial of deficit following neurological impairment stressed the importance of their methods. In addition to neurological examination, patients were administered standard tests and observed in daily activities. Formal interviews were conducted two to three times per week and recorded verbatim. The inter-views included questions regarding the patient's illness and what the patient perceived as their 'main problem'. Information about pre-morbid personality was gathered using structured interviews with relatives and colleagues. Emphasis was placed on how the patient responded in stressful situations. In particular an attempt was made to establish the symbolic ways in which the patient expressed feelings and how the patient derived status. Weinstein and Cole (1963) found that the content of the patient's anosognosia showed considerable correlation with features of their pre-morbid personality. The authors concluded that the same symbolic elements which had been important in the patient's interpersonal relationships prior to illness were used in conceptualizing the lost function. Patients who had verbal anosognosia were reported by their relatives to previously have had a strong tendency to deny illness. The patients had previously construed illness as a sign of weakness or failure. Preservation of the appearance of health was regarded as a personal responsibility. Health, industry and efficiency were ethical values through which the patient maintained a sense of identity. Conscientiousness, compulsiveness, drive, responsibility, stubbornness, perfectionism and insistence on being right were traits which were reported consistently as characterizing these individuals prior to impairment. Patients who developed paranoid (incomplete) verbal denial such as attributing weakness in the affected limbs to being starved or beaten, were also found to have been compulsively driven pre-morbidly and to deny imperfection. This consistent personality pattern was not found in patients where inattention rather than verbal denial predominated.

Weinstein and Cole (1963) point out that the anosognosias are not fixed entities but take on form and meaning in the context in which they are studied. The process of observation and recording are selective. Attitudes of observers and relatives are important in determining the degree and duration of the denial. Some patients would admit that they had difficulties in some contexts but not in others, while other patients would admit that they had impairments to family members but not to the physician.

Another major debate in the literature of the 1950s and 1960s was the degree to which denial of deficit was associated with clouding of consciousness. For example Weinstein and Kahn (1950, 1955) observed that in denial of conditions other than hemiplegia, such as denial of incontinence, anosognosia was always associated with generalized clouding of consciousness. A related issue was whether the lesion responsible for the disorder was focal or diffuse. Gerstman (1958) considered the function of the parietal lobes in regard to body schema to be well defined in each hemisphere. The left parietal lobe was responsible for body image *per se* while the right parietal lobe served to register any deviation of the body itself from the body schema. Anosognosia was therefore the result of a lesion 'in the non-dominant hemisphere blocking or interfering with the correlated commissural and associational formations and thus causing a breach at an integral link in the functional chain of the process of coenaesthesia, or awareness of the somatic self' (p. 501). Gerstman (1958) suggested that damage of the non-dominant parietal lobe was seen as releasing from '... inhibition an inherent instinctive urge or primitive (unconscious) tendency towards maintaining the integrity of the body or the image of it' (p. 509).

Ullman and co-workers (1960) discussed denial of deficit in a limb, a concrete manifestation of impairment, and failed to find unawareness except in association with diffuse brain damage. In structural terms the authors are suggesting a localization plus generalized impairment hypothesis. They saw the unawareness as the result of perceptual alterations occurring against the background of diffuse brain dysfunction. Weinstein and Kahn (1950) noted that anosognosia was accentuated by the administration of sodium amytal. Gerstman (1958) suggests the occurrence of anosognosia depends on the mode and the rapidity of neurological damage rather than on the extent or the severity. The more sudden the onset the greater the likelihood of anosognosia. Sooner or later a physiological and then a psychological adjustment takes place and disorders are abolished.

There was a tendency to see denial as part of a constellation of deficits which included other phenomena marked by the minimization of change. In the series of patients described by Weinstein and Cole (1963), half showed explicit denial and half showed neglect. All showed either disorientation to time and place, reduplicative delusions, other delusions and confabulations or paraphasic misnaming.

By the mid-1950s, two schools of thought had emerged. One position advocated by Denny-Brown and associates (Denny-Brown et al., 1952) and Gerstman (1958) attributed lack of attention directed to one-half of personal and extra-personal space to a disturbance in the ability to synthesize sensory data. They emphasized that this could occur in non-demented patients who apparently had no clouding of consciousness. These authors saw a close link between the anosognosia and the type of function disturbed and they regarded a single focal lesion as responsible for both the dysfunction and lack of awareness of the dysfunction.

The other school of thought argued that there was no fundamental difference between the mechanisms which produce anosognosia irrespective of the affected function. The association of anosognosia with clouding of consciousness is emphasized.

The position advocated below is that a portion of both of these positions is correct and that there are two general types of lack of insight, a predominantly posterior lack of awareness usually associated with discrete sensory or motor functioning and a frontally mediated more general lack of awareness (self-image maintenance). Both variants have associated lesion sites. The two types of lack of awareness may co-occur.

Other associated disorders

Lack of insight and confabulation

Lack of insight involves the failure of the individual to acknowledge that a deficit exists and can be demonstrated in a number of ways. In confabulatory denial the patient attempts to provide a verbal *account* for their apparently changed circumstances or competencies. Confabulation is the production of erroneous explanations which occur in clear consciousness and in the absence of willful prevarication. Kopelman (1987) suggests that certain types of confabulation are a normal response to memory failure and can be elicited from non-neurologically impaired subjects under circumstances in which memory capacity is exceeded.

Confabulation may include misapplication or displacement of real experiences to account for novel unexplained events. For example a patient recognizes that he is in a hospital in a certain town, but displaces the town thousands of miles to his home state (Benson *et al.*, 1976). This type of reduplicative confabulation has been interpreted as a reasonable response to limited or partial recollection of personal historical information (Marshall *et al.*, 1995; Luzzatti and Verga, 1996). However, confabulation can also include bizarre or outlandish explanations. Once generated the bizarre explanations may be held with the conviction of truth. The confabulator is unable to recognize the absurdity of the statements or may recognize their absurdity when his or her attention is directed to it but nonetheless maintain the belief. Individuals who recover may recognize the erroneous quality of their earlier beliefs but report that they really believed in their account at the time.

Confabulation and amnesia do not always occur together. Most individuals with amnesia and who are aware of their memory deficits do not confabulate. In the absence of profound memory impairment confabulation is largely confined to patients who have symptoms of significant frontal lobe impairment such as difficulty in monitoring responses for accuracy and inhibiting the production of ideas which should normally be filtered out and discarded. Confabulation in the absence of amnesia is associated with orbital frontal or ventromedial brain impairment particularly of the right hemisphere. Moscovitch and Melo (1997) have reported a study which sheds light on this issue. They compared confabulating and non-confabulating amnestic subjects with age-matched controls on a personal and historical version of a long-term memory test. In response to cue words such as 'happy' or 'invention' participants had to describe, respectively, a related event from their personal lives or from history before their birth. A subset of amnestic subjects, those with dysfunction of ventromedial frontal cortex confabulated in response to the cues. The results are interpreted as demonstrating impaired strategic retrieval in confabulation but not non-confabulating amnestic subjects. Strategic retrieval processes, unlike automatic cue-dependent retrieval, are essentially problem-solving routines that are applied to the process of recall. The strategic retrieval process, it is suggested, guides the search and helps monitor and organize output. In addition to the finding of confabulation in the amnestic subjects, confabulation was not at all uncommon among young normal controls when describing historical information, although it was absent in describing personal information. A two-factor hypothesis might account for this data. Confabulation may occur in amnesia or in the absence of historical knowledge in the young control group. This factor might be described as the absence of information that would appropriately constrain the response (the design of this study was such as to minimize the occurrence of lack of insight confabulations in the amnestic subjects). A second factor is an impairment in the reconstructive memory processes with an inability to apply potentially available information, resulting in a second source of absence of constraint. This second factor is a failure of the strategic or reconstructive 'with memory' process where recovered 'memories' are compared for plausibility with other known facts about the world. If this account is correct then the often made suggestion that confabulations occur out of a need to fill the gaps in memory to avoid embarrassment is exactly the reverse of the true situation. Confabulation occurs because of a failure to recognize memory failure and to apply appropriate constraining information.

Burgess and Shallice (1996) performed a detailed analysis of the types of memory-related processes that occur in normal autobiographical recollection when memory is stressed. The eight non-neurologically impaired participants were asked questions such as 'describe the last time you had dealings with the police' and 'when was the last time you saw one of your relatives who does not live with you?'. Participants were instructed to respond for 1 min describing the process of recall using telegramatic speech as 'notes' to themselves. This was recorded and then played back to the participants to allow them to elaborate on the process, this elaboration was also recorded. The verbal reports of the remembering processes were then coded and analysed by the researchers. It was hoped that the normal processes of memory reconstruction would provide insights into how failure of these process might give rise to confabulations. The authors describe a three-part process involving what they label as editor, descriptor and mediator processes. The editor is the internalized process of self-correction. It provides a monitoring process for the results of memory search. The descriptor process determines the parameters of the to-be-searched-for memory. The mediator process serves to test hypothesis and to reason when a correct memory is not immediately available. This type of multicomponent or stage model may account for why confabulation may occur in individuals with or without memory impairment and with or without signs of 'frontal' involvement but is most common where both are present. The idea that there may be a retrieval component and an editor component may help in our understanding of denial of deficit.

Many instances of lack of insight appear to be reasonable accounts of events based on inadequate information. The individual attempts to account for their incapacity using explanations which would have been acceptable before the neurological event. However instances, where the individuals' account of the situation utilizes explanations which are outside the individual's personal history, might be considered to be confabulatory lack of insight. It is not known if there is a different natural history of recovery in these two types of lack of insight.

Delusions

Delusions in organic illnesses are often associated with damage to the limbic system, the basal ganglia, thalamus or rostral brain stem. Delusions which involve misperceptions or simplification (Capgrass syndrome, reduplication paramnesia) are most frequently associated with subcortical connections in combination with right sided or bilateral frontal dysfunction (Benson et al., 1976; Cummings, 1985). Delusions may relate to a specific sensory function or are anatomically limited, i.e. delusions involving a hemiplegia may include a belief that the limb is not the person's own or that it belongs to a specific someone else (e.g. the patient's daughter). Ives and Neilson (1937) suggest that delusions relating to a limb should be distinguished from denial of deficits and have distinct associated lesions. Delusions of limb absence may be associated with lesions in the thalamoparietal peduncle.

Recently a number of workers have studied delusions in organic conditions suggesting that they can be understood as an individual's account of bizarre experiences with specific combinations of factors resulting in specific delusional presentations (Luzzatti and Verga, 1996; Young and Leafhead, 1996). For example reduplicative paramnesia for place (which, in the author's experience, is not uncommon if specifically assessed for) typically occurs in the presence of relocation from one location to another, the memory for which is absent due to loss of consciousness or amnesia, and either bilateral or right frontal brain impairment. Typically reduplicative paramnesia represents an apparent 'mental manoeuvre' which minimizes change to the individual's circumstances. Cotard's delusion and Capgrass' syndrome resemble loss of insight to the extent that individuals reject information from others favouring their own, often implausible, accounts of reality. Different patterns of minimization of change and rigidity of explanations are found in conjunction with different patterns of brain damage and different symptom presentations.

The notion that there is a continuum from normal to delusional beliefs is gaining in acceptability (Halligan and Marshall, 1996). Confabulations may appear to become fixed as delusions. In some instances the individual can recognize the bizarre nature of the their own account but be overwhelmed by the feeling of truth that they experience about it. The inability to suppress the judgement of truth about a belief in contradistinction to multiple counter sources of evidence is a type of perseverative disorder.

THE NEUROPSYCHOLOGICAL ACCOUNT OF LACK OF INSIGHT

Behavioural lack of insight

Behaviour may be triggered automatically with or without higher order awareness (Norman and Shallice, 1980). Damage to the ventral frontal cortex may result in deficits in learning from social reinforcement and in changing responses based on new reinforcement contingencies. Patients with damage to the orbital frontal cortex are often described as disinhibited, unconcerned about deficits, displaying fatuous affect and being irritable and impulsive. These patients may have only a tenuous grasp on reality, be confabulatory and delusional and have profound deficits in reality monitoring. Although patients with orbital frontal damage have been shown to perform normally on the Wisconsin Card sort, they have deficits on learning from emotionally relevant feedback and suppressing behaviours which were previously reinforced (Rolls et al., 1994).

Frontal and posterior types of lack of insight (overview)

Damage in different brain areas may result in lack of insight and different areas of damage may result in different manifestation of lack of insight. The association between confusion and lack of insight appears to be straightforward in that when an individual is unable to process information they will also be unable to learn about their own dysfunction. More problematic is how to account for lack of insight in the absence of obvious generalized intellectual impairment (Starkstein et *al.*, 1992). Lack of insight is significantly correlated with amount of brain damage (as measured by a computerized tomography scan) (Hier *et al.*, 1983) although it is clear that size of lesion is not the exclusive determinant (Levine *et al.*, 1991). The proposal advanced here is that there is a system of cortical and subcortical circuits associated with the integration of environmentally available information about the self into a self-schema and that impairment in this complex process is manifested as lack of insight. The circuits and brain structures involved depend on the type of impaired and the type of awareness involved. A schematic presentation of this theory is presented in Figure 10.1. Isolated unawareness of the functioning of sensory motor systems are caused by damage to posterior parts of the system, often in conjunction with reduced efficiency in anterior portions of the system. The predominately posterior form of denial involves damage to secondary (usually parietal) cortex underlying white matter and thalamic projections. Two frontal syndromes are distinguishable, an attentional subtype and a implicational subtype involving the integration of new information into a self-schema.

Posterior denial

Anosognosia for sensory/motor function impairment may occur following both left- and right-sided brain damage but is far more frequent, severe and protracted following right-sided brain damage (Starkstein *et al.*, 1992). Damage is often in the parietal cortex or deep to the parietal lobe (isolating the thalamus from the cortex) (Neilsen, 1938). Theoretically the most likely processes disrupted may be direct sensory or attentional processes (Crick, 1984). Not all patients with anosognosia have neglect but patients with anosognosia have significantly higher frequencies of hemispatial neglect than patients without anosognosia (Starkstein *et al.*, 1992). Predominately posterior denial may involve a disconnection of sensory/motor systems and frontal and subcortical circuits responsible for (1) allocation of conscious attentional processes and (2) the modification of self-image. Lesions of the inferior parietal cortex, deep to the parietal cortex, thalamus and basal ganglia are implicated in denial of specific function impairments such as denial of hemiplegia or denial of visual deficits. These disorders may be considered a form of disconnection in which primary sensory or attentional processes are isolated from frontal structures. LaBerge (1997) has suggested that thalamic circuits may serve to augment responsivity of primary and secondary cortical systems (Levine *et al.*, 1991).

Frontal lack of insight

Many complex human behavioural capacities are believed to depend on frontal brain structures although neither the mechanisms nor the anatomical basis for frontal behavioural control are well understood (Benson, 1994). Two frontal brain functions can be identified which may be related to the capacity to develop insight. These are:

1 The dorsolateral frontal system which is associated with planning, anticipation, shifting response sets, and mental flexibility. The dorsolateral pre-frontal cortex also has a special role in maintaining non-spatial information 'on-line' in

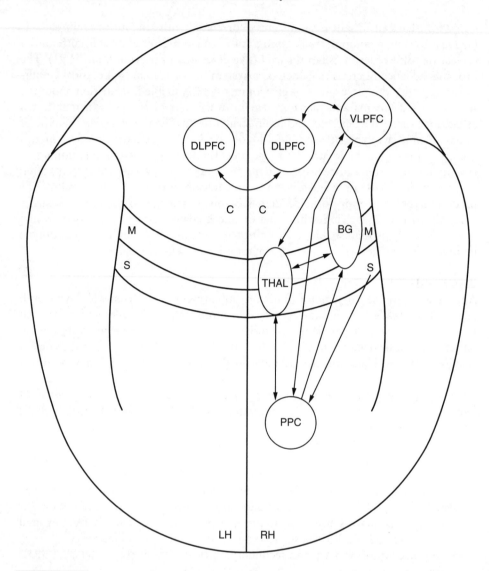

Figure 10.1

Components of a system subserving cognitive awareness.

Posterior components: (a) Primary (S) and secondary sensory cortex (posterior parietal cortex, PPC): registration and modality specific processing, parietal sensory motor cortex. (b) Thalamus (THAL) amplification of awareness via a triangulation system (LaBerge, 1997). Anterior components: (c) Ventral cortex (VLPFC) with connections to the basal ganglia (BG) and anterior cingulate (primarily right hemisphere). Receives input from thalamus and projects to secondary cortical regions. This component of the system is necessary for the participation of conscious attention and attentional control. The pre-frontal cortex both prepares for expected stimuli and underlies the orienting response to unexpected or disconfirming stimuli. (d) Dosolateral pre-frontal cortex (DLPFC) has reciprocal connections with the pre-frontal attentional system. Dosolateral pre-frontal cortex is involved in planning holding information in a working memory store and in the development of 'what ifs' the mental experimentation for action or decisions.

Note: It is not that the above brain areas and circuits are the 'insight centres' it is that the capacity for insight is degraded with impairments of the functions subserved by these areas.

working memory for processing. Patients with damage to this area seem to be unable to incorporate current knowledge in foreseeing future events or in planning future behaviours. They may fail to appropriately constrain responses and once generated be unable to let them go. It is the dorsolateral frontal cortex which performs the integration of emotionally important material into the self-image. Self-awareness is intimately related to the formation and manipulation of imagined constructs. Rumination about future goals or fantasies, mental experimentation with imagined courses of action and planning for the future depend on frontal executive systems (Benson, 1994).

2 The pre-frontal attentional system. There is evidence that tasks involving focused attention involve participation of the pre-motor, pre-frontal and anterior cingulate cortex (Baker et al., 1996). This supervisory attentional system is lateralized to the right hemisphere which accounts for the frequency of attentionally mediated neglect syndromes in patients with right-sided brain injury. The supervisory attentional system involving pre-frontal cortex may be responsible for conscious awareness, a prerequisite for integration of environmental material into a consciously available self-image.

In addition to the above, subcortical circuits may contribute to the allocation of attention to emotionally relevant information. Cummings (1993) describes five frontal-subcortical circuits. Damage to these circuits can produce motor or behavioural abnormalities and damage to any circuit structure may produce symptoms by altering distant structures in the same circuit. The actual systems involved in the emotional weighting have not yet been established however damage to a circuit involving the thalamus and the anterior cingulate gyrus results in apathy and deficits of attention.

The two-factor hypothesis advanced here might account for the majority of the observed anosognosic phenomena. Lack of insight for specific sensory/motor functions might thus result from a primary sensory or attentional disorder associated with parietal/thalamic damage in conjunction with damage to the frontal subcortical systems responsible for updating the self-schema. This hypothesis of a two-stage model for the lack of insight into specific sensory or motor processes has received some support from lesion studies (Starkstein et al., 1992; Ellis and Small, 1997). Prigatano and Altman (1990) report a study in which 64 traumatically brain-injured patients were divided into three groups. Patients in group I overestimated their behavioural competencies, patients in group II showed behavioural ratings similar to relative's report of competencies and patient in group III underestimated their behavioural competencies. Patients with dementia or acute confusion were not included in the study. Ratings focused on the patients ability to perform daily tasks. Initial GCS did not separate groups. Group I patients had greater evidence of bilateral and multiple lesions than groups II or III. A greater percentage of group I patients had frontal lesions but this did not reach significance. Speed of left-hand finger tapping was worse in group I than groups II or III suggesting right frontal involvement. Patients in group I did not show an increased rate of memory or difficulties in abstract reasoning as measured by standard

Table 10.2	Frontal:	Implicational (dorsolateral)
A theoretical schema for understanding forms of lack of insight		Attentional (ventral)
	Posterior:	Sensory/attentional

neuropsychological tests. A study by Starkstein *et al.* (1992) found that patients with denial of hemiplegia or visual deficits showed predominantly right-sided lesions involving the inferior parietal and superior temporal lobes, thalamus and basal ganglia in conjunction with significantly more evidence of frontal subcortical damage.

The current theory suggests that different types of deficits will be observed following sensory/attentional versus frontal lesions. Frontal disorders are less likely to be modality specific. Dorsolateral frontal lack of insight is also more likely to occur in conjunction with poor judgement and planning skills and can be regarded as a generalized difficulty in interpreting the meaning of events to the self (updating self-schema).

THE PSYCHOLOGICAL ACCOUNT OF LACK OF INSIGHT

Some of the phenomena of anosognosia seem to be dramatically outside the realm of normal human behaviour. Other phenomena appear to be exaggerated but recognizable versions of the types of lack of insight that are found among the non-neurologically impaired. If insight is regarded as an active process, then the ability to maintain awareness might gradually deteriorate with damage to the neural networks which subserve awareness and so the post-brain-injury state might appear as an exaggerated version of normal lack of insight. From a cognitive perspective also the deficits which may follow brain injury can lead to grossly exaggerated presentations of normal human processes. Limitations in the person's ability to incorporate new information are discussed below under the same tripartite classification of types of insight used above; behavioural, cognitive and implicational. These are not perceived as different on introspection but are differentiable systems of insight.

Behavioural

Acquisition of behavioural responses can be impaired despite relative preservation of cognitive knowing (Verfaellie and Heilman, 1987). There is evidence for a double dissociation. For example patients can describe what they should be doing on the Wisconsin Card Sort but be unable to do it, i.e. they continue to engage in errorful performance while they clearly state how to perform accurately (Burgess and Shallice, 1996). One patient, seen by the author, would feed himself food that was burning his mouth while at the same time saying 'it is too hot, I should not be eating it'. Patients may acquire behavioural information of which they have no awareness even in the absence of significant memory impairment. The classic example being the hemiplegic patient who confabulates numerous reasons for not standing when asked to do so but denies the true reason. Patients with orbital frontal damage may fail to recognize the social behavioural importance of an event and be unable to learn from social behavioural consequences (Rolls *et al.*, 1994).

Cognitive

In circumstances where an individual has a change in their competencies or when for some other reason they need to revise their view of themselves the following processes would need to occur. First the individual would have to orient to or become aware of a potentially personally relevant event. The perceptual processes of the individual with all of their biases (perceptual and cognitive) would operate a filter on the event and its personal relevance. Probably at this very early stage an emotional evaluation would occur along the continuum 'feels good, feels bad'. The event itself is analysed to see whether it is consistent with the person's view of what is possible or understandable in the context of their view of themselves and the world. This action is performed by the constraint monitor in the model (Figure 10.2) which draws on knowledge of the world and of the self (self-schema). In cases where the information continues to be anomalous (to not fit with the person's view of themself and the world) the information is maintained with continued allocation of attention and is analysed to determine meaning for the self. Outcome in terms of meaning are once again subject to the constraint monitor that draws on the same knowledge basis described above to determine if the analyser's resolution of the anomaly is itself acceptable. In some cases this process requires an alteration in the knowledge base of the individual or the world (self-schema, semantic knowledge). This process of schema revision is intrinsically effortful and mostly aversive. For important changes, loss of a loved one, treasured attributes, etc., the process of revision requires repetition over days or weeks to produce a change in schema. This process is marked by continued reorientation to the loss.

Failures in cognitive self-awareness might occur at any point in this process. Some individuals may fail to attend to environmental events, some may do so and perceive them but fail to analyse them based on their immediate feeling of bad evaluative response. Others may fail to analyse their response and place it in the context of their view of themselves in the world.

The types of processing failures which are suggested to disrupt insight after brain injury also affect many other functions. The problems that result in lack of insight are not caused by damage to an 'insight centre' they are problems in processing and response formulation that affect insight among other complex functions.

After brain injury a person may be egocentric and may not attend to the social interpersonal consequences of behaviour or have a truncated, constricted view of the consequences of their own behaviour (Shallice and Evans, 1978). At its most basic the brain impairment may lead a failure to monitor external social environmental events and so the individual does not have orienting responses to disconfirmatory information about their view of self. The supervisory attentional system may fail to alert the individual to disconfirming events (Shallice and Evans, 1978). The individual may not recognize that an event or behaviour is occurring. The individual's internally generated view of the world may be sufficient to over-ride even profoundly discon-

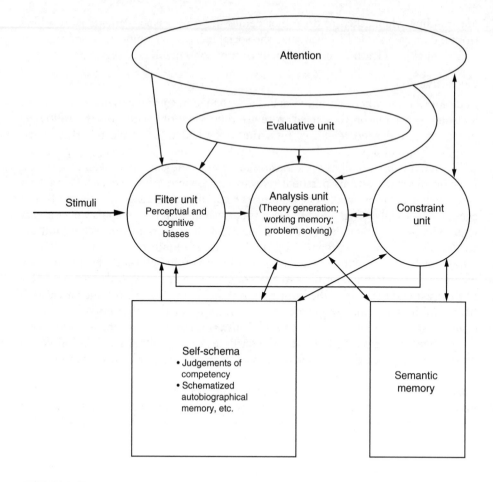

Figure 10.2

A preliminary psychological model of Insight. The model should be read from left to right through the processes cycle through the nodes. Attention must be allocated to an external event, somatic perception or idea to be processed. Orienting responses occur to unexpected non-habituated phenomena. Immediate appraisal along a continuum 'feels good, feels bad' is made by the evaluative unit. The filter is a perceptual/cognitive interpreter of events and is powerfully biased by the self-schema made up of habitual thoughts, reactions and responses to the world, overlearned autobiographical memories, etc. The flow of information to the filter from the constraint unit can retrospectively change the memory of the perception itself. The filter biases perception and interpretation however normally it operates with the constraint unit to control the perceptual experience. The analysis unit serves to reason and form hypotheses, it is identified with working memory and it is here that sense is made of the event and where it is examined and with great effort processed in light of the self-schema and other facts about the world. The constraint unit compares outcomes in terms of meanings for reasonableness and to the self-schema. The constraining unit is powerfully involved in the allocation and whether the process is to continue to cycle through the system in order to change self-schema. There may be no obvious output. Procession may continue, result in the alteration of self-schema or stop.

firming information. That this type of deficit might follow damage to the frontal control function is consistent with the Norman and Shallice model of attention (1980).

Some individuals may attempt to explain the event in a way that is consistent with their self-schema. Other individuals who have damage to the constraint monitor may fail to bring their knowledge of the world and of themselves to bear in constraining their explanation and produce bizarre confabulatory responses. The two types of lack of insight are analogous to the two types of confabulation that have been identified (Kopelman, 1987; Burgess and Shallice, 1996), one is consistent with the individual's established explanatory framework and another type is spontaneously confabulatory and is probably associated with more profound impairment in right-frontal brain systems.

According to Norman and Shallice (1980) tasks that require the deliberate allocation of attentional resources involve: planning or decision making, troubleshooting, they are ill-learned or contain novel action sequences, are dangerous or technically difficult, or require the overcoming of a habitual response or resisting temptation. Following brain damage individuals may not engage in the ruminative mental explorations of their behaviours or potential behaviours that they did prior to injury. There is no comparison or judgement of current behaviour against cherished preferences, goals and ambitions. The result may be a highly constricted or idiosyncratic view of social and behavioural consequences. This constricted mental exploration allows the individual to maintain a complacent attitude about beliefs which are patently implausible to others. Patients may deny the consequences of their behaviour based on poorly grasped understanding of the world. Patients may fail to incorporate known information about the world in making judgements. So, for example, the patient may reason about another patient entering his room uninvited 'When he comes into my room, I hit him, he stops'. The fact that the patient stops is gratifying and there is no consideration given to the long-term inconvenient consequences of hitting people or any thought as to whether the perpetrator wishes to be known as someone who hurts others, etc. The

Table 10.3	Advanced age
Factors associated with lack of insight (controversial factors marked with a question mark: inclusion does not indicate factors are necessary or sufficient)	Recent onset
	Extent of lesion
	Confusion
	Mental impairment
	Sensory deficits
	Attention deficits (neglect)
	Memory impairment
	Delusions
	Non-physical nature of denial (concrete to abstract gradient)
	Pre-morbid factors? Low intelligence? Rigidity?
	Severity of injury
	Presence of denial in family and significant others?

supervisory attentional system does not alert the individual to mismatches between stimuli and goals in terms of meaning (immediate stimulus–response associations are preferred over higher order associations). The individual may not have a cognitive theory of their own influence on others, or if such a theory exists it may be very unrealistic. The cognitive theory itself may be grandiose and implausible as it is not actively compared to all relevant data.

Implicational

In implicational insight an individual's self-schema has been updated and the post-injury limitations are assumed in the person's behaviour, the metacognitive model incorporates the limitations. The individual's perceptual and cognitive biases are set to perceive information about their own deficits and failure to compensate for them, so as to maintain strategies that the individual is using to maintain function.

Assessment

Assessment of insight into current illness can be by direct questioning about a known deficit (known from behavioural observation or neuropsychological testing), questioning regarding the impact of deficits on current functioning and questioning regarding the likely impact of the deficit on future plans. Behaviour should also be observed so as to evaluate its consistency with verbal reports. A number of structured interviews are available. For example Fleming *et al.* (1996) have reported preliminary data on the Self-Awareness of Deficits Interview (SADI). The SADI has three areas in which the individual with brain injury is questioned:

1 self-awareness of deficit
2 self-awareness of the functional implications of deficits
3 ability to state goals.

In each area a number of questions are asked to establish the patient's level of awareness. Latitude is afforded to the interviewer to reward items based on context and to elicit more information. The responses are rated on a four-point scale from 0 (no disorder of awareness) to 3 (severe disorder of awareness).

An alternative method of evaluation is to have the patient and the treatment staff or the patient and the patient's family compare ratings of performance on a structures scale. The differences between the two sets of rating can be considered a measure of the person's denial of deficit. Family ratings are important in determining awareness because in non-hospitalized patients family members may have the most detailed knowledge of the patient's functioning. A number of different scales are available (Fleming *et al.*, 1996) for family/patient ratings but the comparison method is not without problems. It is unclear that non-neurologically impaired people have accurate judgements of competency, so it is unclear at what level lack of insight is pathological. There may also be systematic variation in family members' reports of patient's competencies. Family members may minimize changes early in the patient's recovery and give more accurate information later, so that patient denial can appear to have become more profound through time, whereas actually the relatives' denial has become less marked. It is therefore difficult to know what is actually being measured by the differential response format.

Given the limitations of any individual approach, multiple data collection methods (interview, observation and questionnaire) and multiple sources of information (patient, relative, and staff) should be used to establish a comprehensive picture of the patients degree of insight (Fleming *et al.*, 1996).

TREATMENT

Little empirical evidence exists to demonstrate the efficacy of treatment of lack of insight. Awareness of deficits typically improves with spontaneous recovery. Many people deny deficits early in recovery who are readily able to admit to them weeks or months later. Specific responses to treatment have not been established and so intervention is based on clinical reasoning. Physical problems are likely to be recognized before psychological problems and the implications of the problems for future plans and life goals only recognized late in recovery. The process of adjustment can be seen as falling into three stages: active denial, ambivalence and engagement. In active denial the patient rejects any information relating to deficit and states that there is nothing wrong. The patient is often actively hostile to treatment and denies any similarity between himself or herself and other patients.

In the stage of ambivalence the patient begins to come to terms with some brain-injury related changes and begins to develop a new self-concept. A typical statement at this stage might be 'I can't believe that this is so difficult for me'. In the engagement stage the patient recognizes problems and actively engages with treatment staff in developing an effective and tolerable way of 'being in the world'. The therapist assists the patient in changing the patient's frame of reference or their explanatory stance in order to assist them in understanding how to best cope with a current situation. The importance of emotional support and a positive frame of reference cannot be overstated. The desire to confront the patient into accepting their disability should be resisted.

Youngjohn and Altman (1989) describe a self-awareness group for the treatment of denial. In a group context patients were asked to make predictions of competency on a word-list learning task and a calculation task. Most patients predicted a higher level of accuracy than they actually achieved. Feedback provided to participants lead to a prediction which more closely approximated actual performance on later trials. The effect was maintained at 1 week and the authors report that the patients' experiences in the group were useful in the overall rehabilitation programme as patients had concrete examples of how their self-perception could be inaccurate.

Time is probably the most important factor in developing 'insight' for most patients. Evidence that patients' views of their competencies change through time comes from a study by Tangeman *et al.* (1990) of the response of patients to a 1-month programme of rehabilitation provided at least 1 year post-CVA. The patients demonstrated significant improvement which they retained at 3-month follow-up. Comments from patients indicated that they were not ready to fully make use of acute rehabilitation. Patients stated that a period at home was helpful in giving them the opportunity to experience how the stroke would affect their day-to-day life suggesting that this had not been evident to them in the acute recovery period.

The psychological model advocated here suggests that failure to achieve insight may result from a number of different sources. The goal is to have the patient update their self-schema and develop a metacognitive model that adequately represents the way that they are post-injury (to the extent that this will positively affect functional behaviours). The model suggests that failure can occur in a number of different steps in the process of insight. Interventions might vary depending on the specific processing problem. The patient may fail to attend to the information or evaluate the information so negatively that it is suppressed. They may also fail to adequately constrain the information so that its potential to interact with the self-schema is compromised. Idiosyncratic interpretations of events may not be constrained (i.e. that therapist just hates me). Material is not appropriately analysed and compared with the self-schema.

Given the theoretical position advocated here, what recommendations can be made? Where a deficit is considered to be primarily attentional, therapy should maximize the patient's attention to tasks involving the disturbed function. In addition the efficacy of therapies intended to address attention directly should be explored in the treatment of denial (Vallar et al., 1990; Lin, 1996). However, the long-term efficacy of these types of interventions are unproven. Evaluative suppression should be managed by helping the individual develop an acceptable way of being in the world while providing feedback relating to the impaired functions. Naming and conscious (therapist-guided) reflection and processing of new information may facilitate changes in schemas and developing responses. The therapist often wants the patient to recognize their true deficits, when taken to the extreme this is unnecessary and counter-productive. It is important to obtain very specific information about a problem the patient may be experiencing due to lack of insight. Insight is not an abstract phenomenon but surrounds key conceptualizations of the self and the world. Central issues are those which obstruct key adaptations (rehabilitation goals). As suggested earlier, individuals with damage to the pre-frontal cortex are likely to preferentially attend to immediate and concrete stimulus–response relationships. These patients have profound difficulty in suppressing the response based on an immediate concrete association in favour of higher order associative relationships. These patients do not analyse their own behaviour and that of others to discover relationships. They may also develop an elaborate justification of their own behaviour. Patients focus on pleasure or convenience rather than on the whole interpersonal context and what their actions might mean to others (Sirigu et al., 1995). Similarly they are unable to spontaneously focus on the implications their current actions have for the attainment of their higher order goals.

The following steps are typical of cognitive behaviours approaches and should be followed in working with a patient with lack of insight.

Identify the problematic behaviour for the patient in non-judgemental terms. Patients often experience all interactions around the behaviour as aversive. They therefore try to avoid all engagement with staff around the behaviour, experiencing their interactions with staff as staff picking on them. The patient understands the behaviour in very different terms from the way others do. For example, a patient who believed that all women were sexually attracted to him believed that women who approached him about the problem were jealous of the women who received his attention and the men were jealous of his prowess. The approach should be non-judgemental in order to understand the patient's explanatory model. There needs to be an open exploration with the patient and the interchange itself needs to not become aversive. The collaborative stance allows for an analysis of the cognitive distortions that lead to rigidity, the evidence for the patient's view. The therapist encourages the consideration of consequences, both a comparison of consequences to (1) view of self, and (2) long-term goals. A patient who is repetitively physically aggressive 'if other people get in my way' may focus only on the short-term benefit 'he got out of my way' rather than the long-term disadvantages 'I have to stay in a place like this'. Test the patient's ability to entertain alternative explanations. Individuals always have 'reasons' as to why they engage in a particular behaviour. As in all types of cognitive behaviour therapy it is not necessary that we ascribe the cause of the behaviour to the thoughts. The goal of the therapist is to bring the behaviour under attentional control of the patient. Behaviours that are justified *post hoc* or that are habitually unattended to are unlikely to be suppressed. The therapist needs to enlist the patient's active cooperation to suppress the behaviour. The aim is to have the patient attack their own permissive thoughts and suppress the behaviour. Patients are encouraged to describe the arguments against the beliefs themselves and to iterate the advantages of alternative behaviours. Patients are encouraged to develop alternate responses. Patients may then be trained in and rewarded for implementing alternative responses. Methods for doing so are described at length in Giles and Clark-Wilson (1993). Staff should be encouraged to massively reinforce appropriate behaviours.

SUMMARY AND CONCLUSIONS

Understanding our own behaviour and its causes (our self-explanatory model) is a complex function involving the processing of multiple sources of information and which involves many cognitive processes. Human beings develop a self-concept which includes competencies, potentialities and a metacognitive model. The self-concept is valued by the individual and provides security and a sense of identity. Human beings minimize change which threaten these values. As a result of neurological disease or damage an individual may have difficulty in revising their self-schema and metacognitive models. If there is 'elegant degradation' within this system then the strength of the ability to form higher order associations prior to injury may affect the individuals ability to understand their deficits following injury to the frontal areas. In this chapter it has been argued that:

1 The 'default setting' of human beings is not insight but a stable view of the self. By which it is meant that revision of basic knowledge of the self is an active process of the organism not a passive receptive process. This process can be impaired in a variety of ways. Without the engagement of an active process the self-image is maintained. Certain types of frontal and parietal brain damage may lead to exaggerations of what are very human phenomena. The brain damage constrains the patient's ability to learn certain classes of information (i.e. the capacity to learn about changes in competency is impaired).

2 Insight is a very complex process and damage in various component processes can disrupt it. Any brain damage probably has an effect on an individual's overall capacity for self-analysis however ventral frontal and dorsolateral frontal mechanism are centrally involved in this function (particularly damage to the right frontal region).

3 A two-stage model can account for impairment of insight associated with specific sensory modalities or motor functions.

4 Non-modality specific loss of insight is probably associated most with damage to frontal systems.

5 Denial of hemiplegia, denial of blindness and other unimodal incapacities are associated with damage to parietal cortex and damage to structures deep to the parietal cortex. These deficits only occur following brain damage. Damage to frontal structures results in a type of lack of insight which is on a continuum with the type of lack of insight which is ubiquitous in the non-neurologically impaired.

Other factors such as memory impairment affect insight. Both neurological improvement and structured experience can impact lack of insight. Although the evidence reviewed here suggests that there are different lack of insight syndromes, there are no straightforward evaluation techniques which allow us to distinguish them. It is very likely that different types of lack of insight have different natural histories of recovery or deterioration and might respond to different types of intervention strategies. The boundaries that divide functional (psychogenic) from the organic (neurological) are blurring and the dichotomy itself appears increasingly anachronistic. The theory presented here offers a way to reintegrate neurological and psychological evidence regarding lack of insight and suggests that the dichotomy has been a result of inadequate conceptualization in two levels of explanation.

11 Vocation and occupation

Jo Clark-Wilson

Work is a central aspect of the lives of most people, especially for those in the 16–65 age group. Individuals are guided in their career choices by family, friends and teachers, and are also influenced by their abilities, interests, expectations and ambitions; social circumstances; the economic climate and employment opportunities.

People have differing attitudes towards work. Most people work to earn money in order to survive and gain the lifestyle they prefer. Some people are motivated less by money and more to fulfil their potential and achieve their life ambitions. Many people are interested in working to gain a role in society and status in the community and others want financial independence from their partners or family. Some people are not in the labour market but have established roles in, for example, childcare or household management and have alternative sources of income.

Occupation provides a structure to a person's days and can give rhythm to their life and a sense of security. Work also creates challenges and opportunities for people to gain from new experiences and allows participants to develop social networks. Work occupies people in constructive and meaningful activities. Work is usually paid whereas volunteer work is a service provided for no financial gain. Many individuals who are either unable to work or who do not need to work engage in volunteer work as a way of contributing to the community.

Society has a generally positive outlook towards those who are gainfully employed, with employment conferring 'status'. Status gives people roles, responsibilities and expectations within their community, and, ultimately, society. Those without employment often become increasingly isolated in their community and lose their position in society.

Factors influencing work entry or re-entry after brain injury

Olver *et al.* (1996) followed 103 brain-injured individuals for 5 years post-discharge from a comprehensive rehabilitation programme. Of 68 people who were employed at the time of injury, 34 (50%) had resumed employment by 2 years, but only 27 (40%) remained employed at 5 years. Of those enrolled in higher education at the time of injury, 64% were still studying at 2 years and 12% were employed (6% full time and 6% part time). Olver *et al.* found that brain-injured individuals did not seek help when their jobs were in jeopardy and many were unable to find other work once they became unemployed. At the 5-year follow-up 12% continued studying, 29% were employed full time and none part time, and 59% were unemployed. The authors advocated supported employment to increase long-term employment rates (Olver *et al.*, 1996).

Individual evaluation of work skills is necessary after a mild, moderate or severe brain injury as outcomes vary widely. Factors affecting entry or re-entry to work include age, severity of injury, educational attainment before and after injury, physical and cognitive abilities, personality traits and behavioural control. Social factors, types of employment and work environments can also affect the likelihood of successful return to work.

Age

Younger brain-injured people are more likely to return to employment than older people (Schalen et al., 1994; Ponsford et al., 1995; Teasdale et al., 1997). Teasdale et al. (1997) found that older people had consistently more difficulty finding employment and that educational programmes were not usually open to them. Younger people, who maintain a realistic view of their situation, have adequate social skills and who relate well to their work colleagues are more likely than other brain-injured adults to find employment.

Severity of injury

Prigatano et al. (1987) found that only 23% of traumatically brain-injured persons admitted to a neurosurgical centre with Glasgow Coma Scale (GCS) scores of 8 or less were employed 2–4 years post-injury. Of the moderately injured (GCS 9–12) 50%, and of the mildly injured (GCS 13–15) 62%, were engaged in productive activity.

Longer than average post-traumatic amnesia and hospital stays and lower-prestige occupations post-injury were associated with 'poorer employment status' (Lubusko et al., 1994). Vogenthaler et al. (1989) found that increased severity of injury led to increased long-term impairments but that in relation to work this trend did not always hold true. Mildly injured people were often unable to manage and many severely injured people were able to return to vocational activities.

Educational attainment before and after injury

Asikainen et al. (1996) examined the influence of age and prior educational level on the social and vocational outcomes of a group of 508 people with brain injury. Participants in a rehabilitation and re-employment programme were categorized according to severity of injury on the GCS, 3–8 (severe), 9–12 (moderate) and 13–15 (mild). Age was divided into categories of 7 or younger, 8–16, 17–25 and 26 years of age or older. Those participants who had a higher educational attainment and whose severe injuries were sustained in late teens or early adulthood, usually had a better outcome than those who suffered injuries earlier in life (childhood and early teens) and had poor pre-morbid educational attainment. No relationship was found between moderate and mild injuries, age, pre-injury education and outcome (Asikainen et al., 1996).

Education, skills training and work experience before injury provides background knowledge of work routines, skills for use in the workplace and a direction or focus to the individual's career development. However, these factors can also adversely affect the individual's return to work. If the injured person had highly developed skills and status in a workplace, return to lower paid employment or more routine work may be viewed by the individual as unacceptable.

Cognitive and neurobehavioural factors

Cognitive and neurobehavioural deficits rather than physical disabilities are often the most important factors affecting return to work. Ben-Yishay *et al.* (1987) suggest that poor self-awareness and unrealistic expectations are primary contributors to high unemployment rates among brain-injured people. Factors which may influence work performance include problems maintaining attention, attending to more than one piece of information at a time, coping with distractions, processing information at speed, and understanding and remembering instructions or information relating to work. Planning and initiating activities, organizing time effectively and putting plans into action can be difficult for the brain-injured individual. Individuals with brain injury may have difficulty using problem-solving strategies at work reducing their ability to compensate for deficits and manage new situations. In addition many people have mood instability and irritability as part of the consequences of injury. Headaches and fatigue can affect the brain-injured person's work performance. Many brain-injured people cannot tolerate noise, cope with stress or pressure and become excessively anxious and agitated. Rigidity of thinking, an inability to cope with change and inflexible ways of dealing with all situations make working with some brain-injured people difficult. Persons with brain injury can be egocentric, have limited insight into their condition and believe they are always right, despite evidence to the contrary (see Chapter 10). Such individuals may have difficulty in accepting criticism or coping with their own or others' mistakes. Some brain-injured people express their views without considering how their comments affect others. Poor social and interpersonal skills, an inability to accept criticism and an inability to get on with co-workers are all factors which contribute to an unsuccessful return to work (Cook, 1983; Haffey and Lewis, 1989).

Frontal lobe impairments and work

Individuals with severe frontal lobe disorders often have difficulty in returning to work. Limited insight into their own abilities can lead the individual to mistakenly believe that they have resumed their previous level of skill and, as a consequence, this leads them to set unrealistic goals. These individuals are often unsuccessful in work and do not understand why. They blame others for their failures and have difficulty learning from their own experiences. Brain-injured individuals with these types of problems can be very difficult for rehabilitation professionals to work with. The patient without insight will often focus on unachievable targets and actively reject lesser, but achievable, goals. These individuals feel that professionals are unnecessarily negative and deliberately exaggerating their problems to block their return to work. Some people are unable to understand the significance of rehabilitation for work unless the activities are directly related to the particular job they believe they are capable of, and should be, doing. Any other form of work activity is considered unacceptable. Many of these individuals repeatedly apply for employment without divulging their medical history. The patient may be successful at the interview because they possess an appropriate knowledge base and have good interview skills. Such individuals may be able to work for a period of time before their problems become evident. Maintaining employment is, for many individuals, more difficult than finding employment (Kreutzer *et al.*, 1995).

The needs of the patient to return to work should be considered in relation to the importance or value of work to the family. Additional stress is caused by the need for the main wage earners to return to work or for another family member to take over this role. Family members are often left to cope with their relative's practical and emotional difficulties when attempting to gain some meaningful employment.

CASE STUDY 11.1

Patient 1 (coma of 3 weeks and PTA of 2.5 months) suffered a severe brain injury in a car accident on his way to work. Prior to the accident, Patient 1 worked with his brother as a self-employed building contractor. He built his own home and was independent in running his own business doing building work and gardening. Following the injury Patient 1 had attention and memory deficits, an inability to solve problems and his reasoning abilities were seriously compromised. He lacked insight into his condition and was inflexible in his thinking. He had mood swings which varied from elation, giggling and disinhibition to withdrawal, depression and suicidal thoughts. His thinking centred on himself and he showed no consideration for others. He required continuous supervision from a carer as he was impulsive and unpredictable. In addition to his brain injury he also suffered significant orthopaedic injuries.

Patient 1 asked his brother to write down the jobs which they had previously completed together. Using this information Patient 1 wrote his curriculum vitae and sent a copy to employers in his local area. He did not divulge any information about brain injury or that he could not physically complete the work himself and required assistance from care staff to put activities into a logical sequence. Patient 1 could not draw plans or reliably estimate the number of items required for any building job. Despite repeated feedback about his difficulties he was unable to develop insight into the factors preventing him from returning to his previous vocation.

Social factors

Family dynamics and other social influences affect vocational outcome. People have roles and responsibilities within their family, their home and workplace. After a brain injury many people do not know how to occupy their time and become bored and isolated at home. The pressure for rapid return to work can be increased by factors such as limited financial resources, intolerance to the noise of young children, stress at home and limited role definition in the home. In addition the brain-injured individual's friends and family may have limited understanding of cognitive deficits, not understand why the individual is not returning to work and advocate strongly for an early return to work. Following return to work the individual with brain injury may begin having problems outside the work environment. Excessive fatigue, lack of confidence at work, insecurity in the work role, anxiety, distress and agitation, and the need to resolve issues immediately can greatly increase stress in the home setting in addition to the work environment. Spouses, parents or children may have to provide practical and emotional support during the time when their relative returns to work, whilst also coping with greater responsibilities as the brain-injured person may be unable to fulfil normal family roles.

Employers and work settings

Wilms (1984) surveyed 175 businesses and found that most employers stressed the need for positive work habits and attitudes, and valued the employee's ability to get along with co-workers, and capacity to follow basic instructions rather than specific vocational skills. Unfortunately it is often these positive work habits and inter-personal skills that are most affected by brain injury.

Factors affecting a person's return to work include the availability of appropriate employment, support of the employer, hours of work, level of responsibility, the work environment and the availability of support from services with an understanding of brain injury, for instance, rehabilitation personnel, case manager, disablement employment adviser, job coach and work colleagues.

People with brain injury who are attempting to return to their previous employment often find it difficult to cope with reduced abilities or responsibilities in their existing work. A different job in the same company can lead to reduced status. Finding appropriate employment can be extremely difficult for people with brain injury who are entering the workplace for the first time or who are seeking employment after not working. Factors which reduce the opportunities of brain-injured people to return to employment include: high societal unemployment (i.e. a highly competitive labour market); employers not wishing to take the risk of employing disabled people who have been unemployed; and people with brain injury being unrealistic about the type of work appropriate for them; or the low wages accorded to the job.

Sympathetic employers and support services with an understanding and appreciation of brain injury are difficult to find. Special assistance from an employer is important in achieving a successful return to work for brain-injured people. Johnson and Gleave (1987) found that both the provision of special work conditions and the maintenance of those conditions for a protracted period were associated with a successful return to work. Hours of work (whether full time or part time), and flexible shift systems can influence successful employment as many brain-injured people fatigue easily or need longer to prepare themselves in the morning.

The working conditions and environment may also influence a brain-injured person's return to work. An individual with brain injury may have difficulties working in noisy or distracting environments, in facilities which require continuous high levels of concentration (i.e. potentially unsafe environments), or in work settings where there is excessive stress, for instance, deadlines or constant demands.

West (1995) studied the effect of work environments on return to work for persons with brain injury. Thirty-seven individuals with brain injury were placed into supported employment by six placement agencies. All were assessed using the Vocational Integration Index (VII) an observational instrument for rating the opportunities for integration (job scale) and the extent to which an employee benefits from those opportunities (consumer scale). Individuals who maintained employment for 6 months (19 people) had been rated higher on all subscales and total scores (West, 1995).

Consideration of the factors described above, plus previous educational and work experience, enable rehabilitation professionals to develop a plan which maximizes the brain-injured person's chances for successful return to work.

APPROACHES TO FACILITATE WORK ENTRY

Many brain-injured people return to their previous employment without difficulty. For others, a staged plan of return to work is required. Planned return to work should involve rehabilitation, work retraining and job coaching. Some severely injured people require sheltered work, volunteer placements or individual programmes of activity. The process of return to work varies considerably and depends on the ability of the brain-injured person, support of employers and the availability of resources.

Returning to previous employment

Englander et al. (1992) conducted a telephone survey of the pattern of return to work of 77 individuals with mild traumatic brain injury (GCS scores of 13–15 and PTA of less that 48 h). Each person was contacted 1 and 3 months post-injury to determine the frequency and severity of post-traumatic symptoms and whether or not they had returned to work. Twenty-six per cent of those contacted had subjective complaints; 88% had returned to work or school, 16% of those returning did so with some symptoms (Englander et al., 1992).

For most people who have had a brain injury of any severity returning to work is a high priority. Many individuals with brain injury receive limited advice from medical practitioners and return to work prematurely.

Following mild brain injury the ability to work is influenced by post-concussional symptoms, such as headaches, slowed information processing, attentional deficits, inability to cope with stress or irritability. Many people find themselves in negative cycles, working hard to maintain their standard of work whilst making errors, suffering failure and trying to cope with the symptoms resulting from their brain injury. This leads to a loss of confidence in their ability; limited understanding of the reasons why their skill levels have reduced; excessive fatigue; and an inability to tolerate the normal stresses of a work environment.

Most people need time to recover from the injury, to build stamina and progress back to the work setting. Information and education about the consequences of brain injury and support (usually from staff at brain-injury clinics in outpatient hospital settings) is needed to review the progress and establish realistic goals to aid the mildly injured person's return to work. Individuals need a staged return to employment. Working part time and gradually increasing hours per day and days per week helps adjustment to work and thereby increases the individual's chances of successful return to work. The brain-injured person and their families need help to ensure they have the financial benefits they are entitled to so that they do not rush back to work and risk failure.

Employers vary in both how long they will keep a job open for their brain-injured employee and the support they offer to people returning to work. The employer is motivated to know whether the employee is likely to be able to return to their previous job or alternative work in the same company. Unfortunately it is difficult to give definitive responses to these questions in the early stages of recovery. However it is possible to provide the employer with realistic information regarding the rehabilitation potential of the employee; a general estimate of the timing of any likely return to work (if this is possible); and the support which would be required to facilitate work re-entry. Close liaison needs to be established with the employer regarding the possible options for the employee. The employer may have other work more suitable for the patient within the existing organization or alternative suggestions for how the employee's skills could be used.

An evaluation of the brain-injured person's skills and deficits should be completed and compared with an analysis of the type of work and abilities expected by the employer. This evaluation should highlight realistic goals for rehabilitation of the patient and the training procedures required to improve the patient's work skills. The brain-injured individual should be tested, whenever possible, in rehabilitation facilities or in volunteer settings prior to their return to their previous work. By doing so major problems can be addressed without 'burning out' the prospective employer.

The success of return to work can be affected by the injured person's attitude towards their brain injury and the support of the employer and work colleagues. Discussion with the employer and employee about a gradual return to work could incorporate education about the brain injury and the potential difficulties the employee could have. This would enable the support systems to be established and the risks inherent in return to work to be highlighted. A work trial would allow opportunities for the person to test out their skills in a safe environment. A graded process of work re-entry, for instance, gradually increasing hours from part time to full time, would allow time for the brain-injured person to adjust to their workplace, and increase their confidence and endurance.

Repeated contact with a health professional, for instance, a psychologist, occupational therapist, case manager, disablement employment adviser (UK), a vocational counsellor (USA) or job coach is necessary to ensure consistent advice, support and guidance for the development of strategies to cope in the work setting.

Although many individuals are able to reintegrate into the work environment many do so only tenuously and remain vulnerable. Employers may not be able to accept the employee's work performance or tolerate their altered behaviour. The brain-injured person may have limited resources to draw on during changes in work type, pace of work, or organizational or interpersonal changes. They are often less productive than their work colleagues, reported to be 'difficult' and are often at risk of having their jobs eliminated, if economic circumstances worsen. Brain-injured persons, working in the field of technology, are likely to have greater difficulty in maintaining their jobs, because new skills constantly need to be learned, updated, practised and developed in generating and using new hardware and software.

CASE STUDY 11.2

Patient 2 was working as an engineer for a telecommunications company when he suffered a severe brain injury in a road traffic accident (coma duration and PTA unknown). He had right-sided hemiparesis and cognitive deficits. After the accident he was known at work to be intolerant, he always believed he was right and would not accept comments or constructive criticisms from others. Patient 2 had technical knowledge which was valuable to the company but when the computer systems changed, he was very slow to learn the new software. His work involved troubleshooting and resolving the computer problems as they arose but he could not cope and was offered a compensation package if he would leave the company. Patient 2 believed that his job performance was adequate and that his work colleagues just wanted to 'get rid of him' and this increased his paranoia and agitation. Medical retirement was eventually applied for and successfully obtained. His period of return to work was constructive in that he knew he had been able to maintain a job for a period of time and this increased his confidence and belief in himself. However, over time he also recognized that the stresses in work affected his family life. He tired easily at work and became very irritable with his family. He decided that working caused him too much stress and he decided to limit the amount of pressure he was under so that he could maintain family relationships.

Obtaining new employment

Three stages can be identified in helping brain-injured persons return to work:

1 assessment of work potential and vocational needs
2 work rehabilitation and training for work
3 finding and maintaining open, supported or volunteer work placements.

Many professional disciplines may be able to help brain-injured people return to work, including the Disablement Employment Advisers in the UK or Department of Rehabilitation vocational counsellors in USA, occupational therapists, case managers, psychologists (clinical and occupational), social workers and others.

Assessment of work potential and vocational needs

In the UK people with disabilities who are deemed able to work are referred to the Disablement Employment Adviser. Following an interview the disabled person is referred to an occupational psychologist or work assessment centre for an initial assessment. The occupational psychologist advises the person with brain injury as to whether they are likely to gain from an assessment and work rehabilitation programme.

The assessment methods used to evaluate the person with brain injury will depend on the local services and their expertise in brain injury. In rehabilitation settings neuropsychology, physiotherapy, occupational therapy and speech and language therapy assessments are undertaken. In vocational settings standardized occupational psychology evaluations and work samples (mini versions of real work) are completed. Standardized psychometric tests are used to identify cognitive disorders. An individual's performance on standardized vocational assessments is influenced by the structure of the assessment and the anxiety of the person in the test situation. These assessments cannot predict whether individuals will be able to work in open or sheltered employment (Teasdale et al., 1997) but are often used by occupational psychologists to guide them in their view about whether the brain-injured person would be successful in a work rehabilitation programme.

Vocational rating can be helpful in quantifying work behaviours. These scales describe work performance and behaviour based on observation. Examples of vocational rating scales include the Functional Assessment Inventory (Crewe and Athlestan, 1981) and the Work Personality Profile (Bolton and Roessler, 1986; Tyerman, 1999). Accurate, detailed and, where appropriate, quantified observation over time provides information regarding work performance. Ben-Yishay et al. (1987) found that employability ratings conducted immediately after work trials proved to be accurate predictors of actual employability and that it was likely that observations of clients in work settings contributed substantially to the predictive validity of the employability ratings. These assessments, undertaken in work placements, provide a more accurate picture of the individual's performance in normal settings than can be provided by testing. A true reflection of the abilities of the brain-injured person is obtained in work situations, for instance, abilities to cope in a less structured environment, to maintain drive and motivation, to generate ideas, to plan and organize work, or to sustain attention to tasks for a reasonable period of time. Observation of the individual's interactions with their manager and work colleagues, their performance in work and of their behaviour in that setting is also useful.

The assessment process can also help the brain-injured person, when necessary, find a new career path based on their interests, experiences and skills acquired before and after the accident. Guidance and support from a specialized vocational therapist is often needed to help the brain-injured person in adjusting to the altered situation and in choosing realistic and achievable employment goals suited to their personality and ability profile.

When individuals are injured in childhood or early adolescence it can be more appropriate to refer them to specialized further education colleges, some of which have experience of working with brain-injured adults. They can then be directed towards appropriate training courses as part of the college vocational programme.

Work rehabilitation and training for work

Disabled Employment Advisors (UK) and Department of Rehabilitation (USA)
Disablement Employment Advisors in the UK and the Department of Rehabilitation in the USA support training to obtain employment or other methods to facilitate return to work. In the UK the Disabled Employment Adviser acts as a member of the local Placement Assessment and Counselling Team (PACT). In order to participate in the Department for Education and Employment's employment programme, the brain-injured person has to meet the definition of a 'disabled person' in the 1995 Disability Discrimination Act (a person with a physical and mental impairment which has a substantial long-term adverse effect upon his or her ability to carry out normal day-to-day activities) and meet the employment handicap criteria in Section 15 of the Disabled Person's (Employment) Act 1944.

People have to be considered 'fit for work' by the Disablement Employment Adviser. If they are deemed unfit for work they receive financial benefits, for instance, incapacity benefit or severe disablement allowance. The disability working allowance in the UK is an allowance established to encourage those with a disability to enter the job market. In the USA individuals who are not able to work due to disability may be eligible for social security disability benefits.

Vocational rehabilitation
Prigatano *et al.* (1984) compared the outcomes of 18 traumatically brain-injured graduates of an intensive neuropsychological rehabilitation programme with 17 traumatically brain-injured people from the same referral base who did not participate in the programme. The aims of the neuropsychological rehabilitation programme were to aid the clients' cognitive functioning, increase their awareness about the nature and consequences of their problems and aid their psychological adjustment to life as a disabled person. Although successful in meeting the programme goals, the programme failed to produce meaningful changes in vocational outcome.

Ben-Yishay *et al.* (1987) developed a rehabilitation programme which had three phases: (a) 20-week intensive neuropsychological remediation, (b) guided occupational trials lasting 3–9 months and (c) job placement and follow-up. The authors reported that at the conclusion of the work trials component 84% of the graduates were considered capable of engaging in productive activity (60% competitive work; 3% school; and 21% sheltered or subsidized work). At 6 months follow-up actual employment was consistent with the employability ratings (53%, competitive; 3%, school; and 23%, sheltered). All of the individuals treated had failed to obtain or hold jobs post-injury before entering the specialized vocational rehabilitation programme.

Successful job placement and retention was associated with the following gains observed during rehabilitative programming: (a) improved self-awareness and self-regulation of emotional responses, (b) enhanced efficiency of residual information processing abilities, and (c) increased acceptance of life as a disabled person. Job instability was related to: (a) alcohol abuse, (b) disinhibition, (c) temporary psychiatric complications, (d) failure to accept limitations leading to attempts to return to academic pursuits beyond the person's capabilities or to continued efforts to obtain rehabilitative services for intractable deficits, and (e) financial disincentives to work (Ben-Yishay *et al.*, 1987).

Tyerman (1999) has described a specialized brain-injury community work rehabilitation programme called 'Working Out' in operation in the UK. During the initial process of assessment a work personality profile is developed which considers task orientation, social skills, work motivation, work conformance and personal presentation of each participant. A work preparation group helps the participants re-evaluate their strengths and weakness post-injury, consider the implications of brain injury for retraining and re-employment and explore the issues relating to the brain injury and interpersonal skills in the workplace. The programme incorporates individual project work designed to help the participants develop their skills in work-based interests and follow their rehabilitation objectives. This facilitates further recovery and adaptation to the brain injury, assesses work potential, promotes accurate self-appraisal and fosters positive work attitudes and behaviours. Groups provide opportunities to explore feelings and frustrations related to the brain injury, promotes awareness and understanding of the personal, family and social effects of brain injury, provides guidance and support in coping with these effects and encourages peer group support. This work rehabilitation programme also organizes supported work placements and provides ongoing client support.

An alternative to this type of rehabilitation programme can be provided in supported work placements where specialized training is provided by a job coach at the workplace (see below).

Finding and maintaining open, supported or volunteer work placements

Open employment
Different factors need to be considered depending on whether the brain-injured person is returning to a previous employer or attempting to gain employment with a new employer. New employers do not have any commitment to the person's recovery and return to the workplace. Conversely new employers do not have expectations based on previous knowledge of the person and can therefore view their work performance more objectively.

Those people unable to return to their previous employment need to become 'competitive' in the job market. Unemployment is common and opportunities are limited for individuals with disability. Getting a job is difficult as there are limited jobs available for people who have not worked for a period of time and whose skills and behaviour show sign of impairment. This remains true despite legislation in both the UK and the USA that protects the rights of the disabled.

221

Preparing for work is an essential part of gaining employment. Pre-vocational training ensures that the brain-injured person has adequate work-related behaviours, for example, getting up and being ready for work in the morning, travelling to and from the workplace, working for reasonable periods of time, dealing with fatigue, tolerating noise, using appropriate memory strategies, planning and organizing work, coping with new situations, and working and socializing with others in the workplace. Preparation for employment also involves practice or support in completing job applications, coping with interviews and dealing with the systems or routines in the workplace. A group setting can be invaluable for preparing for work to establish peer support with others in similar positions.

Brain-injured people often require vocational counselling about employment opportunities to suit their personality, medical condition and physical and cognitive skills. Realistic employment goals are essential for success in the work setting. While some people appreciate that they are unable to work in their previous careers, others cannot accept the change in their circumstances. One person who gave evidence in court was questioned why, as a trained nurse he would not accept work as an auxillary nurse (nurse's aid). He responded 'would a barrister work as a sales assistant?'.

People often find that employment constantly highlights the difficulties they have as a consequence of their brain injury. Support is needed when they are employed to help them develop strategies to overcome problems found in the workplace and to establish methods of coping.

CASE STUDY 11.3

Patient 3 worked as a marketing manager before he suffered a severe brain injury (coma duration and PTA unknown). Following his injury he was described as exhibiting the dysexecutive syndrome, i.e. he had difficulty in planning and organizing activity or in managing two tasks at one time, sustaining attention to tasks over time, and monitoring and adapting his activity according to circumstances in the workplace. His communication was slightly disinhibited and very tangential. Patient 3 was known as 'irrelevant Ted' in a temporary work placement, from which he was terminated. When he obtained a job as a shop assistant in a music store, Patient 3 stated 'if I cannot cope with this, what can be expected in life!'. He managed the job for 3 months but could not understand why he constantly made mistakes and put merchandise in the wrong place. His manager gave him feedback but he could not alter or adapt his behaviour to function more effectively. Patient 3 had no help from psychologists or a case manager in the workplace which could have enabled him to develop effective strategies to overcome his difficulties. These opportunities were not open to him and the music store manager could not understand why Patient 3 behaved as he did and could not complete even simple work.

Supported employment

Supported employment provides the opportunity for paid work in real work settings to individuals with severe disabilities, who would be unable to maintain competitive employment without permanent support at the job site (Wehman *et al.*, 1993).

The six assumptions of the sheltered employment model are the following:

1 vocational intervention, job site training and behavioural modification takes place at the job site, not in the therapy room
2 assistance needs to be provided as long as the individual needs it
3 supported employment should only be used with those people with severe disabilities who are unable to gain or maintain employment on their own
4 the work should be real and meaningful and pay received for it
5 individually designed compensatory strategies should be analysed and developed at the job site
6 jobs should occur in integrated work settings with normal co-workers, not sheltered workshops (Wehman *et al.*, 1993).

Disabled Employment Advisers and/or staff at work rehabilitation programmes establish supported work placements in the community. This involves placing the disabled employee in open employment alongside able-bodied colleagues. A number of models are available including individual placement, enclave, mobile work crew and small business models (Giles and Clark-Wilson, 1993). The individual placement model is used most frequently with brain-injured people.

Selection of potential jobs is based on the results of an evaluation of the person's strengths and weaknesses and on the job task analysis. Assessment of the underlying skills needed for the workplace and matching these to the abilities of the brain-injured person can require skill and creativity from those involved in their support.

Wehman *et al.* (1993) reported the results of a supported employment programme which placed 80 severely brain-injured individuals into competitive employment during a 5-year period. The majority of individuals were seen a significant period of time after their injuries (mean 6.1 years) and gained employment in warehouse, clerical and service-related occupations. The monthly employment ratio increased from 13% post-injury with no supported employment to 67% with supported employment services. During the 5 years, 20% of programme participants lost their jobs because employment was terminated. The reasons given for termination of employment were redundancies, employment setting issues, interpersonal relationship issues, mental health/substance abuse/criminal activity and other issues such as attendance, transportation and involvement in litigation. The authors also stated the economic situation (i.e. recession) led to a substantial decrease in work placements, increase in the number of hours required in available employment openings and increased competition for employment by people without disabilities (Wehman *et al.*, 1993).

Job coaches

Employers or managers need to understand the issues involved in supporting their new employees. The job coach educates potential employers, facilitates communication between the client and the employer or manager and liaises with the client, family and the carers. Training in the work setting from a job coach can facilitate success in the workplace. Job coaches need to understand their client's specific problems, have knowledge of the work required by the brain-injured person in the workplace and realistic expectations of the brain-injured person's performance. The job coach ensures that the brain-injured person can structure their work and time effectively, understands the demands of the job and maintains their attention to the job. The job coach provides support and assistance, as required; helps the brain-injured person solve their own work-related problems; provides moral support; and helps the person appreciate other people's expectations of them. Observing the person with brain injury in the work setting and providing regular reviews of job performance help to identify potential problems. The job coach can then provide constructive feedback regarding difficulties and facilitate methods to overcome problems. Kreutzer *et al.* (1991) state that feedback regarding job performance is critical for job success and ongoing assessment is needed to monitor the relevant aspects of the client's work performance (Kreutzer *et al.*, 1991). As the brain-injured individual's confidence grows and they begin to appreciate the structure and systems of the workplace and their own role in this setting, the support system can gradually be reduced to that required to maintain them on a long-term basis (Kreutzer *et al.*, 1991).

Wehman *et al.* (1994) studied staff time, cost and outcome of a supported work programme for individuals with brain injury. Findings indicated that, on average, the job coach was needed for 18 weeks to ensure that the individual achieved job stabilization. The staff input required was 80% of employee's hours over the first 4 weeks of a placement, to less than 5 h per week after 14 weeks of employment, and less than 3 h (on average 2.24 h) per week after 30 weeks of employment for the remainder of the first year (Wehman *et al.*, 1993). Costs for the service were only provided for a 1-year period and the authors stated there was enormous variability in the amount and type of services required to promote long-term employment (Wehman *et al.*, 1994).

Volunteer work placements
Participants of a work training programme can be supported in volunteer work trials, enabling them to gain work experience within a supportive environment. work placements allow time and opportunity for people to establish their skills; obtain an independent assessment of their work potential; identify strengths and weaknesses and identify their residual difficulties in the work setting; and help the participants to re-establish work routines and behaviours. It allows the person with brain injury to gradually increase their work tolerance, rebuild self-confidence and it provides an independent employment reference for job applications. Staff at the volunteer work placement can provide feedback regarding the brain-injured person's overall capability. These work trials and supported placements are linked with a support group, which helps the individual understand and cope with the complexities of work post-brain injury and facilitate adjustment to the new setting.

A volunteer work placement provides the brain-injured person with work experience and there is an incentive for employers to provide these experiences as they receive some additional help at no cost.

Sheltered workshops

Sheltered workshops offer various occupational activities and are usually run by local authorities or voluntary organizations such as Remploy in the UK or Goodwill in the USA. In the past in the UK there were sheltered work environments for people with severe disabilities but these resources have reduced in number and placements are difficult to obtain. Sheltered work placements provide routine factory or light workshop activities in a supported environment on a long-term basis. Sheltered work is not appropriate for many brain-injured people. Unlike people with mental retardation, many brain-injured people have expectations of themselves functioning in the open labour market. Also brain-injured people often fail to identify with others with similar problems. Nonetheless sheltered work may be an appropriate resource for some.

CASE STUDY 11.4

Patient 4 obtained a degree in engineering before starting work for a large manufacturing company in the UK. Patient 4 had worked at this company for 6 weeks when he was involved in a road traffic accident (coma 2.5 weeks, PTA unknown). Patient 4 received outpatient rehabilitation at a large general hospital but as his progress was very slow, he was admitted to an intensive, specialized rehabilitation programme for approximately 6 months.

Patient 4's rehabilitation goals all involved his return to work. It soon became evident that he would have difficulties returning to his previous workplace because of his significant physical, memory and social-skills deficits. He had a contracture in his left elbow and mild right hemiparesis. Patient 4 could not cope with frustration or criticism; was inflexible in his views; intolerant of other people's ideas; and generally lacked consideration. Patient 4 often felt he could not cope in social settings as he could not utilize strategies to analyse social situations or see issues from other people's perspective. He needed constant reassurance and feedback about his performance as he had lost confidence in himself. His main strengths were that he was motivated, keen to learn and would work hard in addressing the problems he had as a consequence of the brain injury.

The rehabilitation programme was directed towards teaching patient 4 the skills he needed to return to the work setting, for example, cognitive and social skills, problem solving in social settings and graded work-oriented projects incorporating cognitive, social and work skills. The programme also included educational sessions on brain injury and psychotherapy to help patient 4 adjust to his change in circumstances and feedback every afternoon to discuss areas of concern.

A staged plan was developed to assist Patient 4 to live independently away from home and to work. Initially he returned to the house that he lived in with two flat-mates for weekends and these visits gradually became longer. Members of the rehabilitation team met with patient 4 and his work manager to discuss the kind of support that he needed to return to work and how this support was to be provided. Patient 4 returned to the workplace in the same role he had before the accident and started work for 3 days a week from 10.00am to 2.00pm. Gradually over a period of 3 months these hours were increased to 5 days a week from 9.00am to 5.00pm.

When Patient 4 returned to work, he became fatigued which adversely affected his social skills. However, he recognized this problem and worked hard to control his outbursts of frustration and tactless comments. He had the support of a clinical brain-injury case manager and telephoned the clinical case manager once or twice a day, to discuss his work problems. Patient 4 had high expectations of himself at work and became frustrated when he made mistakes or could not reach his own standards. He had to concentrate very hard on his work and tired easily whereas previously he had found work very easy. He became extremely concerned about how other people (his manager and work colleagues) viewed his work. He felt these people were criticizing his work and patronizing him and he took all comments as personal slights. Patient 4 had difficulty in relating to other work colleagues because he lacked confidence in himself and sought reassurance from his work colleagues.

As Patient 4 gained confidence at work, his relationships with his flatmates became strained. Trivial domestic issues became exaggerated and he lost his temper on a few occasions. He was possessive about space, accused his flatmates of using or moving his belongings and became agitated if he did not feel people were completing their jobs in the home. The relationship between Patient 4 and his flatmates deteriorated to such an extent that he had to move to alternative accommodation. Eventually, after another two moves, he decided to live alone as he could not live with others or cope with socializing after work or at weekends.

Over the following year the frequency of Patient 4's calls to his clinical case manager gradually decreased. He became more confident in his work and reassured that he was able to manage satisfactorily. However he was still not able to perform to his full capacity and decided to apply for other jobs within the same company. Patient 4 gained a job in the information technology department, inputting data. This type of work was more suitable as it did not require Patient 4 to rely on his memory or to manage people.

Regular reviews of Patient 4 in his work setting continued to be provided by the case manager. Specific situations or issues continued to be raised in conversations with the brain-injury clinical case manager on the telephone. Possible approaches to deal with the issues were discussed and Patient 4 then developed effective strategies to cope with the situation. One example of an issue was when he contacted the clinical case manager to say that his manager was ignoring him and he did not know what he had done wrong. In analysing the situation with him, the case manager established that his manager's father had died the previous week. Patient 4 had not associated the changes in his manager's behaviour with the bereavement but had related it to his own performance. The case manager and Patient 4 discussed 'bereavement' to help his understand his manager's needs and various approaches were developed to enable his to adapt his behaviour accordingly. He was then able to generalize strategies he used in one situation to another.

Patient 4 gained confidence in his work and successfully completed a graduate programme in information technology on a day release course. Although there is ongoing support from the case management if needed this is only required infrequently. Patient 4's social life has improved and he has developed social networks, especially in a church community.

OCCUPATIONAL ACTIVITIES AND LEISURE TIME

People who are unable to return to work need routine and structure in life. The development of a fulfiling life structure assists in the brain-injured person's adjustment to their altered situation. Creating, planning and organizing activity is not easy for many brain-injured people, due to their cognitive deficits, and they often rely on family, friends or support workers to construct an interesting activity programme.

Day facilities for brain-injured adults or for the young disabled are available and many people enjoy a range of activities at these centres. Others refuse to attend as they do not believe they are disabled and see no similarity between themself and the other people that attend. Educational courses and day or night classes can stimulate progress and occupy time in a meaningful and constructive way but often brain-injured people need support initially to cope with these situations. Volunteer work can help brain-injured adults develop a sense of worth but the placement needs to be carefully matched so the brain-injured person can be successful.

Creating new leisure pursuits depends on the brain-injured adult's interests, abilities and the opportunities open to them. Joining special interest groups, for instance, art classes or photography, assists in the acquisition of new skills and enables new social networks to be developed. General everyday activities required for survival, for example, eating, shopping, cooking, household management, cleaning, laundry and gardening, physical leisure pursuits, e.g. swimming, and socializing can provide a basic framework of activity. The activity programme needs to be constructive and balanced.

Many people who have suffered brain injury become socially isolated. Purchasing needed companionship or support is not possible due to limited personal financial resources and limited funding from statutory services. Families are often placed under excessive strain because of providing care to their relative and frequently cannot tolerate the ongoing, excessive demands for care or give extra attention when needed. Many brain-injured people need individual attention for specific activities or to prevent them placing themselves at risk.

Support workers/carers need training to appreciate the needs of the brain-injured person and to provide them with fulfiling activity and a satisfying lifestyle. All programmes of activity need to be matched according to the needs and abilities of the brain-injured person and these people need to be supported so that a positive approach to their occupational activity can be maintained.

CONCLUSION

There are many factors which affect a person's return to work; age, severity of injury, physical, cognitive and behavioural deficits, employers and social factors. Various approaches can be utilized to facilitate return to work but these have to be individually designed to meet the needs of the brain-injured person and others. Vocational assessment and specialized work rehabilitation can facilitate return to work. Supported employment with a job coach enables many brain-injured persons to return to work. Although supported employment is relatively inexpensive the funds are often not available. Alternative forms of structured activity are required if a return to work is not possible and support is needed to help create an alternative lifestyle and adjust to altered circumstances.

12 Problems in implementing an integrated programme for brain-injury rehabilitation

Gordon Muir Giles, Ian Fussey

Many of the chapters in this book contain practical approaches to rehabilitation, supported wherever possible by a theoretical rationale and empirical evidence. Some of the techniques described are specialized, and there may be readers working in some settings who feel that they could not use the techniques described. Although some interventions do require a coordinated and highly trained team, others do not. This chapter describes the basic requirements of a team approach to rehabilitation using a behavioural model and suggests some interventions that can be used in non-specialized programmes with a minimum of staff training.

Every setting imposes limits on the type of interventions that can be used appropriately; nevertheless rehabilitation staff in a variety of settings can apply a functional behavioural model. However, the application of this type of model does have costs. Working with brain-injured individuals can be stressful and at times unrewarding. The application of a functional behavioural model requires a shift in professional attitude which can be challenging in itself. Nonetheless the benefits to the patient outweigh the costs to the rehabilitation team.

The rehabilitation team will be discussed in terms of the way rehabilitation services are provided. A 'user's guide' to techniques of behaviour management will be presented with reference to the constraints imposed by the settings in which brain-injury rehabilitation occurs.

THE REHABILITATION TEAM

Brain-injured individuals often receive rehabilitation from a range of professionals working independently under the overall guidance of a physician: occupational therapists, speech therapists, physiotherapists, nurses, psychologists and so forth. The term 'multidisciplinary team' has been used to describe this type of organization of service provision. The term implies that a group of professionals are working together towards a defined goal, but unfortunately words are not necessarily deeds. Each member of the team may believe that what he or she can provide is more relevant to the patient. Therefore, members of the team may all be doing what they think is appropriate for the patient's needs, but the interventions may not be coordinated into a common goal (Monzzoni and Bailey, 1996). It is important that the professionals work together towards common goals established for the patient (and if possible with the patient).

The functional behavioural approach, which considers functional goals rather than therapist-generated targets, requires that the team work together such that each therapist understands how his or her professional input can be linked to that of colleagues in other disciplines. This approach demands a considerable degree of communication and may require therapists to blur their role boundaries so as to meet the patient's needs.

THE PROBLEM OF ROLE DEFINITION

Ambiguous role requirements are stressful in most work settings. Professionals spend a considerable part of their training and early career developing a professional identity. It is sometimes difficult to recognize that our own view point is not the only one that counts. This is particularly true when we are passionate about what we do. Even if we can recognize that our own discipline does not have all the answers, there is usually someone on the treatment team who has not yet achieved this degree of perspective. However, those who work with people with brain injury need not lose their professional identity in order to belong to a rehabilitation team. Rather the opposite, as each professional brings to the team his or her own expertise there is often an increased respect for the particular strengths of each discipline.

An essential requirement for a rehabilitation team is communication. Ideally, this should include all those who come in contact with the patient. An overall treatment plan needs to be carried out consistently, especially where there are specific behaviour management plans for individual behaviours. The task of learning new ways of responding is difficult enough for the person with brain injury, but may become much more difficult when there is confusion between therapists as to when and how an intervention is to be carried out.

Communication between team members is essential, but poor communication is not the only cause of inconsistency. Staff may rotate between different units causing consistency problems. The ideal situation would be for unit-based staffing. Nursing staff work with the patient 24 h a day, so it is essential for nursing staff to assume some responsibility for programme management. Frequent changes in staff are confusing for patients and increase the problems of implementing behaviour programmes. This arises partly because of the difficulty of training new staff so that they can participate effectively in the behavioural programmes. Unfortunately, many therapists develop the habit of blaming nursing staff when things do not work out, producing a 'them and us' atmosphere. It is important that therapists recognize the constraints under which nursing staff operate. The nursing department in a hospital setting is the largest department, with the most complicated staffing pattern and a very busy schedule of things which must get done. Nursing staff may regard therapists as having a 'holier than thou' attitude, and the situation may deteriorate from there. The development of more tolerance and respect is usually a starting point for solving these problems.

Management decisions are also often difficult for staff to understand. Most of us working in rehabilitation settings will at one time or another have questioned the motives of those who manage rehabilitation facilities. Is it a deliberate attempt to drive us crazy? Although there are, no doubt, some deliberately wilful administrators, by and large the decisions seem bizarre to us only because we do not know the particular constraints within which the administrator is working. The reality is that there will always be staff changes, vacation and sickness and a system needs to be established that can function despite these contingencies.

Discussion of staff training is included throughout this book as adequate education is essential for a team approach to brain-injury rehabilitation. If a rehabilitation approach aimed at functional goals is the treatment of choice, then a close working relationship needs to be established between therapists with open lines of communication to the patient and family members. Although a greater understanding of the methods of therapists of different disciplines can be an advantage, it may also lead to colleagues and family members coming up with new ideas about how to treat the patient. For many professionals this can be a daunting prospect. However new ideas may result in benefits to the patient and professional ego should be allowed to take second place.

Although the idea of cross-training has become a concern for many therapists in the USA, in brain-injury programmes many therapists are routinely trained by other therapists in the rudiments of their skills. This cross-training, for example, allows the physical therapist and occupational therapist to help carry out a programme to teach the patient how to use a communication device and the physical therapist and nursing staff to teach the patient how to dress themselves and so on. Basic orientation and training can be provided to new staff, with inservice training provided to all staff on a continuing basis particularly about new interventions being used with specific patients. A training manual which contains the aims and methods of the unit may also be helpful. Elsewhere we discussed the development of a facility culture as a tool for the patient's treatment, but it is also very important from the staff's perspective. Culture means a set of articulated and implicit practices and assumptions that are the normative behaviours for the group. The development of a culture is difficult, but after a while, the culture can become self-perpetuating. The most difficult period of staff training is the start-up of a programme. Later staff will learn a lot by watching other staff members. Because most facilities will settle on a limited number of interventions which work well for the particular patient population treated, staff members will soak up 'how we do things here'. From the perspective of a clinical manager, it is exciting to watch a staff member execute an intervention that they have never been taught but which they know how to do from participation in the programme culture. However, it can take a great deal of hard work and years for this to happen.

Many brain-injury programmes are relatively small regardless of setting. Usually only a limited number of staff grasp the 'whole picture' and fully understand the goals and methods of the programme. This makes the units difficult to maintain at optimal efficiency. Key managers and therapists can feel overworked and unable to take time off for illness or vacation leading to 'burn out'. This problem can be partly alleviated by the development of a rehabilitative culture. Managers should train all staff in the central philosophy of the programme and empower staff to make decisions consistent with this philosophy. Consideration should be given to how core values in the programme are communicated to staff.

FUNCTIONAL BEHAVIOUR MANAGEMENT: A USER'S GUIDE

The first task in behavioural management is assessment. If performed adequately, this allows a quantitative evaluation of the current state of the patient's behaviour or skill level and facilitates an objective view of the patient's response to intervention. Assessment should include both excesses and deficits of the behaviour or skill, but should also extend beyond the actual behaviour to consider the circumstances of the behaviour. If one takes into account both the antecedent and consequences of the behaviour, then what is measured is a behavioural event. Knowledge of the behavioural event allows the behaviour or skill to be modified by changing the antecedent or consequence of the behaviour, thus the A–B–C recording of behaviour (see Table 12.1).

With the information gained from the A–B–C recording it may be possible to intervene to change a target behaviour. In the case presented in Table 12.1, the target behaviour is the patient screaming, it is possible to change the antecedent (change the therapist, work with the patient in her room, assist the patient to the mat without asking her to do anything), or change the consequences so that the screaming does not result in the patient avoiding therapy. Changing the antecedent or the consequence might significantly impact the target behaviour.

The use of the A–B–C recording will also show whether a behaviour or skill can be performed in one setting or under one set of circumstances but not in another. For example, the patient described in Table 12.1 never screamed and only required moderate assistance from nursing staff when getting into bed. It is often necessary to analyse the patient's ability to function in a range of settings. It is wasteful to devote energy to devise tests said to be similar to real-life tasks when it is possible to assess the patient in the actual real-life situation.

It is often suggested that focus on a behavioural model denies the existence of thoughts and feelings. In fact, in a cognitive behavioural approach, thought may be given as much weight as behaviour in working with an individual to change behaviour and feelings. Nonetheless it is true to say that in a behavioural model thoughts and feelings are not given as much salience as they are in other treatment

Table 12.1

The A–B–C record

Antecedent
The patient has been brought to the therapy department in a wheelchair. The patient is asked to remove the wheelchair arm rests and swing aside the footrests prior to transferring to the therapy mat.

Behaviour
The patient begins screaming and swearing at staff. She refuses to cooperate and any attempt to assist her perform the activities leads to redoubled screaming.

Consequence
The patient is transported back to her room. She stops screaming immediately upon leaving the therapy room. The patient avoids therapy.

approaches. A behavioural event is a behavioural event, regardless of the emotional state of the individual. What is important in assessment is to define the behaviour or skill in such a way that the whole team can agree on its occurrence or non-occurrence. The problem with emotional states or vague terms such as 'getting better' is that they are liable to subjective interpretation and can therefore invalidate measurement. If the treatment team cannot tell whether an individual is getting better or worse, the team cannot know if the intervention is helping. Nonetheless a behavioural approach does not deny the individual's thoughts, feelings or right to express them within socially defined limits.

FUNCTIONAL ASSESSMENT

Each discipline working with individuals with brain injury has methods of assessment – some formal, some informal. The problem with many assessment methods is that they give little indication of the problems likely to be faced by the patient in the natural setting. To the extent that many of the formal tests constrain the patient's behaviour, they may result in the therapist missing the point entirely. For example, following formal evaluation the speech therapist was working with a patient on his tendency to circumlocute and missed the important point that in the community he would stop every woman he found attractive on the street and ask her out on a date.

The results of each discipline's formal assessment are often difficult for other disciplines to interpret. A functionally based assessment of the patient's skills and disabilities can be performed by observing the patient in a variety of settings. Is performance variable? Are there certain settings which cause a change in performance? Are these person specific? What are the minimum interventions necessary for adequate performance? From this type of evaluation it is possible to highlight problem areas. However, formal assessments are often helpful in determining why performance breaks down. Only following a full functional behavioural assessment is sufficient information available to begin meeting with the patient and family and to set treatment priorities, taking into account the likely future physical and interpersonal environment of the patient.

Deciding on priorities

In working with a severely impaired brain-injured individual it is not always possible, or advisable, to try to work on all problems simultaneously. It is necessary for the treatment team – including the patient and family – to decide on priorities. Deciding on the set of problems to address can be difficult where there is no coordination between the disciplines except in those patients who have marked behaviour disorder. Here, unfortunately, it is not unusual for most members of the team to want someone else to take care of the patient's behaviour problem. While each discipline may have individual goals for the patient, it should not be forgotten that the priorities to be considered foremost are those most likely to advance the patient's rehabilitation.

Functional analysis and setting targets

Target setting requires a detailed analysis of what the patient is and is not doing. Often the problem can be broken into parts (task analysis) to facilitate learning of a complex skill or behaviour. Having established a baseline of the targeted behaviour, it is possible to set targets for change. Like behaviours or skills, targets should be clear to all concerned. If the targets are reasonable and likely to be reached, they can enhance motivation for the patient and therapist by charting recovery in a way that is readily apparent. In some cases recovery from brain injury can be slow, and this can be disheartening for patient and therapist: setting targets helps make apparent small improvements which might not otherwise be recognized. Sometimes the top priority will be to manage inappropriate behaviour. When this is the case, a functional behavioural analysis is central to determining what factors are currently maintaining the behaviour (Treadwell and Page, 1996).

A number of techniques can be used to manage problem behaviours and to assist in the learning or relearning of behavioural skills. The principles of reinforcement have been discussed earlier in this book and will not be reviewed here. Remember, however, to reward the occurrence of an appropriate or desired behaviour rather than penalize the patient for inappropriate behaviour. Even when the goal is the elimination of a behaviour, the patient can be rewarded for periods in which the behaviour did not occur. This makes for a more positive attitude on the part of the staff and guards against the development of a punitive attitude towards the patient. Wherever possible, the goal should be to reinforce all desirable behaviours and strenuously ignore all inappropriate behaviours.

However, it may be necessary in cases of extremely undesirable behaviour to use more intrusive forms of management. In most instances, the use of these procedures will be restricted to specialized treatment programmes where special safeguards are in place to protect the patient. However, it is helpful that all those working with brain-injured people understand the principles of their use.

SPECIFIC TECHNIQUES IN FUNCTIONAL BEHAVIOUR MANAGEMENT

Antecedent control

Central to the development of an appropriate retraining programme is an understanding of the features of the environment that elicit behaviour in a patient. Altering the environment is often sufficient to elicit a needed behaviour. Once elicited, the behaviour can be practised and becomes an increasingly available part of the patient's behavioural repertoire. Part of the therapist's overall approach needs to include 'cue experimentation' where the therapist attempts different methods of cueing in order to obtain the desired behaviour. Yuen (1994) described the use of antecedent control to modify personal hygiene behaviours. In Yuen's case report the patient frequently refused to get out of bed in the morning. When he was assisted to get up, he would immediately dress. In order to get the patient to have a shower, staff would have to block his access to clothes and physically redirect him. The physical redirection often resulted in the patient pushing and kicking staff. At times, staff were not able to have the patient shower despite the fact that the patient was capable of being completely independent once the showering had been initiated. Despite the best efforts of the staff, shower frequency averaged once or twice per week. After 3 weeks a new programme was introduced in which the therapist greeted the patient in the morning by saying 'Good morning ... it is time to take a shower and the water will be ready for you' the therapist then turned on the shower so that the patient could hear the water running. The patient rate of showering increased to six or seven times per week. Yuen (1994) comments that due to the simple nature of the intervention, staff training was minimal and a note in the units communication log enabled staff to successfully carry out the programme.

Following brain injury, naturally occurring stimuli may not be sufficient to lead the patient to engage in appropriate behaviour, and it is necessary to introduce new controlling variables. However, as the patient engages in the behaviours over and over again, the availability of the behaviour increases. This reduces or eliminates the necessity of additional cueing (Giles and Clark-Wilson, 1993; Yuen, 1994).

Time-out

In specialist behavioural programmes this procedure may involve taking the patient to a locked, bare room where he or she may remain under close, although discrete, supervision for a period of 2–5 min. Often used following periods of physical aggression, it is designed to remove patients from the reinforcement of the result of their actions, such as the attention which they might otherwise receive, or observing another person suffer. At a practical level, this technique gives all staff a definitive response to situations which could be threatening and which could escalate out of control.

Depending on the severity of the patient's overall impairments, there may be alternatives to using a time-out room. If the patient is severely physically handicapped, simply removing them from the scene may be adequate. Staff may place the patient in the corridor or at the other end of the room if it is safe to do so. If the patient cannot be moved, the staff member can simply walk away from the patient, returning after 2 min as if nothing had happened (difficult to do if one has just been struck). This is necessary to deny the patient the gratification of knowing he or she has caused harm or discomfort. This form of time-out can be refined as described in the next technique.

Time-out-on-the-spot

This procedure involves not reinforcing the patient for inappropriate behaviour in the context of an ongoing activity. This technique, although simple, requires a great deal of staff coordination to be effective. For most staff, not responding to verbal abuse or being hit runs counter to their natural inclination to reprimand and to admonish the patient not to engage in the aberrant behaviour again. Giving the patient attention for inappropriate behaviour may, of course, increase the likelihood of its recurrence. Time-out-on-the-spot can be administered in two ways. One method is to not pay attention to the individual on the production of an inappropriate behaviour for a brief period (20 s) by, for example, moving away and talking to someone else.

A second technique is for the staff member to continue to pay attention to the patient but to ignore the inappropriate behaviour. The latter method is most suitable when an activity is proceeding and should not be interrupted or when the patient's apparent goal in producing the inappropriate behaviour is to end the activity. In the following example, a physical therapist uses the technique in an ambulation programme.

Therapist:	'Grasp the walker and move on the instruction. Push the walker. Step and then shift your weight. Push. Step. Shift.'
Patient (Shouting):	'Is this what you want you stinking whore?'
Therapist:	'Push. Step. Shift.'
Patient:	'You bloody whore!'
Therapist:	'That was a good step, let's try again.'

Note how the therapist ignores the patient's inappropriate verbalization and concentrates on the goal of teaching the patient how to walk.

Task analysis

Task analysis divides tasks into component parts which can be taught. The analysis provides a method of organizing behaviours making them easier to learn. The components of a task analysis may be converted to prompts. For example, a task analysis is required for the use of stimulus control procedures as well as for more straightforward task training such as learning safe street crossing.

Chaining

Functional tasks can be thought of as complex stimulus–response chains in which the completion of each activity acts as the stimulus for the next step in the chain (Kazdin, 1994). Chaining is described in Chapter 6.

Prompts

Prompts (or cues) are events which facilitate the production of a behaviour. In many instances, prompts are available in the environment, but they are no longer sufficient to guide behaviour, or they have lost their meaning entirely (e.g. sitting at a table with a tray of food no longer cues eating behaviour). The therapist adds additional prompts to those already available in the environment. An additional discussion of prompting methods is included in Chapter 6.

Practice

Repetition of a behaviour increases the probability of the behaviour being further repeated (Giles and Clark-Wilson, 1993). This is known as response practice and is the most important aspect of successful behavioural training. As practice is continued, the behaviours can become automatic. Overlearning refers to the practice of a skill well beyond the point where mastery has been achieved. Overlearning increases the chances that a skill is consolidated in the individual's repertoire of skills and reduces the effort required for performance of the skill (Giles and Clark-Wilson, 1993).

Shaping

It is not always possible to reinforce new desirable behaviour because in many cases the desired response does not occur spontaneously. Shaping refers to the reinforcement of closer and closer approximations to the desired behaviour. Tasks are graded in difficulty so they are achievable. As competency is demonstrated, the tasks requirements are increased. For example, when not escorted to a specific location, Patient 1 would pace around the unit in an agitated state. The goal of the intervention was to encourage him to sit with others and engage in appropriate conversation. Initially, a staff member would stand by the doorway to the patient lounge and give Patient 1 praise and a cookie for approaching the doorway. Later Patient 1 was rewarded for entering the room and provided with additional reinforcement for each 30 s he stayed in the room. Later still he was only reinforced when he was sitting down, and still later only for either sitting quietly or engaging in socially appropriate conversation. Inappropriate behaviours were timed-out-on-the-spot (ignored). The programme was rapidly effective with Patient 1 attending the patient lounge independently during scheduled breaks.

Modelling

This term refers to social imitation in the context of behaviour management. This process is the means by which new responses are acquired, reinforced, or extinguished at a distance, through the observation of the behaviour of others. A large proportion of our behavioural repertoire is developed in this way, not through our own first-hand experience but by observing others in particular circumstances and how they fare as a consequence of their behaviour. It follows, therefore, that those in contact with the brain-injured person are all potential models for appropriate or inappropriate behaviour.

The development of a rehabilitative culture relies heavily on modelling. For example, in a transitional living community there were daily group meetings in which patients were conspicuously congratulated and rewarded for working hard on their specific goals. There was a consistent message of unconditional positive regard for patients working on coming to terms with their post-injury self (in an attempt to address denial). Because new patients saw their peers working hard to overcome behavioural and social-skills difficulties, it was easier for the new patients to accept and work on such difficulties in themselves.

Discriminant learning

Discriminant learning is a term borrowed and adapted from animal learning experiments. In helping the brain-injured person to learn a new skill or behaviour, it is important that they are assisted in discriminating between behaviours which have a positive outcome for them and those which do not. When reinforcement is provided for a behaviour, it is important to make it clear to the patient the reason for the reinforcement. For example 'Well done! It is really good to see you go to your room to cool down when you are getting upset'. The reinforcement strongly linked to the behaviour will enhance the learning.

Most behavioural techniques are simply the common-sense application of a number of rules. It should be noted that a frequent criticism of behavioural methods is that they do not last. While it is true that anything which can be learned can be unlearned, recent evidence suggests that brain-injured people's responses to behavioural interventions are maintained over very long-term follow-up (Lloyd and Cuvo, 1994).

WHY BEHAVIOURAL MANAGEMENT MAY FAIL

Unrealistic expectations

Some staff believe unrealistically that a behaviour programme will immediately prevent the patient from engaging in the target behaviour. When the patient does not instantly cease the inappropriate behaviour, the staff believe that the intervention has failed. A related problem is the tendency to set unrealistic targets for the patient, such as progressing from engaging in a behaviour on a hourly basis to not at all. This sets the intervention programme and the patient up for failure. Remedy: provide the staff with another avenue to vent their frustration with the patient and educate about how behavioural interventions work.

Consistency

Lack of staff consistency can seriously jeopardize the success of functional behavioural programmes. Failure to consistently reinforce appropriate behaviours or erratic responses to inappropriate behaviour will also impede learning. A problem may arise when staff dislike a particular behaviour and 'move the goal posts' so that a patient does not reach the target. Staff may find it very difficult to ever reward a patient who engages in a particularly obnoxious behaviour, despite the fact that the patient is doing it much less than a week ago. Remedy: establish clear goals and targets understood by everyone in the treatment team.

Communication

Poor communication among team members will adversely affect consistency. The aim should be to have all members of the treatment team aware of their colleagues' roles and how their own contribution relates to the overall approach. In carrying out a functional behavioural approach, it may be that certain team members disagree with adopted techniques for managing disturbed behaviour. It is better that such disagreements are voiced openly rather than covertly disrupting the consistency of the approach. Remedy: regular team meetings that allow for discussion in an atmosphere of trust.

Flexibility

The behavioural model relies on approaches that are functional and specifically designed to meet the patients' needs rather than textbook guidelines. Flexibility is needed. Remedy: put the patient first.

Institutional constraints

It may be that the model proposed here in its entirety is inappropriate because of institutional constraints. There may be a lack of available resources, or the number of patients treated may be too small to sustain a brain-injury programme. One or two people working together can successfully carry out some programmes with minimal assistance of other staff members (see for example the discussion of stimulus control procedures in Chapter 5). In outpatient settings it is sometimes possible to enlist the assistance of family members and friends and good results may be achieved with apparently intractable problems. Remedy: keep fighting the system and do not give up hope.

Learning constraints

Even the most severely injured patients can learn. However, it may have to be accepted that, due to the profound nature of some patient's injuries, the limits of their learning will be reached before real functional gains can be made. It is necessary to accept that with limited resources it is not possible to continue with rehabilitative efforts beyond the point where learning is not demonstrated. Long-term management using behavioural principles may then be used to maximize the patient's quality of life.

A NOTE ON WORKING WITH THE FAMILIES OF BRAIN-INJURED PEOPLE

Severe brain injury is a catastrophic event for the patient and the patient's family. Many individuals are able to face the profound family crisis with composure and compassion for those around them, but not surprisingly many are not. It is important for all members of the treatment team to remember that family members are facing profound losses. Staff are often a target for families in their grief, and handling the rejection and hostility of family members can be difficult. It is important to remember however that the family is rejecting the diagnosis and is angry at the staff because the staff represent the reality of the potential loss which they must face. The family need honest and straightforward information presented in a way that they can use. Rehabilitation professionals should keep in mind that they are not in the business of taking hope away from people and that a true appreciation of the nature of the loss takes time. Trying to understand the experience of the family can assist staff in working with family members. The following vignette illustrates some of these issues. A family had been labelled by the treatment team as a 'difficult family'. The patient, the only son in the household, was verbally assaultive and would scream at staff if his needs were not met immediately. The family was highly critical of the treatment team and ignored all the rules put in place to control the patient's aggressive behaviour. The patient had a swallowing disorder and was highly impulsive in his eating, necessitating a pure diet. However, the family was unable to follow staff recommendations and insisted on bringing pizza for the patient as that is what he said he wanted. The family believed everything that the patient said and 'sided' with him and against the treatment team. Treatment staff were mystified and exasperated.

Some gentle questioning elucidated the dynamics of the situation. Over recent years the patient and his parents had not been getting along. The patient had been into heavy metal music, ran with a crowd the parents disliked, stayed out late, and drank heavily. The relationship was marked by mutual hostility. Against this background, the son had a severe brain injury. It occurred to his parents that he may die and not realize how much they loved him. Their remorse that they had not expressed their love and their fear that this failure 'caused' their son's accident overwhelmed them with guilt and made them incapable of saying no to him.

A frank discussion of these issues helped the staff have more compassion for the parents and it also assisted the parents in recognizing the source of their conflicts with staff. Gradually, the parents were able to recognize that the best way to help their son was not always doing what he asked.

CONCLUSION

The fundamental question, for this as for any treatment approach, is does it work? The answer is yes but with qualifications. A functional behavioural approach is the most effective set of interventions available, but it cannot resolve all of a patient's problems and it has drawbacks that have already been described. In some cases, it can seem like a miracle. In most cases, it can produce meaningful changes with consistent work from the patient and a dedicated staff and family. It can and should be used in conjunction with appropriately targeted pharmacological interventions.

It will be clear to anyone working in the field of brain-injury rehabilitation that an integrated team approach puts more pressure on staff in an already stressful area. It may appear that many of the factors in the functional behavioural approach to brain-injury rehabilitation seem to exacerbate those areas of practice that we already know to be stressful. However, it is suggested that the advantages gained, in terms of job satisfaction and demonstrable achievements, will more than compensate for these costs. This chapter has attempted a practical look at implementing functional behavioural programmes in rehabilitation environments. No doubt some problems have been missed, but it is left to individual therapists working closely with their colleagues to solve those problems, in the ways most advantageous for themselves and their patients.

13

THE SOCIAL AND EMOTIONAL CONSEQUENCES OF SEVERE BRAIN INJURY: A SOCIAL WORK PERSPECTIVE

Mary Roberts Lees

INTRODUCTION

A decade has passed since this chapter was first written for the first edition, a decade which has seen an increasing number of people survive serious brain injury. More rehabilitation and long-term resources which offer specialist care and management have appeared. None of this alters the fact that severe traumatic brain injury always has serious implications for survivors and their families. The not inconsiderable output of researchers in this field, to which this chapter refers, assists social workers and other professionals to understand the problems of patients and to plan their care. This chapter is intended for clinicians who work in brain-injury services, whether acute hospital or rehabilitation unit based. In addition to the rehabilitation literature there have also been government studies, the latest in the UK of relevance to social workers is the report of the Social Services Inspectorate part of the Department of Health (1996) *A Hidden Disability*. Above all, the arena of brain-injury rehabilitation and services is of paramount importance both to those who have suffered injury and their families, friends and employers.

This chapter continues to focus on the unique and shared reactions of survivors who have suffered severe brain injury and their families. Brain injury inevitably brings changes in personal relationships and to family structures. Families learn, with difficulty, to accommodate to the needs of the brain-injured family member. In commenting on some individual solutions as well as general outcomes, this chapter illustrates how both social work intervention and clinical team involvement can help survivors and their families.

FAMILY NEEDS IN THE ACUTE STAGE OF RECOVERY

Whatever the cause of admission to neurological units; traffic accident; suicide attempts; subarachnoid haemorrhage; or other neurological insult, the event is usually an emergency. This produces an immediate crisis for family and friends. The necessity of spending long periods of time at a hospital means changes to usual family routines. If the injured person is admitted to a regional neurological centre, families have to make arrangements to be away from home. The family is faced with a completely new situation and awesome demand (Tzidkiahu *et al.*, 1994).

Initially, there will be offers of practical assistance for families. The focus is on recovery: parents, children, spouses and parents are involved, even when the patient is in coma. They will talk to the patient about familiar people and events, play taped music and generally feel part of the recovery process. There is a clear role to play and this helps with the initial shock and distress. Future outcome or need for care is unlikely to be discussed fully at this stage even if the length of coma is viewed as a predictor of outcome (Teasdale and Jennett, 1974). Families often state that they did not receive helpful factual information, or advice, at the acute stage of recovery (McMordie *et al.*, 1991). Because they are fully involved in the caring role, families are preoccupied, often highly anxious, and may not comprehend what is being said to them. Often families report that if they were given information, it was unacceptable to them at the time and they ignored it. At the height of distress families will refuse to accept a poor prognosis. They may adopt an aggressive role, believing that if they, and the patient, fight hard enough physical problems can be overcome. They are less likely to acknowledge the outcome of cognitive damage and certainly do not anticipate the psychosocial and emotional difficulties that lie ahead. Each individual family takes on the problems engendered by brain injury with little awareness of the issues involved.

As Lezak (1978) has stated, families need information and guidance, even though they are very likely to be unwilling to accept it at an early stage. Later emotional difficulties often have their root in a family's initial disbelief about the prognosis, and determination to prove the medical staff wrong. This conflict leads, as discussed later in this chapter, to the adversarial alliance between staff and relatives described by McLaughlin and Carey (1991). Relatives who have become deeply involved in caring for their brain-injured family member find it difficult to relinquish a role which has become a way of life, often to the exclusion of usual family activities. If the patient is beginning to make progress in physical recovery of function, the family may well equate this with a generalized recovery. They will expect the person they all knew before the injury to return with previous personality intact.

Outcome is difficult to predict and families are distressed and vulnerable in the acute stage of recovery. Clinical teams may be unwilling to give negative information and families may deny the seriousness of the predicted outcome. It would be helpful nonetheless, at this stage, to convey hopeful but realistic information to the family. They should have access to literature explaining brain injury and details of the voluntary support organizations such as Headway in the UK and their local chapter of the Brain Injury Association in the USA. They may not consult such organizations initially but access should be encouraged at the point when the survivor and the family begin to be aware of the need for informed assistance.

Clinical staff in neurosurgical and intensive care units, as well as community-based medical and nursing services, need also to be knowledgeable about realistic recovery and outcome potential and to consider these when talking to families. Nothing is gained by giving too little or too much hope at the time of injury. Such advice is often remembered and can affect the potential for later working relationships between patients, their families and the clinical teams in rehabilitation units.

When someone has suffered a brain injury it is important that there is systematic monitoring of their progress, and also the progress of the family in coping with the emotional demands of the situation. In some neurological, surgical or intensive care units, social workers are introduced to the family immediately, to offer counselling, practical services and advice. A case manager might also be appointed, through the patient's solicitor (lawyer), who will monitor the care of the patient throughout their recovery.

Family members are in need of information and assistance, but may be unwilling or unable to accept this, so it is often useful if the social worker initially adopts a practical role. With the development of trust and the gradual acceptance of the need for more intensive intervention by the family, the social worker can begin both to provide counselling and to act as a link with the clinical treatment team. The family should be able to meet team members and discuss individual therapies. At this time the family's emotional needs may become evident. Understanding the impact of the patient's disability or family functioning gives some indication of likely future difficulties (Kreutzer et al., 1994) and families already experiencing problems prior to the accident or injury may function even less effectively afterwards as a result.

Social workers need to assess the patient's role within the family and what effect the loss of this role has on both patient and family. Sometimes the process of putting together a patient and family history is helpful in clarifying roles. This can help the family as well as giving the clinical team an understanding of the patient prior to injury. This process can be comforting to the family who is entrusting the care of their relative to comparative strangers. Families need to be advised to care for the emotional and physical health of all members at this stressful time (Lezak, 1978) and the social worker can become a source of support for the whole family. Young children may have to adopt a particularly difficult role in assuming practical, sometimes adult, responsibilities, at the same time as experiencing the loss of a parent. Children can begin to react to this burden long before the uninjured parent is aware of it. The person who is the prime caregiver carries the major burden, but those family members who also depend on the caregiver experience stress (Lezak, 1988).

As the brain-injured patient stabilizes clinically and develops increasing functional independence, transfer from acute hospital units to rehabilitation units will take place. The patient will receive further physical, cognitive, behavioural, or other therapeutic, treatment. Unfortunately, this path of care is not always seen as essential and if a patient makes a good physical recovery they may be discharged home, inappropriately, before the total effect of brain injury on their cognitive and emotional functioning is fully understood. Ideally, the transition from hospital to home should always include the referral to community-based social services by the hospital-based clinical social worker. In the USA the level and length of health insurance availability varies tremendously and does not always allow for adequate access to specialist services. The introduction of the Community Care Act (1993) as a further implementation of the National Health Service and Community Care Act (1990) in the UK has brought a more effective process of discharge planning in physical and mental health services. However, the precise needs of brain-injured survivors are often not fully understood by social services care managers and often the individual or family only receive comprehensive care if a specialist social worker advocates for them. It is not unusual to find families experiencing high levels of stress and depression as a result of attempting to cope with the problems of living with a brain-injured person without any professional social support. The situation is already made stressful by financial loss, inadequate practical assistance, and emotional disturbance (Livingston, 1986, 1987). Community social work services lack specialist skills and knowledge about brain injury but do not always recognize the gap in service. This becomes more apparent when attempts are made to decide which is more appropriate, mental health or physical disability services. The need for long-term individual and family counselling and services is not always recognized. Yet it is when the brain-injured survivor returns home from hospital or rehabilitation unit that these particular problems are highlighted and there is sometimes massive disturbance to family relationships (Lezak, 1978). Caregivers can experience psychological stress for as long as 15 years post-injury (Kreutzer *et al.*, 1994).

What are the specific changes and difficulties experienced by survivors? Each individual has their own pre-injury strengths and weaknesses, different attitudes to life, experiences and personality profile and therefore their approach to difficulties will be unique. Their families, friends and employers will also experience a degree of loss or change in their contact with brain-injured survivors. Survivors of severe brain injury may experience devastating loss yet have limited insight into the change in themselves (Tyerman and Humphrey, 1986; see also Chapter 10). If the patient has recovered well physically the changes in personality may be difficult to recognize. This creates difficulties for a family; to outsiders or peripheral family members little change is apparent; for the spouse or partner, child, parent, or grandparent, there is often an awareness of great change in the behaviour and interpersonal relationships of the brain-injured survivor. This is variously interpreted by family members who sometimes assume that feelings have changed and they are no longer loved. There can be a distant quality to the expression of any emotion, an irritable response to former patterns of family behaviour, and yet the family do not realize these can be a consequence of brain injury. It is particularly important that support for the family continues, and is consistent, so that these issues can be explored and understood.

When a family becomes aware that a full recovery is not possible and relationships within the family become difficult, there is often disappointment, resentment of new roles and even a sense of failure at not achieving a better outcome. This is compounded by the fact that the brain-injured person is often unaware of the problem. They may be genuinely unable to perceive change in themselves and are puzzled by the reactions of familiar people. Pressure from the extended family or community to resume previous lifestyles post-injury can confuse, frustrate and distress close family members who are beginning to realize that relationships have changed to the point where normal life is no longer possible. The major burden is beginning to be carried by the family (Weddell *et al.*, 1980).

Brain injury produces a number of changes for the survivor and family:

1 For the survivor there is an immediate experience of physical disability which may become long term. Previous strengths and capabilities have disappeared and daily life revolves around the progress to be gained and maintained in treatment programmes and activities. This is an acceptable area for the family

to focus on initially. A realization that physical dependency may be permanent may be much more daunting for survivor and family.

2 Severe brain injury causes loss of status. Many survivors are unable to return to full-time work at the level of functioning pre-injury. Those who do return to work often do so in a lesser capacity, or in sheltered work (Weddell *et al.*, 1980). Job coaching can assist return to work but has to be intensive (Skord and Miranti, 1994).

3 Where a wage earner stops work to help look after a brain-injured child at home, the family experiences loss of income and employment. Possibly both parents worked and even if only one can no longer do so, because of the increased responsibility of caring for the child, there will be a commensurate loss of income. Employment also gives the family status and social networks and these are hard to replace in the home environment (Osberg *et al.*, 1997).

4 The family may have to move into more modest accommodation for financial reasons or because their present accommodation does not meet the physical needs of the brain-injured family member.

5 The non-injured spouse or partner may need to assume full financial responsibility for the household. Other caregivers come into the home to look after the survivor and young dependent children. The new caregivers may include in-laws, parents, sisters or friends, part-time or living in the home. There are subtle shifts in family patterns, coupled with a loss of outside activity. Relationships and status change within the family.

6 The brain-injured person loses self-respect and may well be depressed by their physical condition (Lewin *et al.*, 1979). The loss of friendships and contacts outside the family, combined with loss of leisure activities, which reduces contact further, leads to a sense of isolation and loss both for survivor and family (Lezak, 1988).

The family experiences losses similar to those experienced by the survivor. If the wage earner is injured the family also loses status and income. The family has to make adjustments in their behaviour towards, and relationship with, the survivor and family life begins to revolve around the injured person. Children take on adult roles, spouses become main decision makers (instead of being an equal partner in a couple or family team). Parents or survivors may have to resume a caregiver and parental role. All energy is focused on the survivor with significant loss for other dependents and the extended family. There is less time for the usual family social events and activities and the family may becomes isolated.

In addition to the practical problems experienced by the family, the survivor presents them with the consequences of perceptual, cognitive and personality changes (Rafferty *et al.*, 1984). Serious memory problems affect relationships, causing anxiety and irritation for all involved, depriving the brain-injured survivor and family of shared memories. The survivor may have severely impaired recall, forgetting immediate past events and confusing chronological order. It is very difficult to sustain an emotional attachment to someone who has no recollection of your past and present together and it requires strength and loving detachment for a partner to be able to do so.

Children in a family where an adult is brain injured often have to lead an unnaturally restricted life because they can be exposed to irritable verbal, and even physically aggressive behaviour. Children may be afraid of provoking outbursts of temper or even physical abuse. The family begins to tread warily and relationships become strained. The survivor's needs dominate in ways which vary from the subtle to the extreme. Many brain-injured people are very self-absorbed, not able to feel for others and require almost continuous attention. They may be irresponsible, or so it seems, to the family, behaving in casual or inappropriate ways which are greatly at odds with their previous personality. If the survivor is restless and easily bored he or she may demand a greater degree of stimulus or attention which is not easily available within the family. However deep the affection for the survivor it may be increasingly difficult for the family to offer care, when all the giving brings little positive response or return of affection.

These changes within the family system may be apparent whilst the survivor is still in hospital, or rehabilitation unit, or on their return home. Once the initial crisis has passed the family members become aware of the increased dependency and may be less tolerant of changes to usual family routines. Although in a sense the family has suffered a loss, they are not able to grieve. The survivor is different in many ways, but is back in the family, so there is no effective mourning process. The survivor can be demanding at a time when the family is drained of strength and has lost direction. The reality of the situation may be denied because changes in the individual, the family and its relationship to the community are too painful to acknowledge. A period of denial is a protective mechanism and may have to be respected. It is difficult for clinical teams, who may be encouraged by a survivor's physical progress, to acknowledge the family's dilemma (Lezak, 1978; Lewin *et al.*, 1979; Livingston, 1987).

THE SOCIAL WORK ROLE

Whilst the brain-injured patient is still in coma, or a post-traumatic amnestic state, it is difficult for the social worker to establish a meaningful relationship with the patient. Even during post-traumatic amnesia each new contact for the survivor is of the moment and will not be remembered. In the later stages of recovery the social worker may still have difficulty in establishing a counselling relationship with a person who has little motivation towards improvements and change; who can be egocentric and facetious; has little or no insight; and who is locked into obsessional ideas.

It is instead often the family with whom a counselling and supportive relationship is established. The family needs information about the behavioural and emotional changes they can expect and an explanation about the way they relate to the brain injury. Personality changes are the most burdensome aspect for relations (Junquè *et al.*, 1997).

It is difficult for the family to accept a poor prognosis or negative information about likely changes in lifestyle. Professionals often refer to a stage of denial both for survivors and family. It is important to remember that the survivor may be hampered by a myriad of cognitive and perceptual impairments that mimic denial. The family may, at the same time, need a stage of denial as a protective mechanism (Leaf, 1993). It is not helpful to challenge denial or confront the family at too early a stage. They will eventually acknowledge change, when they are able to face the challenges that change has brought with it. The social worker should continue to support the family, give information, and show acceptance both of the difficulties the survivor is causing, and the family's reaction to unexpected and unwelcome stress. If the social worker has specialist knowledge about brain injury, and effective counselling skills, they can reassure the family that certain stages are to be expected in both the patient's and family's emotional recovery, and that they can expect continuing support and guidance with these.

Discharge of the brain-injured person to home should involve a system of continued guidance, advice, and support for the family. The recent legislation affecting discharge procedures in the UK are designed to ensure proper preparation is made for discharge with an assessment of needs by Social Services and a package of care designed to meet those needs. It is helpful to be able to ask for such care packages for survivors and families but it is rare to find an aftercare programme that includes specialist neurological services. The dependence on the hospital or rehabilitation unit can lessen once the patient has been at home for a period and the community-based occupational, speech and physio therapists and social worker enter the picture. If possible, the hospital or unit social worker should ensure that survivor and family do not feel they have been abandoned by the clinical team. A community-based social worker should ideally be introduced and visit the hospital to meet survivor and family prior to discharge, or the hospital social worker should continue making home visits until a positive transfer of responsibility is achieved. This process tends to take place from specialist units on an informal basis. Survivors going home to districts less familiar with brain-injury services have a more difficult time in accessing continuing social work or therapist support. Unlike rehabilitation processes involving people with physical but not cognitive and emotional disabilities, problems for the brain injured and their families begin when they are reunited. This is a vital period when help needs to be offered, not only with practical legal and financial issues, but also to meet both current and future emotional needs of the family. The social worker must try to establish an honest and supportive relationship in preparation for the difficulties ahead. Recovery will continue over several years and appropriate resources need to be available at different stages when progress is made or problems experienced.

In addition to the care management services available now to disabled people in the UK through statutory services, the past 10 years have also seen an increase in the number of private-sector case managers. Unlike government-mandated care managers, case managers are privately funded from compensation awards (and interim payments) to monitor the brain-injured person's complex needs from the point of injury and acute hospital admission until, if necessary, suitable long-term care has been found.

Case managers usually have an occupational therapy or social work professional background. The case manager can access a range of services, including government social services, if appropriate, but the client's financial status is still assessed by social services care managers and they may have to contribute to this care provision. National Health Service treatment is still without charge but community services are no longer free in most areas of the UK. The care manager, conversely, can buy in private services for clients if local social services provision is not available. Both case management and care management can, therefore, access similar services but are not necessarily seen as complementary service provision, either can include social work and counselling services in the package of care designed for the client.

In the USA the insurance company case manager operates in the same way as the private-sector case manager in the UK. However, this service is only available to a small proportion of severely brain-injured individuals in the USA, those with private health insurance. Unfortunately, those who are most at risk of brain injury are also the most likely to be underinsured. With limited service continuity a coherent long-term plan of care is the exception rather than the rule. It is also less likely that they will have social workers with specialist brain-injury knowledge and experience.

The UK's Carers (Recognition and Services) Act 1995 was intended to give carers rights to assessment of their needs in the caregiver role and to provide the services they need to carry out their tasks. A survey carried out 9 months after the Act came into force showed that although the rights of carers had been promoted at the level of policy, this had failed to filter down to the level of practice (George, 1997). In particular, older carers were unsure that their formal caregiver role would fit eligibility criteria. Neither this Act nor the care management services available under the Community Care Act focus particularly on the needs of people with brain injury, who are a small group among a wide range of people with physical or mental health disabilities in need. Problems begin when the same criteria are applied to all groups.

COUNSELLING

The counselling process is necessary, in addition to the comfort, friendship and advice offered by relatives and friends. The spouse or partner, parent or child of someone with severe brain injury needs someone to whom it is safe to talk and who has no vested emotional interest in the situation. They need to express negative feelings and will have fears and anxieties, resentments and difficulties to share. Spouses and partners have lost the one person with whom they would previously have shared problems, the survivor. The wider group of family and friends may not want, or be able to hear, the negative feelings that close relatives need to express, as those feelings may conflict with their own needs and reactions. For the family the brain-injured member needs to be integrated and accepted in a new way. This may be difficult to accept by those who do not live closely with the situation. The wider family can maintain a level of denial not possible for close family members.

With the loss of an important role within the family, that previously occupied by the brain-injured person, family function may be disturbed (Lezak, 1988; Leaf,

1993). There may be a need for family or individual therapy, perhaps provided conjointly with a psychiatrist or psychologist. Clinical treatment may be needed when the survivor's return home causes anxiety and depression in family members (Livingston, 1987). Pharmacological treatment for family members should not be provided in isolation. Consistent support from a social worker, who is accepted by the family as someone who is accessible and helpful, and to whom feelings can be ventilated, should be offered in conjunction with pharmacological treatment.

The health care worker, or clinical social worker, must be able to accept feelings of anger and resentment from survivors and relatives, support them in their distress and act on behalf of all parties. This is important in preparation for a later stage, when it becomes necessary, for the family's emotional health, to redefine responsibilities and roles within the family. If the social worker is seen as being equally committed to both the brain-injured individual and family members, it is easier for the family to accept advice about the necessary changes to family functioning without feeling disloyal. The family sometimes have to disregard the survivor's perception of how they should live in favour of a plan which accommodates the needs of the whole family. This produces a sense of guilt with which the family may need help. The social worker acts as a moderator, embracing the viewpoints of all family members but with necessary detachment and objectivity, and plans for, and protects, the emotional well-being of the whole family.

There are difficulties inherent in any assumption that families will continue to remain involved with brain-injury survivors. Families are involved in a grieving process and need their own emotional rehabilitative therapy once the acute stage of their relative's brain injury is past. The losses experienced by family and friends are as significant as those of the brain-injured person. The clinical therapy team needs to support and understand family reactions and be prepared for the disintegration of some families. In counselling the family the social worker should facilitate decision making about the future, by helping family members to consider alternative arrangements for the survivor's care. Families are unique and coping skills vary tremendously – expecting them to be fully involved in the activities of rehabilitation can add to the family burden. Many well-intentioned attempts at family therapy can be counter-therapeutic and cause guilt and anxiety, for example, to a spouse or partner who cannot contemplate a continuation of a life together when the survivor is so changed (Maitz, 1993). Families have to be allowed to make decisions based on a reasonable understanding of the likely difficulties ahead. Paradoxically, allowing people to contemplate separation of the family from the survivor, or a divorce for spouses, can prevent this from happening. Showing acceptance and concern for the family, as well as the survivor, and indicating a non-judgemental approach to any decisions they make can give people time to think their problems through and make more informed decisions. Families should not be expected to continue untenable relationships. Sometimes the non-injured partner is able, following separation, to become a close friend to the survivor, playing an important and protective role in their life without having to pretend they feel an emotional depth of feeling or relationship.

Sexuality is a difficult and sensitive issue in the counselling process with partners of the brain injured. Partners often say they feel they are making love to a stranger. Considerable trust in the counsellor may be needed before sexual problems can be discussed. Elliott and Biever (1996) comment on the lack of information available about sexual dysfunction after brain injury. Their article provides valuable information and clarifies some direct relationship between organic damage and sexual function. They also describe the depression and social isolation felt by partners attempting to resume a sexual relationship with someone who can be sexually inappropriate, excessively demanding and publicly embarrassing. As a result of their brain injury some patients can be flirtatious and sexually inappropriate and sexually demonstrative towards other people, even propositioning complete strangers, and using sexually disinhibited language in social situations (Miller *et al.*, 1986). Conversely, where a couple had a close, loving, relationship the injured partner may show no sexual interest, and this unemotional distance may cause pain and a real sense of loss. The spouse or partner of someone with a severe brain injury may no longer feel able to respond emotionally or sexually, when they previously had a close, loving, relationship and this can lead to marital friction.

It is not unusual to find the brain-injured partner displaying jealousy and also becoming obsessionally possessive, limiting their partner's freedom and causing disruption to family life. Partners of the brain injured should be given the opportunity to discuss sexual problems on their own and, with the sensitive approach of a counsellor, be able to lessen guilt and anxiety about their own or their partner's loss of sexual response. If couples do not separate they may be able to change their relationship into one of loving friendship rather than sexual intimacy. This may happen more readily if the effect of the injury is a decrease in libido (Lezak, 1978) rather than in the presence of hypersexuality. If there has been a change in sexual relationship the survivor may well express sexual frustration, and some anger, which may need the intervention of the therapy team, both in providing management strategies for the survivor and to protect the family. Jealousy and sexual frustration provide more risk than indifference, but any change of sexual behaviour can be distressing to partners. When couples stay together there can be so much emphasis on practical care and strategies, that rediscovering an intimacy pleasurable to both partners may not be given any importance. Blackerby (1993) discusses possible methods for enabling intimacy. He suggests a renewal of courtship in which a couple examine the differences between their pre- and post-brain-injury relationship and adjust to new and different expectations of each other. If this process is successful sexual tensions can be lessened as a different, but valuable, intimacy is discovered. Fostering this process requires skilled counselling and a focus on communication of needs by each partner. This may succeed where both partners are interested and where there is a great level of tolerance towards the survivor by the uninjured partner. Both partners have to agree to make changes in their expectations of each other and to adapt to those changes before the process of rediscovery of intimacy can take place.

THE EXPERIENCE OF READJUSTMENT – SOME FAMILY PROFILES

Although each family is unique, and each family's pattern of recovery is different, there are enough similarities to allow the formulation of management strategies. In reviewing family responses where a family member had been severely brain injured, all families felt their lives had changed irrevocably, to the detriment of their usual lifestyle. Where there has been marital or family conflict and problems before injury, family breakdown is often inevitable. Pre-injury problems may have revolved around financial worries, child-rearing difficulties, unemployment, loss of affection and many other factors. It can be particularly stressful for anyone to contemplate leaving a brain-injured partner, and guilt may prevent them from doing so. If a couple had hidden their relationship problems from their children and extended families prior to injury, a separation from the brain-injured partner will seem to be exceptionally disloyal. All partners find extreme difficulty in separating from injured spouses. When the marriage had been a secure and affectionate one the departing partner considered themselves to be callous and cruel. Often the separating partner wanted to remain involved in a caring and active way, and was more able to handle their guilt and grief for the lost partner by remaining a friend, and acting as an advocate. This was surprisingly quite possible for couples where the survivor was unable to remember the partner or spouse and family life. It was less possible where the injured partner was unable to see themselves as having changed, or understand why their relationships had broken down. Survivors can sometimes strongly deny any problems in themselves, or their relationships, and will manipulate separating partners into experiencing considerable emotional distress about their decision to leave. Marriage breakdown is widespread in modern society, not only for people with disability. The guilt and remorse associated with leaving a disabled partner can be compounded if that person, consciously or unconsciously, uses their disability to hold on to their relationship. Those with a strong religious background and commitment to marriage may not be able to contemplate separation or divorce. Where a partner is disabled, but is not suffering brain injury, relationships continue because, despite the need for physical care, the partnership is still viable with no loss of personality or affection (Brooks and McKinlay, 1983).

Family profiles

The young wife with a brain-injured husband

Recent marriages do not often survive the problems caused by changes in personality, emotional response and physical abilities of the brain-injured partner. When the young brain-injured husband is discharged home after rehabilitation, and there are young children in the family, the wife often finds that her husband's position within the family has changed, and he has become another child to be cared for. However, he may be irritable and aggressive, unable to monitor his own behaviour. He becomes demanding, vying with his own children for his wife's attention. The young wife no longer has an adult partner to share child-care and family responsibilities, just when financial problems increase. The family unit becomes isolated, especially if financial pressures cause a move to a new home, away from friends and neighbours, and the children's schools and friends. Caring for pre-school-age children in a new area can be a lonely experience, especially if the presence of a brain-injured husband makes ordinary social contact difficult. The additional stress of coping both with young children, and stubborn and destructive behaviour in a partner with whom one has had a relationship of only a few years, may lead to marriage breakdown. Initial participation by the family in the acute stage simply postpones the appreciation of the extent of the problem. When young partners become aware that complete recovery is not possible, that their partner is no longer the same person, disillusionment and despair leads to a breakdown in the marriage. With a partner in long-term rehabilitation, and with an awareness of a loss of affection coupled with major problems, it is not unusual to find young partners gradually separating. Visits are less often and families adjust to the loss. Partners may even be able to make new emotional relationships, although it is notable that there is an ongoing sense of grief for the lost partner. Partners often report the feeling that someone who was loved has died but a new and different person has appeared, in the same body. Counselling for young partners, as indeed for wider family relationships, has to build in an acceptance of a bereavement on these two levels. Grief needs to be expressed for the personality which has been lost. The relationship with the survivor is a different one, and this loss has to be mourned as well. Young people, with limited life experience, may present special difficulties to the counsellor. They have less experience of relationships and are less able to realistically accept both the change in their partner and impact on their marital and family life. It is often not reasonable to expect young partners of people with brain injury to continue the marital relationship, and it is necessary to allow them to separate and form, eventually, new relationships to help them and their young children resume a family life.

Families with adolescent children and brain-injured father

Unlike wives in new marriages, those who have been married for some years and have adolescent children may react to the problems of brain injury with a more positive attitude and outcome. The marriage may have been successful and have weathered difficulties. The wife may, therefore, feel a strong commitment to her brain-injured spouse. Older children are able to offer practical and emotional support and a family life continues despite financial loss. The wife may be able to work, if children are school age, and therefore have a stronger network of social relationships. Becoming the major decision maker and family head may need guidance but if the wife can assume some control of the situation it may be more tolerable. Difficulties arise if the wishes of the brain-injured individual, with limited insight and stubborn egocentricity, are not in the interests of the whole family. The wife will need to give her partner choices and a degree of control over his life, the right to make some decisions whenever possible or reasonable but not at the expense of herself and children. It can be difficult for a loving partner and family to accept that allowing the survivor to dominate, out of sympathy or loyalty, is not always reasonable or possible. Compensating for these losses may create a tyrant –

or lead to a loss of activity for a family trying to accommodate someone who is very unmotivated. Violence towards the family cannot be tolerated and wives should seek professional help to ensure home life remains stable for the children. During the rehabilitation process, family roles will have altered and adjusted to a different lifestyle. Adolescents will have assumed adult roles. This can be particularly difficult for boys when their brain-injured father returns home and expects to reassert authority. Adolescents change a great deal in a few years. This may place the father in a confrontational situation competing with adolescents to re-establish a superior and controlling position (Lezak, 1978). Adolescent children experience emotional upheaval in the most ordinary of families, as a normal process of adolescence. Extra conflict will be engendered if a child's new role as an adult family member is downgraded by the return home of a parent who is unable to understand his children have matured. It is also difficult for the wife to promote the return to a parental role of a survivor who may display childish embarrassing and obsessional behaviour, who is irritable with the children, and who insists on instant compliance with his wishes. Adolescents may be unwilling to bring friends home because of their father's behaviour. Their school work suffers and failure, especially at school examination time, can have far reaching effects. Adolescents may need the opportunity of individual as well as family counselling as they are often unable to admit they are not able to cope with conflict because they are loyal to both parents (Morton and Wehman, 1995).

Families cope better where behavioural problems are under control and physical recovery is reasonable (Brooks and McKinley, 1983), where pre-injury family bonds were strong and when the family can adopt a tolerant, more relaxed, attitude towards the survivor's difficulties. If the father has an important role within the family, and does not display the more obvious consequences of severe brain injury, it is possible to integrate him into the family's new life. Wives are often adamant that there is no other solution but to continue as a family. This is very evident in marriages where religious faith underpins family life.

Older partners with brain-injured husbands

In long-established marriages with husband and wife playing very traditional roles, it is more possible that a relationship will survive. The wife adopts a caregiver role towards her brain-injured husband. She may have adult children who can provide practical assistance and acknowledgment of stress, together with a system of shared care, which allows the wife some respite. If the couple have established social contacts in a familiar neighbourhood there is less likelihood of social isolation. Again, wives may need some assistance in taking on a more dominant head of family role but many respond to new challenges and are unwilling to let the injured partner remain in hospital or nursing home care. Residential care is no longer financed by the UK social security system and can be very expensive. Families are unwilling to see family homes sold to meet the cost of long-term residential care. Social Services may be able to provide care at home services to support the couple.

If a couple retired and moved to a new area prior to the brain injury, and do not have an established circle of friends, it may be less easy for a wife to care for her husband. If her partner has socially unacceptable and disturbed behaviour the caregiver role can be isolating and lead to depression. The possessive and obsessional characteristics caused by brain damage can cause the caregiver to feel imprisoned, restricted in all usual activities.

The difficulties experienced are similar to those of families caring for an elderly member suffering from Alzheimer's disease. Alzheimer's disease is increasingly a topic of media attention but services are underdeveloped despite this and the distress involved in caring for sufferers can be very debilitating. Partners of people with Alzheimer's disease usually find ways of keeping the sufferer at home for as long as is possible, often explaining that they have a loyalty to a previously affectionate long marriage which prevents them considering any alternatives. Local Alzheimer's disease societies offer companionship and services to support couples and families. The older woman is more used to the housekeeping, nursing and care giving role which enables her to continue supporting a loved partner. Women have stated that a husband with an acquired brain injury is entitled to the same care from their wives as would have been necessary if they had developed dementia in old age (Corcoran, 1992).

The husband of a brain-injured woman

There is currently less available research and information about what happens to families where young married women suffer from brain injury. The ratio of women to men acquiring brain injury is one in three. Experience suggests that the marriages of young brain-injured women rarely survive the separation caused by lengthy hospitalization and rehabilitation. These young women once again become the responsibility of their parents. Efforts to involve young or recently married husbands in the rehabilitation programme may postpone the breakdown of the relationship but men have to resume employment and are less able to remain closely involved. They are less likely to be able to look after their brain-injured wives at home. Young men return, during the wife's hospitalization, to a bachelor existence, or home to their own parents in order to be able to continue in employment. If the wife remains in a rehabilitation unit for some years the young husband will be in need of companionship and may form new relationships. New emotional alliances are not without complication. There is enduring guilt involved in separating from a brain-injured partner and the husband may have to deal with a lack of understanding, resentment or anger from the wife's relatives. They may feel he is walking away from a situation whilst they are taking on responsibilities as a result of his action. It can be painful to face such criticism when separation has become inevitable and where the marriage had not been problem free or secure prior to the incident causing brain injury to the wife.

In more established marriages, perhaps where there are young children, husbands of brain-injured women have more need to remain involved, and do so, often supporting them in quite testing situations at home with surprising ease and tolerance. This may be because they are expected and helped to bring in domestic assistance whereas women expect to be the major caregivers (Corcoran, 1992). The wider family may provide respite care, housekeeping and child care. This enables husbands to remain with a brain-injured partner and their children and to continue to cope with the changed domestic situation. Employment does not necessarily provide men with social networks, in the way women perceive these, but it provides activity, company and financial viability which makes the family situation more tolerable. There is a somewhat better chance of the family continuing to live together.

The brain-injured individual and the extended family

Grandparents and grandchildren are often more tolerant of difficult behaviour and the different post-injury personality of a brain-injured individual, and can find ways of supporting and assisting the immediate family. As is often evident in family life, the relationship between grandparent and child is more relaxed, and one step removed from the emotional bond and interaction between parent and child. This distance can be helpful. The relationship between the brain-injured person and a grandparent or grandchild may not be as confronting as that between parent and child. Help is offered to the major family caregivers by the extended family, who may live in the neighbourhood and are therefore able to give practical help and respite care. Sometimes families need advice from counsellor or social workers to develop care routines, offering help with domestic tasks, or simply giving those most closely caught up with daily care to have some time for relaxation and recreation. Their acceptance of the brain-injured individuals opens the way to provide stimulus and entertainment and add positively to their lives.

The single brain-injured individual

This review has portrayed some frequently encountered family scenarios. The outcome for single people is more serious, because they have no family to be involved in their rehabilitation process. The range of people who suffer brain injury includes single people, single parents and those who are widowed or divorced. Because of the absence of family involvement the rehabilitation team becomes the support of the single survivor. As with physical and mental illness it is the social worker in the clinical team who takes the lead in planning a survivor's community discharge, this places a particular responsibility on professionals where the single patient is especially vulnerable, may not be able to make decisions, and has no family to guide the team and protect the patient's interests. Single people lose their homes, jobs and friends and are at risk of suicide post-discharge, if they are depressed and socially isolated. Often an attachment forms to the clinical team, more than to other patients, as the team approach indicates tolerance of problems and inappropriate behaviour. If the rehabilitation unit offers an active, constructive programme and the individual enjoys a sense of belonging to groups who share therapy and entertainment, the patient begins to identify with staff and patients as within a family. Prior to admission to specialist rehabilitation units, patients may have been inappropriately placed on acute surgical or orthopaedic wards, or in psychiatric hospitals. Their acting out, disturbed and aggressive, behaviour may have resulted in sedating drug therapy as the only treatment approach. It is not surprising that after arriving at an appropriate brain-injury unit, the survivor may sense they are understood and accepted. This results in an entirely natural anxiety at the prospect of having to leave the security of the unit and attempts at discharge planning are seen as a threat. It is not inconceivable that some patients interrupt progress and resort to more acting out behaviour to demonstrate their lack of preparedness to move on. The social worker needs to have developed a relationship with the survivor – to help the transition to the community. Having identified possible resources, in conjunction with a community key worker, the social worker, ideally, should introduce the individual to the residential unit and arrange several visits there before discharge and continue to visit, if possible, until they feel the patient has settled into the new environment. If a compensation award is available, a case manager can be involved and can continue a long-term monitoring of the individual's needs. Where family support is not available the brain-injured individual needs an advocate to protect their interests and, if case management is not appropriate, a disability social worker should be appointed to carry out this role.

Children with severe brain injury and their parents
If a child suffers a severe brain injury, both parents and child become locked in a time warp. Parents will feel a high degree of responsibility, especially if they feel they played any part in the incident leading to the brain injury. They may adopt a continuing role as parent, making this a life-long burden. If appropriate help is not available or acceptable to parents, they focus on the injured child, sometimes to the exclusion of other children or family members. Brain injury inhibits emotional growth and with an emphasis on physical rehabilitation, it is usual for the injured child to mature at a much slower rate than their peer group (Gratten and Eslinger, 1992; Thomsen, 1992). The brain-injured child may have difficulty in relating to others, or be unable to feel or express concern or affection. They may be unmotivated and unable to achieve independence. It is not surprising that usual childhood and adolescent stages are not achieved and parent and child become caught in a pattern of mutual emotional dependency. Parents become afraid to let the brain-injured child explore their environment in case an accident causes further injury. They fear the child's irresponsible and immature behaviour may get them into trouble, especially if the child is sexually disinhibited. Parents can have difficulty in managing irritability and temper outbursts in the child, or dealing with demands for instant affection or gratification. Conciliatory strategies reinforce the child's unacceptable behaviour. Concentration on the child's needs, to the exclusion of other family and friends, can cause serious marital disharmony and resentment by siblings. It is not unusual to find unhappy adults managing the care of a young brain-injured person who dominates their lives. There is a need for far more provision for brain-injured children to assist their families. In the UK this is provided by only a few centres, geographically unavailable to most families needing specialist care for their brain-injured children. Parents sometimes eventually separate, with the mother usually taking the major responsibility for the welfare of the child. If a family does remain together the stresses they experience because of the demands of the brain-injured child can produce tension and interpersonal

hostility which reflects on the lives of other children. Parents need advice, and help, to balance protection and care of their brain-injured child, with the acknowledgement of that child's needs to grow and develop into an independent individual, as far as is possible. Eventually, the child will need to leave the security of home, as they would have done if not injured. Instead of college, employment or marriage, these young people may move into hostels or residential communities, if they have achieved behavioural control, which offer some independence and peer groups. It is difficult for a parent to relinquish the main caregiver role, even if they appreciate not bearing the whole responsibility for the child's behaviour. If the child stays at home there is less opportunity for individual growth, for the parents as well. Parents may still wish to be responsible for their child but need to be encouraged to do this at a distance, giving love and encouragement, but letting the young person experience living in their own way. There will be opportunity for family celebrations and visits home, but the parents begin to lead a life of their own.

It should be emphasized that the family profiles described in this chapter are based on the experiences of a social worker and clinical team working with the survivors of severe brain injury and their families. Individual family difficulties common to those living with people who have suffered mild head injury are not discussed here, nor the problems of brain injury inflicted on babies and young infants by abusive parents. Interest is now shown by community family and child care social workers in evaluating the consequences of pediatric or juvenile brain injury on later individual or family functioning. This topic deserves further research and is not examined in this text.

THE FAMILY AND THE REHABILITATION TEAM

A rehabilitation team should establish ongoing contact with family and friends from the point of admission to planning the brain-injured person's care on discharge. This can be achieved by regular reviews of progress, and in working together on key issues. A family's experience of acute hospital care may not have been positive. Family members are often so deeply involved in the patient's physical care they find it difficult to stand back and let the clinical team do their work. Families can also be reluctant, even if they have had to live with major behavioural difficulties, to allow the brain-injured individual to be involved in a programme designed to help them achieve behavioural control. They may find it difficult to accept that without such programmes their relative may have to stay within locked environments, such as psychiatric hospitals. If extreme behavioural problems are ignored the family may eventually suffer breakdown and separate. Conversely, families may feel such relief at the admission to rehabilitation of their relative that they begin to withdraw entirely. Sometimes families hope that admission to hospital will achieve improvement in areas which were problematic pre-injury, so that eventual return home will be of an individual who is easier to live with (McLaughlin and Schaffer, 1985).

It is important that clinical and rehabilitation teams achieve a non-judgemental attitude to relatives. It is easy to perceive families as being difficult if they seem either overinvolved or do not immediately go along with the teams recommendations. Families may be very disillusioned by previous experiences of unsuccessful treatment or rehabilitation. They may equally be depressed by slow or negligible progress. They may not be able to believe any rehabilitation approach will achieve a more positive outcome. They may in fact be afraid to hope. Ordinary families experience extreme anxiety and stress as a result of brain injury to a member and may not be able to present themselves well to a new team under such conditions. Families may have developed their own coping strategies as discussed earlier in this text (see for example the family described in Chapter 12). These strategies may be caring but conciliatory and the brain-injured person has been able to dominate family life. The family may have become particularly concerned with the appearance, dress and physical health of the brain-injured person as these are areas over which they can have some control. They are, therefore, less than enthusiastic about team efforts to encourage self-care and independence. Families become critical about the patient's physical care and appearance in rehabilitation and get into conflict with the clinical team (McLaughlin and Schaffer, 1985; McLanghlin and Carey, 1991).

The family may also view anything less than a full recovery, for which they have been fighting, as a failure. All these family roles are hard to relinquish and the rehabilitation team should be careful in helping the family understand and accept realistic hopes for future progress (Birley and Hudson, 1983). Sometimes when a patient appears, to the clinical team, to be making considerable progress, it is disappointing if the family does not seem to appreciate the change. The family may not view gradual improvement as being sufficient and it is important to understand what role the brain-injured person played in the family before injury. The family, as well as the patient, need to be understood in their whole emotional and social context. The family has to find a new role for the survivor which is acceptable within the family.

THE SOCIAL WORKER AND THE REHABILITATION TEAM

The social worker is often the first member of the team to be deeply involved with the family of someone in rehabilitation. By finding out about the family and conveying the aims of the rehabilitation team to them, a working relationship develops. It can be helpful to gather a full individual and family social history, soon after the patient is admitted, but when family members have had some respite and are able to relax. It is comforting and helpful for the family to give information so that the team will understand something about the patient's personality and interests prior to injury. The need for social work services can be assessed and counselling and practical services can be offered, not only to the survivor but to their family and other individuals significant in the life of the brain-injured person.

Admission to a rehabilitation unit often allows the family an opportunity to take some time out for themselves, often for the first time since the injury which changed their lives. Partners, children, other relatives and friends, can begin to assess their own emotional reactions and anxieties about the future. The social worker has to be prepared for the fact that some families are still caught up in a process of grieving. If rehabilitation includes a reassessment and reduction in drug therapy, with resultant increase in activity and more acting out and dangerous behaviour, it may cause families real concern. They may feel progress is being lost.

An increase in physical mobility and functioning is welcomed as lessening the family's responsibility for care. At the same time it is possible that the family does not know how to relate to this independence, as they are unused to allowing the brain-injured individual freedom to make choices about their lifestyle. People who have become mobile may also appear less predictable and more dangerous. The family need information and advice about managing this new behaviour and need to feel involved with the team in rehabilitation. They need access to members of the team, the doctor and psychologist, physiotherapists, speech therapists, and occupational therapists, and nurses, as well as the social worker, and will need to be helped to understand physical, cognitive, and perceptual difficulties experienced by the survivor. This is most easily arranged in small family meetings with team members, but can involve family members attending some rehabilitation sessions to learn practical day-to-day management. It is also important that the family are encouraged to take time off from their problems, to take holidays, find recreational activities, to be free for at least some period of time from responsibilities and anxieties, perhaps for the first time for some years.

The social worker will also be considering some alternatives for future care and linking the family with community social services care management or independent case management, to begin to plan with the patient, as much as is possible, for a viable living situation in a community setting. If there are suitable resources in the survivor's home area, social services may well be able to carry out their responsibilities under the Community Care Act. The clinical team's social worker has to educate and inform colleagues in the community about which kind of services would best meet the survivor's needs. Encouraging innovative solutions that allow the survivor as much control over their own life as any limitations permit, is sometimes more difficult, but should remain the prime goal. Each brain-injured person is unique in their potential for recovery, personality, family relationships and life experience and the social worker needs the expertise of the rehabilitation team to support the family, and resources offered by community social services, to achieve the best possible outcome.

PLANNING FOR FUTURE NEEDS

Although social workers in both hospital- and community-based settings are familiar with the outcome of brain injury for the patient, the necessity for individual solutions for their families is less well understood.

Many patients with severe brain injury do not regain their full pre-morbid intellectual and social functioning and goals of rehabilitation need to be set which allow adjustment to a new way of life (Thomsen, 1981). Social workers, family and marital therapists traditionally expect to work towards the preservation of a family system, and it may be difficult for social workers, planning for the brain injured, to accept that to live apart from the family may be an option which is helpful to the family. In the UK most specialist brain-injury rehabilitation units have wide catchment areas and may not find it possible to offer extensive aftercare services. Support for the survivor and family should be life-long – not always intensive – but available when needed. Social workers who will be supporting survivors and families in the community should aim to become involved with them well before discharge into the community becomes an option. Reviews should include the patient, family and clinical team and all those who will be the community support team. This will aid in the transitional phase when options are becoming clearer and decisions are to be made. Survivor and family will decide if they are going to live together or independently. If the latter, then a choice has to be made. Is the survivor going to live semi-independently with appropriate levels of care, or with live-in carer, in a hostel or group home or a residential community? With an increasing emphasis on community care or transitional living facilities in the UK and USA large hospitals or residential homes, especially those designed to care for people with developmental disabilities, should not be considered an appropriate resource for those who have survived brain injury. If survivors are not going to live with family or independently with carers, they need small residential units. With as much individual space and privacy as can be managed, the survivor still needs a planned daily routine with activities and recreation designed to stimulate and encourage them, but within a home-like atmosphere. Staffing ratios need to be sufficient for daily needs but also to manage occasional residual difficult behaviour. Despite the continuing need to monitor behaviour and supervise activities, there has to be an emphasis on as much choice and freedom for the survivor as is possible, given their individual limitations. Where possible, and if acceptable to the survivor and family, sheltered or supported employment may be a worthwhile option. Job coaches and sympathetic employers may make employment possible and this will improve the individual's sense of self-worth and negate feelings of rejection (Skord and Miranti, 1994).

Survivor and family need to be given a great deal of assistance by the team social worker, and care manager or case manager, in considering and deciding upon the most ideal living arrangement for the brain-injured individual post rehabilitation. For many an acceptable outcome is to establish the survivor in a home of their own with live-in carers. Sometimes these carers will need to be qualified nurses, where physical disabilities demand that level of care, but residential care assistants can also provide excellent care. They do, however, need assessment, training and super-vision. The survivor needs a social worker or case manager to coordinate their care and provide continuity and the maintenance of good practice and high standards. Before the Community Care Act, in the UK care at home was usually only possible for survivors who had been awarded realistic levels of compensation awards. Now it is possible for social services in the UK to provide housing and care packages to allow the survivor to leave hospital. Social services care management assessment procedures do not always allow for accurate interpretation of the needs of individuals with brain injury and social workers specializing in this area tend to work only in or near neurological treatment or rehabilitation units.

If finance is available, through compensation for injury, the survivor can purchase their own home. This can be adapted, equipped and furnished for the survivor and they should be involved in these activities, making choices and enjoying the move into the community with as much participation as possible. If the survivor does not have their own home, and lives with the family, care must be taken to monitor the stress that care can produce (Lezak, 1988). Looking after an individual with a brain injury for months on end without respite or support will inevitably lead to a deterioration in all the relationships within the family. Behavioural problems and personality changes produce a higher level of stress than physical disability alone, and relatives report this does not improve with time (Brooks et al., 1986a). If a separate living arrangement is possible this stress can be removed, and if there are opportunities for a reasonable level of visiting by the family, guilt is not as evident. Both the survivor and their family will need considerable support in setting up and maintaining this kind of more physically distant relationship. Clinical or community social workers may be able to achieve this but much will depend on the personalities and strengths of those involved. Many severely impaired survivors are able to tolerate this type of more distant relationship possibly because the capacity for emotional response and their depth of feeling for the family is damaged (Weddel et al., 1980). If the survivor remains jealous and possessive, or hostile, such separate living arrangements and less intense relationships may not be so well tolerated. It may be necessary to encourage separate living accommodation for survivor and family but continuation of a friendly relationship may not be possible and the separation will have to be complete.

CONCLUSION

One in 300 families has a member with persistent disability and this is apt to cause secondary morbidity in family members, sometimes resulting in permanent disruption of relationships (Lancet, 1983). Severe brain injury is usually the result of unanticipated, sudden, events which radically change family life. Survivors continue to have perceptual and cognitive problems as well as physical disability and may not be able to express themselves as they would wish. They misinterpret and misperceive the reaction of the world towards them. Survivors experience frustration and become depressed and they are often socially isolated (Lezak, 1988). Survivors do not always understand that it is the consequences of brain injury that change their present personal and family relationships and reduces their capacity to make new ones. Successful emotional recovery after injury requires insight into problems and clear avenues of communication with others. The survivor may have difficulty in relating to family and friends, demonstrating their emotions in childish or overdemonstrative ways, causing grief and embarrassment to loved ones.

The report of the Royal College of Physicians (1986) described the then current crisis in the provision of care, treatment and rehabilitation for the brain injured. At the time the incidence of major brain injury in England and Wales was estimated as being about 7500 annually. The prevalence of severe brain injury was 150 per 100 000 population. Similar statistics apply in the USA and there has not been a significant reduction in the incidence of injury. Serious accidents happen to innocent bystanders, bicyclists and passengers in vehicles, as well as to those engaged in dangerous work or recreational activities. The report recommended the establishment of specialist services and recognized the need for urgent evaluation of services and research into the optimum organization of brain-injury rehabilitation, and into the techniques of cognitive and behavioural rehabilitation. It made little reference to the need for community residential facilities. It recommended day-care centres, employment and follow-up opportunities and referral to Headway (the UK equivalent of the United States Brain Injury Association).

In 1992 the Department of Health announced funding of £1 million pounds a year for 5 years to be allocated to 12 programmes involved in brain-injury rehabilitation. This was focused on people between 16 and 64, whose brain injury was caused by accident trauma, rather than medical conditions. The Department of Health reviewed five of these programmes in 1996 (Social Services Inspectorate, 1996). The purpose of these visits was to evaluate the contribution of personal social services to the work of the Department of Health funded rehabilitation teams enabling brain-injured people to re-enter their local community. The report highlighted the continuing problems of brain-injury survivors and their families, despite the increase in options and provisions.

Significantly, also in 1996, the United States House of Representatives passed the Traumatic Brain Injury Act. This legislation is intended to provide nearly $25 million over a 3-year period to monitor state grants for services, education and research into prevention treatment and rehabilitation (Goodale, 1997). The optimism in the 1980s and the emergence of more specialist rehabilitation services have been undermined in the 1990s by political change and budget constraints (Giles, 1994a; Leri, 1995). Periods of rehabilitation funded by health authorities in the UK are no longer open-ended. There is pressure on teams and patients to push rehabilitation programmes at a pace which may not be helpful to patient recovery. Families experience the pressures also and are made anxious by the financial pressures imposed by funding authorities. Survivors, despite their myriad problems, work in collaboration with therapists, with a level of determination that deserves support,

In the UK and the USA voluntary associations take a lead in providing support services. Headway is the main support and the major advocate for brain-injury survivors and families in the UK, and in the USA a similar role is played by the Brain Injury Association. The consequences of brain injury are life-long, and services need to be designed, and funded, to offer care in sufficient regional centres so that people can remain close to family and social networks. Ongoing professional services should include the maintenance of physical recovery and the monitoring of care and counselling services provided by outpatient therapists, case managers and specialist community social work teams.

14 COMMUNITY REINTEGRATION AFTER BRAIN INJURY

Catherine Johnson

BACKGROUND

Services for individuals who have suffered a brain injury have developed dramatically in the past 20 years. A paucity of resources post-surgery/injury and an increasing demand for rehabilitation, led to the development of acute rehabilitation services across the Western world but most particularly in the USA. As these services developed and more and more individuals benefited from acute rehabilitation, it became obvious that intensive rehabilitation followed by discharge and the dramatic plunge back into everyday life often led to a rapid loss of the gains made in a rehabilitation environment. Experts argued that intensive rehabilitation should be followed by a slow transitional move back into the community enabling the individual with a brain injury, his family and his community to plan and prepare for community re-entry and future life.

As a result, transitional rehabilitation units or subacute units began to develop providing cognitive, functional and behavioural treatment in a non-medical environment which concentrated on generalizing skills to everyday life in the outside world. However, increasing experience showed that for the severely damaged individual even this was not enough. More and more individuals who had received rehabilitation at both levels regressed because of the lack of follow-up, support and structure when they moved out of the rehabilitation environment. The concept of community reintegration driven by case management began to be developed as a way of trying to ensure and maintain the best quality of life for brain-injury survivors.

Return to the community is not a new concept. Over the years the majority of people with a brain injury have returned (often all too rapidly) to their homes and family; often, it must be agreed, following a Friday afternoon ward round in order to empty beds in busy neurosurgical or medical wards. A telephone call to arrange an ambulance, a handwritten discharge letter and if necessary a referral to the district nurse and *voilà* – the discharge is planned and executed. The individual with a brain injury is home and back in the community.

This chapter is not designed to provide a checklist of how to 'community reintegrate' nor is it intended to identify the components which make up a successful and good return to life in the community. The concept of community reintegration is too complex and too individual to be divided down into a set of components which would indicate to those without experience, or insight or imagination that if we combine (a), (b) and (c) then we get (z) (successful community reintegration). Instead, the chapter will concentrate on central issues and problems that any professional must face in trying to ensure the best community reintegration for the individual with a brain injury and his or her family.

What is community reintegration?

Community reintegration means different things to different people.

Neurosurgeon
An empty bed.

Therapist
The patient has reached a clinical plateau.
An end to their need to be involved.
A time to pass the patient to someone else.

The individual with a brain injury
The achievement of the goal to go home.

The family
The beginning of a new life.
Initial hope and euphoria, then rapid realization of the new reality of unfamiliar new problems and little support.

Family doctor
Who?
A lack of knowledge about the patient pre-injury.
Lack of knowledge/training about the long-term effects of brain injury leading to confusion and frustration.
Don't worry, we can still fix it.

Community reintegration does not mean returning to the pre-injury status quo. Yet often, when discharge is not planned supported and monitored, brain-injury survivors assume that they can return home to their families, their work and their hobbies and all will soon be 'back to normal'. They are reinforced in this by many sources including: their relatives' often stated belief that 'he will be all right' once he gets home, pressure from the employer to return to work as quickly as possible, pressure from friends to get out and about and enjoy themselves, pressure from spouses to take up the relationship where it left off.

Unplanned community reintegration does not work. Marital relationships break down; children of the family opt out of home life; return to work is usually unsuccessful and demoralizing; and friends rapidly disappear. The brain-injury survivor is left a stranger in his own land, misunderstanding, miscommunicating, and frustrated and angry.

Family members usually sooner or later realize that community reintegration is not about returning home as quickly as possible. It is not about picking up the old existence before it becomes a memory. Brain-injury survivors do not always realize this, and that realization, if it comes, may take a very long time.

Community reintegration is about planning and structuring a new way of life; keeping the aspects of the old life which have survived; holding on to hopes and dreams of the way life could be in the future while making the most of the services, resources, friends and family who may be here today.

COMMUNITY REINTEGRATION – HOW TO DO IT?

To construct a realistic approach to community integration after brain injury, it is useful to break down the process of integration into the key areas which must be considered rather than looking at the practical elements of integration. The practical elements vary so widely from individual to individual, that any simple 'how to do it' checklist is likely to be idiosyncratic, simplistic and unhelpful. Instead, the chapter will identify the process involved, the stages to go through, and the problems likely to be experienced by the professional trying to ensure best-quality community reintegration.

The mnemonic CAPTIVES is a useful way of capturing the central elements, while also describing the way many people with a brain injury feel about their life:

C   costs
A   assessment
P   planning, politics
T   teamwork, togetherness and time
I   information
V   viable and vulnerable
E   excellence
S   sabotage.

Costs of service provision – funding available

Successful community integration is not a cheap option. It can be more expensive than institutional living in financial, personal and emotional terms, although the precise financial costs are often spread widely across different 'suppliers' (health, social services, voluntary/charitable sector) and are therefore very difficult to estimate precisely. Community reintegration may be seen as impossible if funds are not available (e.g. from a compensation award) and, in that case, those responsible for the injured person may consider that the easy option is to allow him or her to remain where they are without considering the costs (often very high in real terms) of this decision.

There are services in the community which will have little or no direct cost to the individual, for example services provided by local social services, local education departments, local health services, religious organizations and voluntary groups. However the network of services which these groups provide is inevitably limited and is usually not focused upon the needs of the person with brain injury. Using such services will undoubtedly involve a significant cost to the 'purchaser' in terms of education of the service provider, without which, the services will not be able to support someone with a brain injury. Furthermore, such services are usually only an ancillary part of the full range and network of support required to facilitate community reintegration.

So, there are several cost questions which the professional must ask and answer satisfactorily;

1 what are the 'real' and the total costs of services which are needed to facilitate high-quality community reintegration for the individual with a brain injury?
2 where does this funding come from?
3 is the available funding sufficient to provide support and facilitate community integration?
4 if not, what then?
5 what are the 'hidden' costs to the family, carers, community?
6 how can costs be controlled and maintained at an economic level while maintaining quality?
7 'economic' to whom?

Assessment

In order to answer the above questions and to plan successful and quality reintegration, there must be an appropriate and informed assessment. This must address:

1 the current situation
2 previous background, activities and behaviour
3 future aspirations, needs and costs.

A good and full assessment is an essential first step in successful community reintegration. It should be completed by someone who is experienced in the field of brain injury and their experience should include resettling individuals into the community. Perhaps most importantly this assessor should be the key individual in the injured person's community reintegration. This puts an obligation on the assessor to ensure that the assessment recommendations are achievable and realistic. An analysis of the costs involved should be an integral part of the assessment. An informed assessment ensures that the professional:

1 has a clear picture of the individual with whom he or she is working
2 has identified the important people and things in that individual's life, and
3 can trace a path to where the individual is today, and
4 give a choice of directions which the person may wish to take.

Clinicians have developed a variety of assessment tools which relate specifically to their professional expertise. Frequently such assessments are focused on symptoms (impairment) rather than disabilities or handicaps. Yet the key issue for community reintegration is functional competence and the services which are necessary and available to facilitate that competence. The assessment for community reintegration should be specific to the needs of the brain-injured individual.

The results of the assessment must be incorporated into any 'multidisciplinary' assessment which may have been carried out to give a global and holistic overview of the problems which an individual may encounter, the strengths they may have and the ways these may best be approached.

Planning

Planning the move back in to the community is crucial, and the assessment should enable specific plans to be constructed. Too often people with brain injury are launched from the acute hospital or even acute rehabilitation facility into the apparent service vacuum which is the community. Planning is essential to ensure that the statutory services, voluntary and charitable services, and community activities are available, and that the personnel likely to be involved are trained and in place before the individual returns to the community.

Making a plan

The plan should contain clear and practical answers to the following central questions of community reintegration:

1 accommodation
   (a) should the individual return to the care of their family?
   (b) should they return to their own home if they were living alone previously?
   (c) does this accommodation still exist?
   (d) is group accommodation an option or perhaps a stepping stone?
   (e) if so, who pays?

2 care
   (a) how much care/supervision/support is needed?
   (b) who will provide that support or care?
   (c) who pays?
   (d) who will supervise and train the people providing this?
   (e) what does the individual want in terms of care?
   (f) will they have a choice?

3 daily activity
   (a) can the individual return to full-time employment?
   (b) in the same job?
   (c) in the same company?
   (d) for the same amount of time?
   (e) if not, are they capable of other employment?
   (f) on their own?
   (g) with support?
   (h) if they cannot work what are the options for meaningful and satisfying day-to-day activities?
   (i) is the individual happy to consider these?

4 family and friends
 (a) what is the role of the family?
 (b) who in the family is prepared/able to provide support?
 (c) is this acceptable to the individual themselves?
 (d) have previous friends disappeared?
 (e) are there any other social support networks?
 (f) does everyone involved truly have the injured person's best interests at heart?
 (g) if not, what then?

5 aids and adaptations
 (a) what does the individual expect to do in the community?
 (b) what therefore will be needed in the way of equipment such as wheelchairs, hoists, transport, computers to facilitate community integration?
 (c) will the equipment help to maximize independence?
 (d) will the accommodation of choice need to be adapted?
 (e) can it be adapted?
 (f) is the accommodation, equipment, etc., acceptable to the individual?
 (g) can/should current equipment in the accommodation be adapted to enable the individual to use it easily and safely?

6 what's missing?
 (a) is there anything I have missed?
 (b) every individual has different needs and aspirations, what are the extras particular to that person which are necessary to facilitate their unique integration?

Politics

P is also for 'politics' which can have a dramatic effect on community integration. In the macro sense, national and local politics influence the funding and resources available in the fields of health, social services and education. The move to 'Care in the Community' in the UK illustrates the changes which can be politically led and influenced. Similarly the unification of Germany has influenced the availability of resources available across the board in Germany in the field of brain-injury rehabilitation. In the USA, there has also been political influence on health-care provision.

In the micro sense, professionals, families and people with a brain injury can also exert a 'political' influence on service provision. A UK example is the continuing tension between the public sector services of 'socialized medicine and the independent (private companies, and charities who make a charge for their services) sector. There is still a reluctance in some public sector areas and by some public sector professionals to use independent sector resources even if the public sector services are unable to meet the needs of a particular individual. Such reluctance can be deeply and emotionally held, and very difficult to change. Yet change it must if the person with a brain injury is to have the best possible chance of highest quality community reintegration. Resolving such conflicts and reducing such reluctance will often need external intervention such as that by a case manager.

Teamwork, togetherness and time

Teamwork and togetherness

Successful community reintegration can only be achieved if everyone involved – the individual, the family, professionals, and other employed staff – work together and agree the 'plan' mentioned previously. They should form an *ad hoc* team with the injured person as the central member of that team.

Communication between team members is essential to ensure continued and appropriate liaison with all involved so that no one, especially the individual with the brain injury, feels isolated, marginalized, or resentful. Open and honest communication also acts as a check or balance to help all those involved to understand their own roles and the roles of everyone else; and to prevent the 'knee-jerk' reactions to events or actions which are common, often driven by professional rivalry, and potentially destructive to the well-being of the person with a brain injury.

Honest communication and successful teamwork are an uphill battle, an ongoing issue and a constant struggle. Communication and teamwork are not once-and-for-all activities and they do not 'just happen'. Setting up and training the team which includes the individual and their family requires constant ongoing input and review to ensure that they all continue to work together; to make any changes which may be needed; to provide support to individual team members; and to make plans for the future. Successful teamwork is not a case of 'letting them get on with it'!

Time

Time is an ally in the recovery process. Clinical improvement may continue for a prolonged period despite the gloomy predictions of acute medical staff who have a time perspective of days or weeks rather than months or years. With time can come increased awareness for the person with a brain injury.

Community reintegration takes time. Time for assessment and planning. Time to acquire accommodation and to adapt that accommodation. Time to find services and appropriate professionals. Time to talk and find out what the individual needs, wants or requires.

The importance of time is usually underestimated. Professionals are used to managing their time, and rationing the time that they are able to give to the individuals with whom they work. An individual returning to a new life in the community needs more time than most professionals realize in order to make sense of their new life. That individual will have fears, anxieties, concerns and hopes that the professional must take time to identify, articulate and manage.

Information

> *'Knowledge is power'*

Access to information empowers individuals to make their own decisions to take control of their life. This 'taking control' is a central key to reducing frustration and increasing self-esteem and life satisfaction.

Information is not solely the property of professionals, and part of the professional role is education, enabling people with brain injury and their families to have the information/knowledge which is necessary for them to make informed decisions about their future life. The words 'I don't know but I shall find out for you' should be a routine part of the professional vocabulary enabling a 'win–win' in which the professional person's knowledge is increased, and the brain-injured person's choices are increased and better informed

Access to information also gives rise to 'ideas' and 'initiatives'. The person who does not know what is available or what is possible will not realize that there may be many alternative opportunities open. The brain-injured person or family member who knows what the options are may be able to take an 'initiative' or at least have an 'idea' about what they wish to do

For example, an individual with a brain injury may be frustrated that his family goes on holiday while he has to go into respite care. If he knows that he can go on holiday with his care staff, and hire the aids and equipment to enable him to do so, he can take the initiative and plan a holiday for himself. The person with a brain injury begins to put power and control back where it belongs – in his or her own hands.

Viable and vulnerable

Any plan for community integration must be viable and realistic. The process of accessing, costing, funding, communicating and working together will fall apart if the planning process is working towards an unrealistic goal – for example the goal of walking in a person who's neurological damage is such that they will never walk again. All too often professionals collude together in hiding unpleasant realities from a person with a brain injury, and such miscommunication prevents high quality community reintegration.

The viability of every aspect of planning and implementing community integration must be assessed at every stage, discussed openly and honestly and then, and only then, can the plan be put into action.

V also stands for vulnerability. A person who has had a severe brain injury is exceptionally vulnerable, particularly so when large sums of money may be involved. The person who is a 'patient' under the terms of the 1983 Mental Health Act in the UK is, to some extent at least, automatically protected. However, many very badly damaged people are not competent to manage their own affairs, yet are not considered to be a 'patient', often because the examining medical practitioner is inexperienced in brain injury. Vulnerability exists in all areas of the brain-injured person's life – financial, social, sexual, emotional and physical. Any community reintegration plan should explicitly recognize this vulnerability and put in place systems to protect the injured person.

Excellence

Professionals have an obligation to provide a service which is committed to excellence. Professionals have an absolute obligation to provide the highest quality of service. They have an obligation to provide for others the service they would expect for themselves or members of their family.

Professional standards and accreditation do address this issue by giving professional staff a standard to live up to and to measure themselves by. However the commitment of providing an excellent service is also very much a personal one. Standards cannot account for the way individual professionals relate to the people with whom they/we work, whether they/we like the patient/client or not; and whether they/we are prepared to go the 'extra mile' to ensure the success of their community integration beyond the limits of our professional standards.

E also stand for 'eye on the ball' which relates back to the issue of teamwork. The process of community reintegration is dynamic and for many people with a severe brain injury it will continue for the rest of that person's life. Routine and normal life events can influence the success of this process from the basic problems of a leaking washing machine to the serious distress which may occur at the death or separation of a family member. it is crucial to consider community reintegration as an ongoing process which demands constant vigilance to be successful. The person with a severe brain injury is a very vulnerable person.

Sabotage

Successful community reintegration is achieved through an intricate, and often delicate, web of services and support. It can easily be damaged, often unintentionally and often in unforeseen ways, by anyone involved in either providing or receiving these services, with long-term consequences. Teamwork and communication are essential in order to ensure that all those involved (the person with the injury, the family, professionals and volunteers) are working together, in the same way and towards the same goal. Differences of opinion about, for example, going to a nightclub with a carer; who makes the choice of care staff; daily timetables; return to work; or even contraception, can undermine the support system for an individual in the community and lead to failure.

However there is also the possibility of intentional sabotage, perhaps for all the right reasons, in a situation where professionals, volunteers, families or indeed the person who has had an injury disagree about the way forward.

CONCLUSIONS

Community reintegration after brain injury is a complex process requiring careful planning from the first day after an individual has suffered a brain injury. It requires knowledge of the problems that people experience after injury and also a flexibility to deal with these problems on an individual basis. It requires access to resources and to funding for those resources; and it requires patience and tenacity from all those involved.

However it is not a one-off activity moving an individual from hospital to home. Community reintegration is a continuous process which needs constant monitoring throughout the rest of the injured persons' life – it never ends.

15 FUTURE DIRECTIONS IN BRAIN-INJURY REHABILITATION

Gordon Muir Giles

INTRODUCTION

Since the first edition of this book there has been considerable progress in the prevention of brain injury and in the care of brain-injured people. However, 50% of all deaths from trauma involve brain injury, which remains the leading cause of death in people under 25 years of age. Persistent public education, enforcement efforts and media attention has made driving while intoxicated socially unacceptable and the use of cycle and horse-riding helmets acceptable or, in some places, mandatory. The use of seatbelts has, in many parts of the world, been mandated by law and airbags are becoming more widespread with an associated decrease in mortality. Advances have continued in early medical management with more people surviving brain injury. Advanced imaging techniques help in the management of the complications which can follow brain injury. Functional imaging technology such as functional magnetic resonance imaging (MRI) and single positron emission computed tomography (SPECT) have not yet been used for routine diagnostic purposes but show great promise, while computerized tomography (CT) and MRI have become routine. Protocols have been developed to reduce the effects of secondary injury and are receiving more widespread application. There is an initial focus on ensuring oxygenation and perfusion, intubation when necessary and aggressive management of intracranial pressure (Silvestri and Aronson, 1997).

New imaging techniques and new theories of how the brain functions are providing increased insight into the neurophysiology that underlies the disorders which follow brain injury. The discipline of cognitive neuroscience has increased our understanding of cognitive functioning and offers the prospect of greater precision in the diagnosis and the development of treatment targeted to specific syndromes (see Chapter 10). The boundary between the study of cognitive processes and neuroscience has been breaking down. As a result, our understanding of cognitive processes are increasingly informed by our beliefs about how the brain works. In the 1970s and 1980s the dichotomy between thought and brain was captured by the analogy with software and hardware in computing. This distinction is now recognized as artificial as real-time brain imaging allows the observation of the brain activity correlates of cognitive operations (Smith, 1997) and there is increased recognition of the plasticity of adult brains in response to experience.

The development of models of cognitive processes can be misleading if this is separated from the understanding of how brains actually perform functions. The development of logical or mathematical models should be constrained by the structural and processing nature of brains. Logic and mathematics while essential to the construction of computers do not in any direct way characterize 'the machine language' of brains. While therapeutic protocols based on these computer-like models of mind may be helpful their effect is most likely by imposing a secondary regulatory structure (a metacognitive regulatory routine).

There has recently been considerable attention paid to the hypothesized evolutionary advantages of consciousness (Edelman, 1992; Churchland, 1995; Deacon, 1997). From the perspective of the rehabilitationist the role of conscious processing is central in learning. Conscious awareness allows for accelerated mapping of environmental events. It allows events that are distant in space and time to constrain current behaviours (this capacity is thought to be subserved by the frontal lobes and is therefore often termed somewhat indiscriminately 'frontal lobe functioning'). The selective focus provided by conscious attention may also accelerate learning as it allows for rapid changes in patterns of responding. Conscious attention is however capacity limited and effortful and could be seen as a stage in the development of less capacity-limited and more automatic-association systems. Its rapidity and the degree of abstraction in relationships which it is capable of mapping also make it very prone to error (i.e. the mapping of relationships that do not exist). This mapping of erroneous relationships is not confined to conscious learning processes (see, for example, Skinner, 1948).

Dennett (1991) has described the 'user illusion' of consciousness, i.e. any being capable of describing its internal states or accounting for its own behaviour would believe itself conscious (pp. 310–311). A similar phenomenon might be considered to exist in regard to learning and could be called a 'learner illusion'. A person intent on learning will believe that it is the attempt to learn that allows learning to occur. New learning may involve effortful attention but there has been, in the author's view, an overemphasis on conscious learning in skill development. Most conscious and highly skilled performance (reading, speaking, playing tennis) is performed without conscious awareness of the subprocesses involved. When a skilled reader reads, the process of reading is effortless with conscious processing only of the content. Conscious learning processes are very important in most people's acquisition of skills but more as 'stage setters' and facilitators. The majority of learning occurs elsewhere. In highly skilled performance, conscious awareness may impede performance (see, for example, Deacon's theory of the importance of poor episodic memory in language acquisition, Deacon, 1997). Multiple systems, only some of which are cognitively mediated, are involved in the development of skilled human behaviour. These various processes are not distinguished by users and are experienced as seamless in most learning tasks (people habitually disregard the common disjunction between cognition and behaviour). Our awareness of the cognitive processes results in their relative contribution to learning being overemphasized. The implicit/explicit distinction is increasingly recognized in studies of awareness but is only now being addressed in practical approaches to skill development in brain-injured people.

There are many instances of double dissociation of learning and awareness (Weiskrantz, 1997). Information can be grasped consciously but does not influence behaviour and information can be neglected consciously but result in changes in behaviour. We have described a number of patients with brain damage who have been taught very complex practical tasks which they have been able to perform successfully but of which they have no awareness (Giles and Clark-Wilson, 1993; Giles, 1998). Conscious processes can also impede learning. Patients who fail to recognize their deficits or those who believe that the rehabilitation specialist is in error, does not like them or are just getting at them, are unlikely to learn new skills even when they engage in the tasks. The individual's perceptions of the process of rehabilitation should be a deliberate focus of the therapist's interventions.

Future studies will reveal more about how experience changes human brain functions and structure. We will hopefully learn more about how best to potentiate these changes.

DEVELOPMENTS IN REHABILITATION

Wade *et al.* (1997, 1998) have demonstrated the importance of providing support services to individuals with mild to moderate brain injury after hospital discharge. The authors found significant reduction in post-concussive symptoms and problems in psychosocial functioning in response to limited support services. The studies by Wade *et al.*, and a study reported by Powell and Greenwood (1998), are significant because they are the first prospective randomized control trials in brain-injury research and they show that adding outreach services to patients after discharge from rehabilitation can improve psychosocial outcome and some aspects of community functioning (Wade *et al.*, 1997, 1998) but they are not studies of rehabilitation effectiveness. To date there have been no comparable studies of the effectiveness of rehabilitation following severe brain injury. Although outcome studies are important many new treatment techniques have come from small-scale or multiple baseline designs which are neither financially or logistically prohibitive. The subspecialty of brain-injury rehabilitation is beyond the stage of development where it is expected that one type of treatment will be effective with all people at all stages in the recovery process (Chapter 4 makes this point explicitly in regard to behaviour management in the acute stage of recovery).

New medications have become available (antidepressants, antiseizure and antipsychotics) and a marriage of pharmacological and behavioural interventions holds the prospect for helping patients who have previously proved to have intractable neurobehavioural disorders. Behavioural interventions have become more sophisticated and new positive approaches allow for management of behaviour disorders with less stress on the patient, family and those providing care (Chapter 4). Although errorless approaches have been used extensively with individuals with learning disabilities (Jones and Eayrs, 1992) it has taken advances in our theoretical understanding of learning for these approaches to become widely used in neurological rehabilitation (but see Giles and Clark-Wilson, 1988a, b; Giles and Morgan, 1989). What are essentially errorless approaches to behavioural control (Burke *et al.*, 1988), compliance training (Slifer *et al.*, 1997) and specific skills training (Wilson *et al.*, 1994; Giles *et al.*, 1997) have been developed for use in neurological rehabilitation. In errorless approaches the training techniques used minimize the potential for the patient to propagate errors (Giles and Clark-Wilson, 1988a, b; Giles *et al.*, 1997). Individuals who possess intact episodic memory can use their recall of a failed strategy to suppress it and to try and alternate strategy (trial-and-error learning). For individuals with amnesia or impaired memory functioning the propagation of an error actually increases its availability and so increases the likelihood that it will be repeated (Giles and Clark-Wilson, 1993). A behaviour or thought increases in availability based on the frequency with which it is rehearsed (this is a central principle of cognitive behaviour therapy).

While implicit learning has been demonstrated experimentally using these methods the patient's ability to spontaneously engage in the task appears related to overlearning of the response. In cases where this is achieved the patient becomes aware of the information, an implicit-to-explicit recall threshold is crossed (Giles and Morgan, 1989; Kime *et al.*, 1997 and commentary by Giles and Hausmann, 1997). Wilson and Evans (1996) have demonstrated the superiority of errorless learning over traditional methods for training amnestic subjects to recall word lists and also report superiority of errorless learning in the training of functional tasks (Wilson *et al.*, 1994).

In the staging of interventions a number of recommendations can be made. As a rule of thumb, antecedent or stimulus control strategies will predominate in the very acute stage of recovery or with the profoundly impaired client (although the desired behaviour once elicited can be reinforced). Behavioural training techniques focusing on habituation and priming will also be used. As the stage of acute confusion resolves a stimulatory approach may assist patients to function at the highest level permitted by their degree of neurological-driven recovery. Where patients continue to demonstrate significant deficits in functional behaviours a specific skills building approach may be adopted. Even profoundly memory impaired people can acquire important functional behaviours through well-designed and obsessively executed skills training programmes. Behavioural control can also be considered a skill which is in many cases susceptible to training. Even following the stage of early rehabilitation the management of behaviours by antecedents continues to be important. However, as rehabilitation progresses patients are able to map regularities in their environment and operant and cognitive behavioural approaches assume greater importance. At all stages of recovery, if a skill is to be maintained, it must be complete (i.e. really functional) and supported by spontaneously occurring environmental reinforcers (or the subject of a maintenance programme). Where these conditions apply, skills acquired by behavioural training have been found to be extremely robust (Lloyd and Cuvo, 1994).

For individuals with mild to moderate impairment, addressing the individual's metacognitive model of their own cognitive processes assumes increased importance. An incongruent metacognitive model may often thwart a well-designed behavioural training programme. Cognitive behaviour therapy is the most clearly articulated system for changing specific unhelpful explanatory models. However, when changes in cognition are considered to be an important part of the intervention, these changes should be clearly defined and specific. Most of the interventions described in this book contain a 'cognitive overlearning element', 'inconvenience training', 'motivational interviewing' or some other means to address the patient's skill-related cognitions. In some instances the primary goal of the intervention is to alter the patient's cognitions in a specific domain. An example of this is cognitive behaviour therapy for lack of insight. Here, as in every other training intervention, the goals of the interventions should be specific and address areas where lack of insight produces specific functional or behaviour problems. In most instances understanding what is important to the patient, an exploratory rather than a punitive or demanding approach, and knowing how the patient construes their situation is important to the success of the rehabilitative effort. People remember what they think, not what the therapist says. If the way individuals recovering from brain injury think about themselves and their place in the world is not a focus of rehabilitative efforts, therapeutic interventions are less likely to be effective.

Central to the production of any cognitive or behavioural change is practice. Any behaviour (or thought) increases in its availability to the individual depending on the frequency with which it is repeated (the more an individual thinks something the more likely they are to think it again) (Ross, 1977). Patients (and therapists) tire of practising a task long before the practice has ceased to be beneficial. It is part of the skill of the therapist to identify the essential components of a task and to maintain the patient's motivation to practice. Learning is difficult, so it is essential to minimize the amount of learning that needs to take place.

Little recognition is typically given to the manipulation of the interpersonal environment in rehabilitation. Partly this is because the effects of the interpersonal environment are difficult to quantify and potential effects on outcome even more difficult to demonstrate. Much can be communicated to a patient via the rehabilitative culture. This culture can be seen as the container or background against which therapy takes place. It can serve as a support structure for staff as well as patients. Giles and Clark-Wilson (1993) have described a therapeutic community for brain-injured people. The aims of this social/interpersonal environment were to provide a secure and accepting milieu which focused on patient achievements, maintain focus on rehabilitative goals, the development of a personally relevant way to talk about the problems experienced after injury, and the maintenance of a positive attitude towards concrete therapeutic outcomes (see also Ponte-Allan and Giles, in press).

The most effective interventions following brain injury continue to be practical, in that they address real world tasks directly. Newer evaluation instruments attempt to be 'ecologically valid' and many of these are excellent for identifying the nature of patient problems (Wilson, B.A. et al., 1991; Robertson et al., 1994). However fundamental problems are often still only revealed by real world assessment procedures (Sirigu et al., 1995). At the time of the publication of the first edition of this book there was a great deal of excitement about computer-based cognitive retraining. The use of computers continues, but it is not the panacea initially envisioned (Chen et al., 1997). There is very little evidence supporting the belief that rehabilitative efforts need to address cognitive skills prior to addressing functional skills (Chen et al., 1997). There are some attempts to use computers to remediate real world deficits but most rehabilitation needs to address day-to-day problems encountered by brain-injured people in the real world in a way not possible using computers. As noted in Chapter 1, even when cognition is the central focus of post-acute rehabilitative efforts it is real world functioning, rather than cognitive functioning, that improves (Mills *et al.*, 1992; Giles and McMillan, in press). The development of measures which address the types of deficits which hamper community integration and direct attention to real functional goals is necessary for progress in post-acute rehabilitation. One of the editors of this book (GMG) has developed the Neurobehavioural Performance Scale, an adaptive behaviour rating scale for use with persons with traumatic brain injury. The scale is valid and reliable and can be completed by different disciplines and it is hoped that this measure can fill this gap in available measures.

THE STRUCTURE OF SERVICE PROVISION

Conditions for rehabilitation are often less than perfect and resources available to provide rehabilitation are often meagre. For many patients the funding of even minimally acceptable services remains problematic. There is a disjunction between the natural history of recovery following brain injury and the duration of services that third-party payers will fund. In the USA there is an accelerating trend for aggressive cost containment in brain-injury services and a contraction in the number of commercial service providers (Giles, 1994a) but in the absence of a central registry of providers this is difficult to quantify. California is recognized as the bell-wether for provision of health services in the USA. In the period 1991–1997 (the last year for which data are available) the number of programmes listed in the Brain Injury Associations directory for California fell by 50%. In the same time period providers of residential post-acute services fell by over 40% (National Head Injury Foundation, 1991, 1992, 1993, 1994, 1995; Brain Injury Association, 1996, 1997). In the absence of robust outcome data insurance carriers and particularly managed care providers are increasingly reluctant to fund post-acute services for the brain-injured survivor. The environment plays a key role in influencing behaviour. Continuing support for even severely brain-injured individuals is often lacking. Social isolation continues to be a major problem for many and community support services are in many places minimal or absent. Anything which can be learned can be unlearned, any insight which can be gained, can, if not supported, be lost. Rehabilitative and supportive interventions for many severely brain-injured people need to be long term and even life-long in many cases. Who pays for rehabilitation and care of the expanding group of patients with acquired neurological impairments remains a 'hot potato' amongst many agencies both public and private.

Both the efficacy and the cost-effectiveness of brain-injury rehabilitation may still reasonably be called into question (McGregor and Pentland, 1997; Giles and McMillan, in press). All might agree that some services need to be provided to brain-injured people but it is in each agency's interests for someone else to pay for them. Increasingly it is recognized that many services for brain-injured people need to be provided on a very long-term basis (Giles, 1994a–c). Brain-injured people continue to be vulnerable and many require a continuum of support in order to function on a day-to-day basis. Patients may need services increased periodically due to life events and the spontaneous variability of neuropsychiatric disorders following brain injury (Ben-Yishay *et al.*, 1987). Case management is recognized in the USA as an essential component of care however the impact of case management is under researched. In a study of acute case management in the UK, Greenwood and co-workers (1994) evaluated the effects of early case management for patients with severe traumatic brain injury (TBI). Although the case management increased the probability of contact with services and increased the range of services contacted, the actual duration of contact with therapy services was not increased. Outcome was not improved in the case management group on a range of measures from cognitive functioning to family burden. It is possible that the case management provided was unable to modify routine practices sufficiently to provide patients with any more effective treatment or that the actual services provided were so far below the level of service provision that would have made a difference that the case management was irrelevant. Greenwood *et al.* (1994) conclude from their study that case management cannot replace skilled specialist rehabilitative interventions. Long-term overall case management by a professional knowledgeable about traumatic brain injury is the exception rather than the rule.

The practice of TBI rehabilitation is affected by organizational and staff training issues. There is no single approach to brain-injury rehabilitation, and many of the models used by therapists tend to be discipline specific with different implications for treatment. Skills which most authorities in the field would agree are essential such as those of goal selection, observation, task analysis, behavioural management techniques, etc. may be absent entirely or covered only minimally in occupational therapy, physical therapy, speech therapy and nursing schools. There continue to be only a limited number of people with the requisite skills and there is limited experience or training hierarchy within brain-injury rehabilitation.

The development and implementation of interdisciplinary goals may be unfamiliar to staff, who may in addition have idiosyncratic notions of what constitutes appropriate treatment. Mozzoni and Bailey (1996) studied therapists whose patients were not progressing on the discipline specific goals identified for treatment on the functional independence measure. Therapists were given specific instruction and monitored on 14 treatment elements, such as prompting and reinforcement. Therapists were given feedback based on structured observation of their interventions. Despite some resistance from staff, the intervention was effective in modifying staff behaviour and led to improved goal attainment in patients. Interestingly a significant proportion of therapists were providing process skill activities rather than specific skills training in target skills (e.g. table-top perceptual motor tasks rather than actual training in skills such as dressing or bathing). Despite participation in multidisciplinary treatment planning and observation of patients failing to improve, staff were unable to independently modify their interventions. Three out of five therapists in the study of Mozzoni and Bailey (1996) were not working on outcome-related activities. The expertise and time is often not available to provide adequate supervision to staff. The institutional and hospital systems are usually constructed in a way which fractionates service provision and reduces the opportunity to develop a cadre of staff with a high level of expertise. The need for increased training in brain-injury rehabilitation is widely appreciated (Becker *et al.*, 1993). The need is recognized for both professional and paraprofessional staff, with educational content areas including cognitive deficits, behaviour modification techniques and family, psychological and social issues (Becker *et al.*, 1993).

Conventional service delivery models are often (if not always) inadequate in rehabilitation following traumatic brain injury and specialized services are preferable. Nonetheless improved outcome from specialized services is difficult to demonstrate. Given the evidence available it is perverse to deny the effectiveness of interventions with some patients but unfortunately despite our best efforts rehabilitative interventions may fail. Clinicians are very poor at distinguishing those individuals who are most likely to respond to treatment and this should be a focus of future research.

Patients should be referred directly to rehabilitation as periods of time in the community may cause lasting problems in regard to patients independence and self-confidence (Eames *et al.*, 1995; Stilwell *et al.*, 1998). Treatment should be provided in the context of a strongly led interdisciplinary team, with a clearly articulated philosophy, a structured treatment planning approach with goal setting and feedback regarding progress towards goal attainment on a regular and frequent basis. Goals set should be realistic and practical and if the intervention is not working it should be stopped (Stilwell *et al.*, 1998). Wherever possible services should be 'seamless' in so far as patients should be transferred to progressively less restrictive environments with continued support and the opportunity to have the level of support increased if they should begin to have difficulties. The disciplined design and obsessional application of functional interventions, that consider both the person and environmental context, can help those with brain injury lead meaningful and productive lives.

REFERENCES

Adams, J.H., Mitchell, D.E., Graham, D.I. and Doyle, D. (1977). Diffuse brain-damage of immediate impact type. Its relationship to 'primary brain-stem damage' in head injury. *Brain*, 100, 489–502.

Adams, J.H., Graham, D.I., Scott, G., Parker, L.S. and Doyle, D. (1980). Brain damage in fatal non-missile head injury. *Journal of Clinical Pathology*, 33, 1132–1145.

Aitken-Swan, J. and Easson, E.C. (1959). Reactions of cancer patients on being told their diagnosis. *British Medical Journal*, 1, 779.

Alderman, N. and Knight, C. (1997). The effectiveness of DRL in the management and treatment of severe behaviour disorders following brain injury. *Brain Injury*, 11, 79–103.

Alderman, N., Knight, C. and Morgan, C. (1997). Use of a modified version of the Overt Aggression Scale in the measurement and assessment of aggressive behaviors following brain injury. *Brain Injury*, 11, 503–523.

Aldwin, C.M. (1994). *Stress, Coping and Development*. New York: The Guilford Press.

Allen, R., Safer, D. and Covi, L. (1975). Effects of psychostimulants on aggression. *Journal of Nervous and Mental Disease*, 160, 138–145.

Anderson, C.V., Bigler, E.V. and Blatter, D.D. (1995). Frontal lobe lesions, diffuse damage and neuropsychological functioning in traumatic brain-injured patients. *Journal of Clinical and Experimental Neuropsychology*, 17, 900–908.

Andrews, T. K., Rose, F.D. and Johnson, D.A. (1988). Social and behavioural effects of traumatic brain injury in Children. *Brain Injury*, 12, 133–138.

Ansell, B.J., Keenan, J.E. and De la Rocha, O. (1989). *Western Neuro Sensory Stimulation Profile. Manual*. Tustin, CA: Western Neuro Care Center.

Arts, W.F.M., Van Dongen, H.R., Van Hof-Van Duin, J.V. and Lammens, E. (1985). Unexpected improvement after prolonged posttraumatic vegetative state. *Journal of Neurology, Neurosurgery and Psychiatry*, 48, 1300–1303.

Asikainen, I., Kaste, M. and Sarna, S. (1996). Patients with traumatic brain injury referred to a rehabilitation and re-employment programme: Social and professional outcome for 508 Finnish patients 5 or more years after injury. *Brain Injury*, 10, 883–899.

Avery-Smith, W. and Dellarosa, D.M. (1994). Approaches to treating dysphagia in patients with brain injury. *American Journal of Occupational Therapy*, 48, 235–239.

Avorn, J. and Langer, E. (1982). Induced disability in nursing home patients: a controlled study. *Journal of the American Geriatrics Society*, 30, 397–400.

Azrin, N.H., Sneed, T.J. and Fozz, R.M. (1974). Dry-bed training: rapid elimination of childhood enuresis. *Behavior Research and Therapy*, 12, 147–156.

Babinski, M.J. (1914). Contribution a l'étude des troubles mentaux dans l'hémiplégie organique cérébrale (Anosognosie). *Revue Neurologique*, 12, 845–848.

Bach-y-Rita, P. (Ed.) (1980). *Recovery of Function: Theoretical considerations for Brain Injury Rehabilitation*. Baltimore, MD: University Park Press.

Bach-y-Rita, P. (1983). Introduction: Rehabilitation following brain damage: some neurophysiological mechanisms. *International Rehabilitation Medicine*, 4, 165.

Bach-y-Rita, P. and Bailliet, R. (1987). Recovery from stroke. In P.W. Duncan and M.B. Badke (Eds) *Stroke Rehabilitation: The Recovery of Motor Control*. Chicago, IL: Yearbook Medical Publisher.

Badke, M.B. and Di Fabio, R.P. (1991a). Sensory information and movement: Implications for intervention. In P. Montgomery and B. Connolly (Eds) *Motor Control & Physical Therapy: Theoretical Framework and Practical Application*, pp. 99–10. Hixon, TN: Chattanooga Group Inc.

Badke, M.B. and Di Fabio, R.P. (1991b). Facilitation: A change in theoretical perspective and in clinical approach. In J. Basmajian and S.L. Wolf (Eds) *Therapeutic Exercise*, 5th Edn, pp. 77–92. Baltimore, MD: Williams & Wilkins.

Bakchine, S., Lacomblez, L., Benoit, N., Parisot, D., Chain, F. and Lhermitte, F. (1989). Manic-like state after bilateral orbitofrontal and right temoroparietal injury: Efficacy of clonidine. *Neurology*, **39**, 777–781.

Baker, S.C., Rogers, R.D., Owen, A.M., Frith, C.D., Dolan, R.J., Frackowiak, R.S.J. and Robbins, W.T. (1996). Neural systems engaged by planning: A PET study of the Tower of London task. *Neuropsychologia*, **34**, 515–526.

Bandura, A. (1986). *Social Foundations of Thought and Action: A Social Cognitive Theory*. Englewood Cliffs, NJ: Prentice-Hall.

Barrett, K. (1991). Treating organic abulia with bromocriptine and lisuride: four case studies. *Journal of Neurology, Neurosurgery and Psychiatry*, **54**, 718–721.

Barry, P., Clark, C., Yaguda, M., Higgins, G. and Mangel, H. (1989). Rehabilitation inpatient screening of early cognitive recovery. *Archives of Physical Medicine and Rehabilitation*, **70**, 902–906.

Basmajian, J.V., Gowland, C.A., Finlayson, M.A.J., Hall, A.J., Swanson, L.R., Stratford, P.W., Trotter, J.E. and Brandstater, M.E. (1987). Stroke treatment: Comparison of integrated behavioral–physical therapy vs. traditional physical therapy programs. *Archives of Physical Medicine and Rehabilitation*, **68**, 267–272.

Batchelor, J., Shores, E.A., Marosszeky, J.E., Sandanam, J. and Lovarini, M. (1988). Cognitive rehabilitation of severely closed-head-injured patients using computer-assisted and noncomputerized treatment techniques. *Journal of Head Trauma Rehabilitation*, **3**, 78–85.

Bear, D.M. (1983). Behavioral symptoms in temporal lobe epilepsy. *Archives of General Psychiatry*, **40**, 467–468.

Becker, D.P., Miller, D., Ward, J.D., Greenberg, G.R.P., Young, H.F. and Sakalas, R. (1977). The outcome from severe head injury with early diagnosis and intensive management. *Journal of Neurosurgery*, **47**, 491–502.

Becker, H., Harrell, W.T. and Keller, L. (1993). A survey of professional and paraprofessional training needs for traumatic brain injury rehabilitation. *Journal of Head Trauma Rehabilitation*, **8**, 88–101.

Bell, K.R. and Tallman, C.A. (1995). Community re-entry of long-term institutionalized brain-injured patient. *Brain Injury*, **9**, 315–320.

Bellack, A.S., Hersen, M. and Lamparski, D. (1979). Role-play tests for assessing social skills: Are they valid? are they useful? *Journal of Consulting and Clinical Psychology*, **47**, 335–342.

Bennett-Levy, J. and Powell, G.E. (1980). The Subjective Memory Questionnaire (SMQ). An investigation into the self-reporting of real-life memory skills. *British Journal of Social and Clinical Psychology*, **19**, 177–188

Ben-Yishay, Y., Silver, S.M., Piasetsky, E. and Rattok, J. (1987). Relationship between employability and vocational outcome after intensive holistic cognitive rehabilitation. *Journal of Head Trauma Rehabilitation*, **2**, 35–48.

Benson, D.F. (1994). *The Neurology of Thinking*. New York: Oxford University Press.

Benson, D.F., Gardner, H. and Meadows, J.C. (1976). Reduplication Paramnesia. *Neurology*, **26**, 147–151.

Benton, A.L. (1969). Disorders of spatial orientation. In P.J. Vinken and G.W. Bruyn (Eds) *Handbook of Clinical Neurology*, Vol. 3, pp. 212–228. Amsterdam: North-Holland Publishing Company.

Benton, A. (1979). Behavioural consequences of closed head injury. *Central nervous system trauma status report*. Washington, DC: National Institute of Neurological and Communicative Disorders and Stroke.

Berger, M.S., Pitts, L.H., Lovely, M., Edwards, M.S. and Bartowski, H.M. (1985). Outcome from severe head injury in children and adolescents. *Journal of Neurosurgery*, **62**, 194–199.

Bernstein, N. (1967). *The Coordination and Regulation of Movement*. London: Pergamon Press.

Berrol, S. (1983). Medical Assessment. In M. Rosenthal, E. Griffith, M.R. Bond and J.D. Miller (Eds) *Rehabilitation of the Head Injured Adult*, pp. 231–239. Philadelphia, PA: F.A. Davis.

Berrol, S. (1986). Evolution and the persistent vegetative state. *Journal of Head Trauma Rehabilitation*, 1, 7–13.

Binder, L.M. (1986). Persisting symptoms after mild head injury: a review of the post-concussive syndrome. *Journal of Clinical and Experimental Neuropsychology*, **8**, 323–346.

Birley, J. and Hudson, B. (1983). The family, the social worker and rehabilitation. In F.W. Watts and D.H. Bennett (Eds) *Theory and Practice of Psychiatric Rehabilitation*, pp. 171–188. Chichester: John Wiley.

Black, P., Markowitz, R.S. and Cianci, S.N. (1975). Recovery of motor function after lesions in the motor cortex of monkey. In CIBA Foundation Symposium 34. New Series. *Outcome of Severe Damage to the Central Nervous System*. Amsterdam: Elsevier.

Blackerby, W.F. (1993). Rediscovering intimacy after head injury. National Head Injury Foundation Publication. *TBI Challenge!* Issue 1, Number 4, Fall, 4–9.

Blanchard, M. K. (1984). *Counseling Head Injured Patients: Guidelines for Community Mental Health Workers*. New York: New York State Head Injury Association.

Blumer, D. (1970). Hypersexual episodes in temporal lobe epilepsy. *American Journal of Psychiatry*, **126**, 1099–1106.

Blumer, D. and Migeon, C. (1975). Hormone and hormonal agents in the treatment of aggression. *Journal of Nervous and Mental Disease*, **160**, 127–137.

Bobath, B. (1978). *Adult Hemiplegia: Evaluation and Treatment*. London: William Heinemann.

Bolton, B. and Roessler, R. (1986). The work personality profile; factor scales, reliability, validity and norms. *Vocation Evaluation and Work Adjustment Bulletin*, **19**, 143–149.

Bond, M.R. (1975). Assessment of the psychosocial outcome after severe head injury. In CIBA Foundation Symposium 34. New Series. *Outcome of Severe Damage to the Central Nervous System*, pp. 141–157. Amsterdam: Elsevier.

Bond, M.R. (1979). The stages of recovery from severe head injury with special reference to late outcome. *International Rehabilitation Medicine*, **1**, 155–159.

Bour, H., Tutin, N. and Pasquier, P. (1967). The central nervous system and carbon monoxide poisoning. 1: Clinical data with reference to 20 fatal cases. In H. Bour and I. McA. Ledingham (Eds) *Carbon Monoxide Poisoning, Progress in Brain Research*, Vol. 24, pp. 469–470. Amsterdam: Elsevier.

Boyeson, M.G. and Harmon, R.L. (1994). Acute and post-acute drug-induced effects on rate of behavioral recovery after brain injury. *Journal of Head Trauma Rehabilitation*, **9**, 78–90.

Brain Injury Association (1996). *Directory of Brain Injury Rehabilitation Services*. Southborough, MA: BIA.

Brain Injury Association (1997). *Directory of Brain Injury Rehabilitation Services.* Southborough, MA: BIA.

Brocklehurst, J.C., Andrews, K., Richards, B. and Laycock, P.J. (1978). How much physical therapy for patients with stroke? *British Medical Journal*, 1, 307–310.

Brooks, D.N. and McKinlay, W.W. (1983). Personality and behavioural change after severe blunt head injury – a relative's view. *Journal of Neurology, Neurosurgery and Psychiatry*, 46, 336–344.

Brooks, D. N., Campsie, L., Symington, C., Beattie, A. and McKinlay, W. (1986a). The five year outcome of severe blunt head injury: A relative's view. *Journal of Neurology, Neurosurgery and Psychiatry*, 49, 764–770.

Brooks, D.N., Hosie, J., Bond, M.R., Jennett, B. and Aughton, M. (1986b). Cognitive sequelae of severe head injury in relation to the Glasgow outcome scale. *Journal of Neurology, Neurosurgery and Psychiatry*, 49, 549–553.

Brotherton, F.A., Thomas, L.L., Wisotzek, I.E. and Milan, M.A. (1988). Social skills training in the rehabilitation of patients with traumatic head injury. *Archives of Physical Medicine and Rehabilitation*, 69, 827–832.

Burgess, P.W. and Shallice, T. (1996). Confabulation and the control of recollection. *Memory*, 4, 359–411.

Burke, W.H., Wesolowski, M.D. and Lane, I.M. (1988). A positive approach to the treatment of aggressive brain-injured clients. *International Journal of Rehabilitation Research*, 11, 235–241.

Burke, W.H., Zencius, A.H., Wesolowski, M.D. and Doubleday, F. (1991). Improving executive functioning disorders in brain-injured clients. *Brain Injury*, 5, 241–252.

Butter, C.M. and Kirsch, N.I.L. (1992). Combined and separate effects of eye patching and visual stimulation on unilateral neglect following stroke. *Archives of Physical Medicine and Rehabilitation*, 73, 1133–1139.

Butter, C.M., Kirsch, NIL. and Reeves, G. (1990). The effect of lateralized dynamic stimuli on unilateral spatial neglect following right hemisphere lesions. *Restorative Neurology and Neuroscience*, 2, 39–46.

Calvin, W. H. (1996). *The Cerebral Code: Thinking a Thought in the Mosaics of the Mind.* Cambridge, MA: MIT Press.

Cannon, W.B. and Rosenblueth, A. (1949). *The Supersensitivity of Denervated Structures.* New York: MacMillan.

Carey, R.G., Seibert, J.H. and Posavac, E.J. (1988). Who makes the most progress in inpatient rehabilitation? An analysis of functional gain. *Archives of Physical Medicine and Rehabilitation*, 69, 337–343.

Carr, J.H. and Sheperd, R.B. (1980). *Physiotherapy in Disorders of the Brain.* Rockville, MD: Aspen Publishers.

Carr, J.H. and Sheperd, R.B. (1987). *Movement Science: Foundations for Physical Therapy in Rehabilitation.* Rockville, MD: Aspen Publishers.

Carroll, W. R. and Bandura, A. (1982). The role of visual monitoring in observational learning of action patterns: Making the unobservable observable. *Journal of Motor Behavior*, 14, 153–167.

Cassidy, J.W. (1990a). Neurochemical substrates of aggression: towards a model for improved intervention, part 1. *Journal of Head Trauma Rehabilitation*, 5, 83–86.

Cassidy, J.W. (1990b). Neurochemical substrates of aggression: towards a model for improved intervention, part 2. *Journal of Head Trauma Rehabilitation*, 5, 70–73.

Casson, J.R., Siegel, O., Sham, R., Campbell, E.A., Tarlau, M. and Di Domenico, A. (1984). Brain damage in modern boxers. *Journal of the American Medical Association*, 251, 2663–2667.

Catalano, J.F. and Kleiner, B. M. (1984). Distant transfer in coincident timing as a function of variability in practice. *Perceptual and Motor Skills*, 58, 851–856.

Cattelani, R., Lombardi, F., Brianti, R. and Mazzuchi, A. (1998). Traumatic brain injury in childhood: Intellectual, behavioral and social outcome into adulthood. *Brain Injury*, 12, 283–296.

Chen, S.H.A., Thomas, J.D., Glueckauf, R.L. and Bracy, O.L. (1997). The effectiveness of computer-assisted cognitive rehabilitation for persons with traumatic brain injury. *Brain Injury*, 11, 197–209.

Cherney, L.R. and Halper, A. (1989). Recovery of oral nutrition after head injury in adults. *Journal of Head Trauma Rehabilitation*, 4, 42–50.

Cherney, L.R., Cantieri, C. and Pannell, J.J. (1986). *Clinical Evaluation of Dysphagia.* Rockville, MD: Aspen Publishers.

Chestnut, R.M., Carney, N., Maynard, H., Patterson, P., Mann, N.C. and Hefland, M. (1999). *Rehabilitation for Traumatic Brain Injury. Evidence Report No. 2.* Rockville, MD: Agency for Health Care Policy.

Childers, M.K. and Holland, D. (1997). Psychomotor agitation following gabapentin use in brain-injury. *Brain Injury*, 11, 537–541.

Churchland, P.M. (1995). *The Engine of Reason, the Seat of the Soul.* Cambridge, MA: MIT Press.

Cicerone, K.D. and Giacino, T.J. (1992). Remediation of executive function deficits after traumatic brain injury. *Neurorehabilitation*, 2, 12–22.

Clark-Wilson, J. (1988). The use of a computer in aiding functional skills training: a single case study. *Clinical Rehabilitation*, 2, 199–206.

Clifton, G.L. (1988). Controversies in the medical management of head injury. *Clinical Neurosurgery*, 34, 587–603.

Clifton, G.L., Hayes, R.L., Levin, H.S., Michel, M.E. and Choi, S.C. (1992). Outcome measures for clinical trails involving traumatically brain injured patients: report of a conference. *Neurosurgery*, 31, 975–978.

Cohen, R.E. (1985). Behavioral treatment of incontinence in a profoundly neurologically impaired adult. *Archives of Physical Medicine and Rehabilitation*, 67, 833–834.

Cole, J.R., Cope, N. and Cervelli, L. (1985). Rehabilitation of the severely brain injured patient: A community based, low cost model program. *Archives of Physical Medicine and Rehabilitation*, 66, 38–40.

Cook, J.V. (1983). Returning to work after traumatic brain injury. In M. Rosenthal, E.R. Griffith, M.R. Bond and J.D. Miller (Eds) *Rehabilitation of the Adult and Child with Traumatic Brain Injury*, 2nd Edn, pp. 493–505. Philadelphia, PA: F.A. Davis.

Cope, D.N. (1985). Traumatic closed head injury; status of rehabilitation treatment. *Seminars in Neurology*, 5, 212–220.

Cope, D.N. (1994). Integration of psychopharmacological and rehabilitation approaches to traumatic brain injury rehabilitation. *Journal of Head Trauma Rehabilitation*, 9, 1–18.

Cope, D.N. (1995). The effectiveness of traumatic brain-injury rehabilitation – a review. *Brain Injury*, 9, 649–670.

Cope, D.N. and Hall, K. (1982). Head injury rehabilitation: benefit of early intervention. *Archives of Physical Medicine and Rehabilitation*, 63, 433–437.

Cope, D.N. and O'Lear, J. (1993). A clinical and economic perspective on head injury rehabilitation. *Journal of Head Trauma Rehabilitation*, 8, 1–14.

Cope, D.N., Cole, J.R., Hall, K.M. and Barkan, H. (1991a). Brain injury: analysis of outcome in a post-acute rehabilitation system. Part 1: General analysis. *Brain Injury*, 5, 111–125.

Cope, D.N., Cole, J.R., Hall, K.M. and Barkan, H. (1991b). Brain injury: analysis of outcome in a post-acute rehabilitation system. Part 2: Subanalysis. *Brain Injury*, 5, 127–139.

Corcoran, M.A. (1992). Gender differences in dementia management plans of spousal caregivers: implications for occupational therapy. *American Journal of Occupational Therapy*, 46, 1006–1012.

Corrigan, J. D. (1989). Development of a scale for assessment of agitation following traumatic brain injury. *Journal of Clinical and Experimental Neuropsychology*, 11, 261–277.

Corrigan, J.D., Arnett, J.A., Houck, L.J. and Jackson, R.D. (1985). Reality orientation for brain injured patients: Group treatment and monitoring of recovery. *Archives of Physical Medicine and Rehabilitation*, 66, 626–630.

Corrigan, P., Yudofsky, S. and Silver, J. (1993). Pharmacological and behavioural treatments for aggressive psychiatric inpatients. *Hospital and Community Psychiatry*, 44, 125–133.

Cowley, R.S., Swanson, B., Chapman, P., Kitik, B.A. and Mackay, L.E. (1994). The role of rehabilitation in the intensive care unit. *Journal of Head Trauma Rehabilitation*, 9, 32–42.

Crane, A. and Joyce, B.G. (1991). Cool Down: a procedure for decreasing aggression in adults with traumatic head injury. *Behavioral Residential Treatment*, 6, 65–75.

Crewe, N. and Athlestan, G. (1981). Functional assessment in vocational rehabilitation; A systematic approach to diagnosis and goal setting. *Archives of Physical Medicine and Rehabilitation*, 62, 299–305.

Crick, F. (1984). Function of the thalamic reticular complex: The searchlight hypothesis. *Proceedings of the National Academy of Sciences*, 81, 4586–4590.

Criswell, H., Mueller, R. and Breese, G. (1992). Pharmacologic evaluation of SCH-39166, A-69024, NO-0756 and SCH-23390 in neonatal-6-OHDA-lesioned rats. *Neuropsychopharmacology*, 7, 95–103.

Croog, S., Shapiro, D. and Levine, S. (1971). Denial among male heart patients. *Psychosomatic Medicine*, 33, 385–397.

Crovitz, H.F. (1979). Memory rehabilitation in brain damaged patients: The airplane list. *Cortex*, 15, 131–134.

Cummings, J.L. (1985). Organic delusions: phenomenology, anatomical correlations and review. *British Journal of Psychiatry*, 146, 184–197.

Cummings, J.L. (1993). Frontal-subcortical circuits and human behavior. *Archives of Neurology*, 50, 873–880.

Davidoff, G., Morris, J., Roth, E. and Bleiberg, J. (1985). Closed head injury in spinal cord injured patients: Retrospective study of loss of consciousness and post-traumatic amnesia. *Archives of Physical Medicine and Rehabilitation*, 66, 41–43.

Dawkins, R. (1976). *The Selfish Gene*. Oxford: Oxford University Press.

Deacon, T.W. (1997). *The Symbolic Species: The Co-Evolution of Language and the Brain*. New York: W.W. Norton.

De Houwer, J., Baeyens, F. and Eelen, P. (1994). Verbal evaluative conditioning with undetected US presentation. *Behavior Research and Therapy*, 32, 629–633.

Del Rey, R. (1971). The effects of video-taped feedback on form, accuracy and latency in an open and closed environment. *Journal of Motor Behavior*, 3, 281–287.

Dennett, D.C. (1991). *Consciousness Explained*. Boston, MA: Little, Brown and Co.

Denny-Brown, D., Meyer, J.S. and Horenstein, S. (1952). The significance of perceptual rivalry resulting from parietal lesions. *Brain*, 75, 433–471.

DeRuyter, F. and Becker, M.R. (1988). Augmentive communication: Assessment, system selection and usage. *Journal of Head Trauma Rehabilitation*, 3, 35–44.

DeRuyter, F. and Lafontaine, L.M. (1987). The nonspeaking brain-injured: A clinical and demographic database report. *Augmentative and Alternative Communication*, 3, 18–25.

Devor, M. (1982). Plasticity in the adult nervous system. In L.S. Illis, E.M. Sedgwick and H.J. Glanville (Eds) *Rehabilitation of the Neurological Patient*. Oxford: Blackwell Scientific Publications.

Diller, L. and Weinberg, J. (1993). Response styles in perceptual retraining. In W.A. Gordon (Ed.) *Advances in Stroke Rehabilitation*, pp. 162–182. Boston, MA: Andover Medical Publishers.

Diller, L., Ben-Yishay, Y., Gerstman, L.J., Goodkin, R., Gordon, W. and Weinberg, J. (1974). *Studies in Cognitive Rehabilitation in Hemiplegia*. Rehabilitation Monographs, 50. Institute of Rehabilitation Medicine, New York: University Medical Center.

Dobson, K.S. (1988). The present and future of the cognitive-behavioral therapies. In K.S. Dobson (Ed.) *Handbook of Cognitive Behavioral Therapy*. New York: The Guilford Press.

Dodds, T.A., Martin, D.P., Stolov, W.C. and Deyo, R.A. (1993). A validation of the Functional Independence Measurement and its performance among rehabilitation inpatients. *Archives of Physical Medicine and Rehabilitation*, 74, 531–536.

Dolan, M. and Norton, J. (1977). A programmed training technique that uses reinforcement to facilitate acquisition and retention in brain damaged clients. *Journal of Clinical Psychology*, 33, 496–501.

Dombovy, M.L. and Olek, A.C. (1996). Recovery and rehabilitation following traumatic brain injury. *Brain Injury*, 11, 305–318.

Ducharme, J.M. and Popynick, M. (1993). Errorless compliance to parental requests: Treatment effects and generalization. *Behavior Therapy*, 24, 209–226.

Ducharme, J.M., Lucas, H. and Pontes, E. (1994). Errorless embedding in the reduction of severe maladaptive behavior during interactive and learning tasks. *Behavior Therapy*, 25, 489–501.

Duncan, P.W. (1990). Physical therapy assessment. In M. Rosenthal, M.R. Bond, E.R. Griffith and J.D. Miller (Eds) *Rehabilitation of the Adult and Child with Traumatic Brain-Injury*, pp. 264–283. Philadelphia, PA: F.A. Davis.

Duncan, P.W. and Badke, M.B. (1987). Determinants of motor control. In P.W. Duncan and M.B. Badke (Eds) *Stroke Rehabilitation: The Recovery of Motor Control*, pp. 135–159. Chicago, IL: Yearbook Medical Publishers.

Eames, P. (1977). Feeling cold: An unusual brain-injury symptom and its treatment with vasopressin (letter). *Journal of Neurology, Neurosurgery and Psychiatry*, 67, 198–199.

Eames, P. (1992). Hysteria following brain injury. *Journal of Neurology, Neurosurgery and Psychiatry*, 55, 1046–1053.

Eames, P. and Wood, R. Ll. (1985a). Rehabilitation after severe brain injury: A follow-up study of a behaviour modification approach. *Journal of Neurology, Neurosurgery and Psychiatry*, 48, 613–619.

Eames, P. and Wood, R. Ll. (1985b). Rehabilitation after severe brain injury: a special-unit approach to behaviour disorders. *International Rehabilitation Medicine*, 7, 130–133.

Eames, P., Cotterill, G., Kneale, T.A., Storrar, A.R. and Yeomans, P. (1995). Outcome of intensive rehabilitation after severe brain-injury: A long-term follow-up study. *Brain Injury*, 10, 631–650.

Edelman, G.M. (1987). *Neural Darwinism*. New York: Basic Books.

Edelman, G.M. (1992). *Bright Air, Brilliant Fire*. New York: Basic Books.

Ehrlich, J.S. (1988). Selective characteristics of narrative discourse in head-injured and normal adults. *Journal of Communication Disorders*, 21, 1–9.

Eisler, R.M., Hersen, M., Miller, P.M. and Blanchard, E.G. (1975). Situational determinants of assertive behavior. *Journal of Consulting and Clinical Psychology*, 43, 330–340.

Elliott, M.K. and Biever, L.S. (1996). Head injury and sexual dysfunction. *Brain Injury*, 10, 703–717.

Ellis, S. and Small, M. (1997). Localization of lesion in denial of hemiplegia after acute stroke. *Stroke*, 28, 67–71.

Elliss, H.D. and Szulecka, T.K. (1996). The disguised lover: A case of the frugoli delusion. In P.W. Halligan and J.C. Marshall (Eds) *Methods in Madness*. Hove, East Sussex: Psychology Press.

Englander, J., Hall, K., Stimpson, T. and Chaffin, S. (1992). Mild traumatic brain injury in an insured population: subjective complaints and return to employment. *Brain Injury*, 6, 161–166.

Evans, C.D., Bull, C.P.I., Devenport, M.J., Hall, P.M., Jones, J., Middleton, F.R.I., Russell, G., Stichbury, K.C. and Whitehead, B. (1981). Rehabilitation of the brain-damaged survivor. *Injury*, 8, 80–97.

Evarts, E.V., Shinoda, Y. and Wise, S. P. (1984). *Neurophysiological Approaches to Higher Brain Function*. New York: John Wiley.

Finger, S. and Stein, D.G. (1982). *Brain Damage and Recovery*. New York: Academic Press.

Fitts, P.M. and Posner, M.L. (1967). *Human Performance*. Belmont, CA: Brooks/Cole.

Fleming, J.M., Strong, J. and Ashton, R. (1996). Self-awareness of deficit in adults with traumatic brain injury: How best to measure. *Brain Injury*, 10, 1–15.

Flint, A. (1991). Delusions in dementia: a review. *Journal of Neuropsychiatry and Clinical Neurosciences*, 3, 121–130.

Fordyce, D.J., Roueche, J.R. and Prigatano, G.P. (1983). Enhanced emotional reactions in chronic head trauma patients. *Journal of Neurology, Neurosurgery and Psychiatry*, 46, 620–624.

Freeman, E.A. (1993). The clinical assessment of coma. *Neuropsychological Rehabilitation*, 3, 139–147.

Freeman, E.A. (1997). Community-based rehabilitation of the person with a severe brain injury. *Brain Injury*, 11, 143–153.

Freeman, T. and Karson, C. (1993). The neuropathology of schizophrenia – a focus on the subcortex. *Psychiatric Clinics*, 16, 281–293.

Freeman, J.A., Hobart, J.C. and Thompson, A.J. (1996). Outcome-based research in neurorehabilitation: The need for multi-disciplinary team involvement. *Disability and Rehabilitation*, 18, 106–110.

Freud, A. (1967). *The Ego and the Mechanisms of Defense. Writings of Anna Freud*, Vol. 2. New York: International Universities Press.

Froese, A., Hackett, T.P., Cassem, N.H. and Silverberg, E.L. (1974). Trajectories of anxiety and depression in denying and nondenying acute myocardial infarction patients during hospitalization. *Journal of Psychosomatic Research*, 18, 413–420.

Fryer, L.J. and Haffey, W.J. (1987). Cognitive rehabilitation and community readaptation: Outcomes from two program models. *Journal of Head Trauma Rehabilitation*, 2, 51–63.

Fujikawa, T., Yamawaki, S. and Touda, Y. (1995). Silent cerebral infarction in patients with late-onset mania. *Stroke*, 26, 946–949.

Fukuyama, H., Kameyama, M. and Harada, K. (1986). Thalmic tumours invading the brain stem produce crossed cerebellar diaschisis demonstrated by PET. *Journal of Neurology, Neurosurgery and Psychiatry*, 49, 524–528.

Fulcher, E.P. and Cocks, R.P. (1997). Dissociative storage systems in human evaluative conditioning. *Behavior Research and Therapy*, 35, 1–10.

Fuller, G., Marshall, A., Flint, J., Lewis, S. and Wise, R.J. (1993). Migraine madness: recurrent psychosis after migraine. *Journal of Neurology, Neurosurgery and Psychiatry*, 56, 416–418.

Fussey, I. and Giles, G.M. (1988). *Rehabilitation of the Severely Brain Injured Adult: A Practical Approach.* London: Croom Helm.

Fuster, J.M. (1995). *Memory in the Cerebral Cortex.* Cambridge, MA: MIT Press.

Gajar, A., Schloss, P.J., Schloss, C. and Thompson, C.K. (1984). Effects of feedback and self-monitoring on brain trauma youth's conversational skills. *Journal of Applied Behavior Analysis*, 17, 353–358.

Galski, T., Ehle, H.T. and Bruno, R.L. (1990). An assessment of measures to predict the outcome of driving evaluations in patients with cerebral damage. *American Journal of Occupational Therapy*, 44, 709–713.

Garland, D.E. (1980). Heterotopic ossification: Incidence, location and management. In *Rehabilitation of the Head Injured Adult.* Downey, CA: Professional Staff Association of Rancho Los Amigos Medical Center.

Garza-Trevino, E.S., Hollister, L.E., Overall, J.E. and Alexander, W.F. (1989). Efficacy of combinations in intra-muscular anti-psychotics and sedatives – hypnotics for control of psychotic agitation, *American Journal of Psychiatry*, 146, 1598.

Gazzaniga, M.S. (1978). Is seeing believing: notes on clinical recovery. In S. Finger (Ed.) *Recovery from Brain Damage: Research and Theory.* New York: Plenum Press

Gennerelli, T.A., Thibault, L.E., Adams, J.H., Graham, D.I., Thompson, C.J. and Marcincin, R.P. (1982). Diffuse axonal injury and traumatic coma in the primate. *Annals of Neurology*, 12, 564–574.

Gentile, A.M. (1972). A working model of skill acquisition with application to teaching. *Quest*, 17, 3–23.

George, M. (1997). Into the unknown. *Community Care*, 12–18 June.

Gerstman, J. (1958). Psychological and phenomenological aspects of disorders of the body image. *Journal of Nervous and Mental Disease*, 126, 499–512.

Gianutsos, R. (1980). What is cognitive rehabilitation? *Journal of Rehabilitation*, 46, 36–40.

Giles, G.M. (1989). Demonstrating the effectiveness of occupational therapy after severe brain trauma. *American Journal of Occupational Therapy*, 43, 613–615.

Giles, G.M. (1991). Shifting responsibility: Who should care for people with brain injuries? (letter). *Journal of Head Trauma Rehabilitation*, 6, xi–xii.

Giles, G.M. (1994a). The status of brain injury rehabilitation. *American Journal of Occupational Therapy*, 48, 199–205.

Giles, G.M. (1994b). Illness behavior after severe brain injury: Two case reports. *American Journal of Occupational Therapy*, 48, 247–250.

Giles, G.M. (1996). *Coping with Brain Injury: A Guide for Family and Friends.* Bethesda, MD: American Occupational Therapy Association.

Giles, G.M. (1998). A neurofunctional approach to rehabilitation following severe brain injury. In N. Katz (Ed.) *Cognition and Occupation in Rehabilitation. Cognitive Models for Intervention in Occupational Therapy.* Bethesda, MD: American Occupational Therapy Association.

Giles, G.M. and Clark-Wilson, J. (1988a). The use of behavioural techniques in functional skills training after severe brain injury. *American Journal of Occupation Therapy*, **42**, 658–665.

Giles, G.M. and Clark-Wilson, J. (1988b). Functional skills training after severe brain injury. In I. Fussey and G.M. Giles (Eds) *Rehabilitation of the Severely Brain Injured Adult: A Practical Approach.* London: Croom Helm.

Giles, G.M. and Clark-Wilson, J. (1993). *Brain-Injury Rehabilitation: A Neurofunctional Approach.* London: Chapman and Hall.

Giles, G.M. and Fussey, I. (1988). Models of brain-injury rehabilitation: From theory to practice. In I.Fussey, and G.M. Giles (Eds) *Rehabilitation of the Severely Brain-Injured Adult: A Practical Approach*, pp. 1–29. London: Croom Helm.

Giles, G.M. and Haussman, P. (1997). Use of a comprehensive program of external cueing to change procedural memory in a patient with dense amnesia (letter). *Brain Injury*, **11**, 466–468.

Giles, G.M. and McMillan, T. (in press). The effectiveness of neurobehavioral rehabilitation. In R.L. Wood and T. McMillan (Eds) *Neurobehavioral Disability and Social Handicap.* Hove, East Susssex: Psychology Press.

Giles, G.M. and Morgan, J.H. (1989). Training functional skills following herpes simplex encephalitis: A single case study. *Journal of Clinical and Experimental Neuropsychology*, **11**, 311–318.

Giles, G.M. and Shore, M. (1989a). A rapid method for teaching severely brain-injured adults to wash and dress. *Archives of Physical Medicine and Rehabilitation*, **70**, 156–158.

Giles, G.M. and Shore, M. (1989b). The effectiveness of an electronic memory aid for a memory-impaired adult of normal intelligence. *American Journal of Occupation Therapy*, **43**, 409–411.

Giles, G.M., Fussey, I. and Burgess, P. (1988). The behavioral treatment of verbal inter-action skills following severe head injury: A single case study. *Brain Injury*, **2**, 75–79.

Giles, G.M., Ridley, J., Dill, A. and Frye, S. (1997). A consecutive series of brain injured adults treated with a washing and dressing retraining program. *American Journal of Occupational Therapy*, **51**, 256–266.

Giuliani, C.A. (1991). Disorders in motor synergies, initiation and termination of movement. In P. Montgomery and B. Connolly (Eds) *Motor Control and Physical Therapy: Theoretical Framework and Practical Application*, pp. 111–120. Hixon, TN: Chattanooga Group Inc.

Glick, S.D. and Greenstein, S. (1973). Possible modulatory influences of frontal cortex on nigro-striatal function. *British Journal of Pharmacology*, **49**, 316–321.

Glisky, E.L. and Schacter, D.L. (1988). Long-term retention of computer learning by patients with memory disorders. *Neuropsychologia*, **26**, 173–178.

Glisky, E.L., Schacter, D.L. and Tulving, E. (1986). Computer learning by memory impaired patients: acquisition and retention of complex knowledge. *Neuropsychologia*, **24**, 313–328.

Godfrey, H.P.D., Knight, R.G., Marsh, N.V., Moroney, B. and Bishara, S. (1989). Social interaction and speed of information processing following very severe head-injury. *Psychological Medicine*, **19**, 175–182.

Goldiamond, I. (1965). Stuttering and fluency as manipulable operant response classes. In L. Krasner and L.P. Ullman (Eds) *Research in Behavior Modification: New Developments and Implications*, pp. 106–156. New York: Holt Rinehart and Winston.

Goldstein, L.H. and Oakley, D.A. (1983). Expected and actual behavioral capacity after diffuse reduction in cerebral cortex: A review and suggestions for rehabilitative techniques with the mentally handicapped and head injured. *British Journal of Clinical Psychology*, 24, 13–24.

Goodale, G.S. (1997). TBI Act signed into law. *TBI Challenge*. Southborough, MA: Brain Injury Association.

Goodglass, H. and Kaplan, E. (1963). Disturbances of gesture and pantomime in aphasia. *Brain*, 86, 703–720.

Goodglass, H. and Kaplan, E. (1972). *The Assessment of Aphasia and Related Disorders*. Philadelphia, PA: Lea and Febiger.

Goodman-Smith, A. and Turnbull, J. (1983). A behavioral approach to the rehabilitation of severely brain injured adults: an illustrated case history. *Physiotherapy*, 69, 393–396.

Gordon, J. (1987). Assumptions underlying physical therapy intervention: theoretical and historical perspectives. In J.H. Carr, R.B. Shepherd, J. Gordon *et al.* (Eds) *Movement Science: Foundations for Physical Therapy in Rehabilitation*, pp. 1–30. Rockville, MD: Aspen Publishers.

Graham, D.I. and Adams, J.H. (1971). Ischaemic brain-damage and fatal head-injury. *Lancet*, i, 265–266

Gratten, L.M. and Eslinger, P.J. (1992). Long term psychological consequences of childhood frontal lobe lesion in patient D.T. *Brain and Cognition*, 20, 185–195.

Gray, J.M. and Robertson, I. (1989). Remediation of attentional difficulties following brain injury: Three experimental single case studies. *Brain Injury*, 3, 163–170.

Greenwood, R.J., McMillan, T.M., Brooks, D.N., Dunn, G., Brock, J., Murphy, L.D. and Price, J.R. (1994). Effects of case management after severe head injury. *British Medical Journal*, 308, 1199–1205.

Greer, S., Morris, T. and Pettingale, K.W. (1979). Psychological response to breast cancer: effect on outcome. *Lancet*, ii, 785–787.

Groher, M.E. (Ed.) (1992). *Dysphagia: Diagnosis and Management*, 2nd Edn. Boston, MA: Butterworth.

Gronwall, D. and Wrightson, P. (1981). Memory and information processing capacity after closed head injury. *Journal of Neurology, Neurosurgery and Psychiatry*, 44, 889–895.

Groswasser, Z., Cohen, M. and Keren, O. (1998). Female TBI patients recover better than males. *Brain Injury*, 12, 805–808.

Gualtieri, C. (1990). Traumatic brain injury: The neuropsychiatric sequelae of traumatic brain-injury. *Journal of Child and Adolescent Psychopharmacology*, 1, 149–152.

Guerco, J., Chittum, R. and McMorrow, M. (1997). Self-management in the treatment of ataxia: A case study in reducing ataxic tremor through relaxation and biofeedback. *Brain Injury*, 11, 353–363.

Hackett, T.P., Cassem, N.H. and Wishnie, H.A. (1968). The coronary-care unit: an appraisal of its psychological hazards. *New England Journal of Medicine*, 279, 1365–1370.

Haffey, W.J. and Lewis, F.D. (1989). Programming for occupational outcome following traumatic brain injury. *Rehabilitation Psychology*, 34, 147–159.

Hagen, C. (1982). Language disorders in head trauma. In A.L. Holland (Ed.) *Language Disorders in Adults*. San Diego, CA: College Hill Press.

Hagen, C., Malkmus, D. and Durham, P. (1972). *Levels of Cognitive Functioning*. Downey, CA: Rancho Los Amigos Hospital.

Hagen, C., Malkmus, D. and Durham, P. (1977). Levels of Cognitive Functioning. Paper presented at the Head Trauma Rehabilitation Seminar. Los Angeles, CA: Rancho Los Amigos Hospital.

Hall, K., Cope, N. and Rappaport, M. (1985). Glasgow Outcome Scale and disability rating scale: Comparative usefulness in following recovery in traumatic brain injury. *Archives of Physical Medicine and Rehabilitation*, **66**, 35–37.

Hall, K.M., Hamilton, B.B., Gordon, W.A. and Zasler, N.D. (1993). Characteristics and comparisons of functional assessment indices: Disability rating scale, functional independence measure and functional assessment measure. *Journal of Head Trauma Rehabilitation*, **8**, 60–74.

Halligan, P.W. and Marshall, J.C. (1989). Laterality of motor response in visuo spatial neglect: a case study. *Neuropsychologia*, **27**, 1301–1307.

Halligan, P.W. and Marshall, J.C. (1996). *Methods in Madness*. Hove, East Sussex: Psychology Press.

Halligan, P.W., Manning, L. and Marshall, J.C. (1991). Hemispheric activation vs. spatio-motor cueing in visual neglect: a case study. *Neuropsychologia*, **29**, 165–176.

Hannay, H.J., Ezrachi, O., Contant, C.F. and Levin, H.S. (1996). Outcome measures for patients with head injuries: Report of the outcome measures subcommittee. *Journal of Head Trauma Rehabilitation*, **11**, 41–50.

Harrick, L., Krefting, L., Johnston, J., Carlson, P. and Minnes, P. (1994). Stability of functional outcomes following transitional living program participation: 3 year follow up. *Brain Injury*, **8**, 439–447.

Harris, J.E. (1980). Memory aids people use: Two interview studies. *Memory and Cognition*, **8**, 31–38.

Hart, T. and Jacobs, H. (1993). Rehabilitation and management of behavioral disturbances following frontal lobe injury. *Journal of Head Trauma Rehabilitation*, **8**, 1–12.

Hartman, J. (1987). Alteration in patterns of urinary elimination. In L.J. Carpenito (Ed.) *Nursing Diagnosis*. Philadelphia, PA: J.B. Lippincott.

Havik, O.E. and Maeland, J.G. (1988). Verbal denial and outcome in myocardial infarction patients. *Journal of Psychosomatic Research*, **32**, 145–157.

Hefferline, R.F., Keenan, B. and Hartford, R.A. (1958). Escape and avoidance conditioning in human subjects without their observation of the response. *Science*, **130**, 1338–1339.

Heilman, K.M. and Watson, R.T. (1978). Changes in the symptoms of neglect induced by changes in task strategy. *Archives of Neurology*, **35**, 47–49.

Heinemann, A.W., Linacre, J.M., Wright, B.D., Hamilton, B.B. and Granger, C. (1994). Prediction of rehabilitation outcomes with disability measures. *Archives of Physical Medicine and Rehabilitation*, **75**, 133–143.

Hier, D., Mondlock, J. and Caplan, R. (1983). Behavioral abnormalities after right hemisphere stroke. *Neurology*, **33**, 337–344.

Hillier, S.L. and Metzer, J. (1997). Awareness and perceptions of outcomes after traumatic brain-injury. *Brain Injury*, **11**, 525–537.

Holland, A.L. (1980). *Communicative Abilities in Daily Living*. Baltimore, MD: University Park Press.

Hooper-Roe, J. (1988). Rehabilitation of physical deficits in the post acute brain-injured: Four case studies. In I. Fussey and G.M. Giles (Eds) *Rehabilitation of the Severely Brain-Injury Adult: A Practical Approach*, pp. 102–116. London: Croom Helm.

Horak, F. B. (1991). Assumptions underlying motor control for neurologic rehabilitation. In M. Lister (Ed.) *11 STEP Contemporary Management of Motor Control Problems*, pp. 11–28. Richmond, VA: Foundation for Physical Therapy, Inc.

Horak, F.B., Anderson, M., Esselman, P. and Lynch, K. (1984). The effects of movement velocity, mass displaced and task certainty on associated postural adjustments made by normal and hemiplegic individuals. *Journal of Neurology, Neurosurgery and Psychiatry*, 47, 1020–1028.

Horn, S., Shiel, A., McLellan, L., Campbell, M., Watson, M. and Wilson, B. (1993). A review of behavioural assessment scales for monitoring recovery in and after coma with pilot data on a new scale of visual awareness. *Neuropsychological Rehabilitation*, 3, 121–137.

Hornsdean, A., Lennerhan, L., Sellinger, G., Lichtman, S. and Schroeder, K. (1996). Amphetamine in recovery from brain-injury. *Brain Injury*, 10, 145-148.

Hoshmand, H. and Brawley, B.W. (1970). Temporal lobe seizures and exhibitionism. *Neurology*, 9, 1119–1124.

Hull, C.L. (1952). *A Behavior System: An Introduction to Behavior Theory Concerning the Individual Organism*. New Haven, CT: Yale University Press.

Hutchins, B.F. (1989). Establishing a dysphagia family intervention program for head-injured patients. *Journal of Head Trauma Rehabilitation*, 4, 64–72.

Illis, L.S. (1983). Determinants of recovery. *International Rehabilitation Medicine*, 4, 166–172.

Ives, E.R. and Neilsen, M.D. (1937). Disturbance of body scheme: Delusion of absence of part of body in two cases with autopsy verification of lesions. *Bulletin of Los Angeles Neurological Society*, 2, 120–125.

Jackson, J. (1994). After rehabilitation: Meeting the long term needs of persons with traumatic brain injury. *American Journal of Occupational Therapy*, 48, 251–255.

Jacobs, H.E. (1988). The Los Angeles head injury survey: Procedures and initial findings. *Archives of Physical Medicine and Rehabilitation*, 69, 425–431.

James, W. (1890). *The Principles of Psychology*. New York: Henry Holt.

Jennett, B. (1975). *Epilepsy After Non-Missile Head Injuries*, 2nd Edn. London: Heinemann.

Jennett, B. (1983). Scale and scope of the problem. In M. Rosenthal, E. Griffith, M.R. Bond and J.D. Miller (Eds) *Rehabilitation of the Head Injured Adult*, pp. 3–8. Philadelphia, PA: F.A. Davis.

Jennett, B. and Bond, M. (1975). Assessment of outcome after severe brain damage : A practical scale. *Lancet*, i, 480–484.

Jennett, B. and Plum, F. (1972). Persistent vegetative state after brain damage. *Lancet*, i, 734–737.

Jennett, B. and Teasdale, G. (1981). *Management of Head Injuries*. Philadelphia, PA: F.A. Davis.

Jennett, B., Teasdale, G., Galbraith, S., Grant, J.P.H., Braakman, R., Avezaat, C., Maas, A., Minderhound, J., Vecht, C.J., Heiden, J., Small, R., Caton, W. and Kurze, T. (1977). Severe head injuries in three countries. *Journal of Neurology, Neurosurgery and Psychiatry*, 40, 291–298.

Jennett, B., Snoek, J., Bond, R. and Brooks, D.N. (1981). Disability after severe head injury: Observations on the Glasgow Outcome Scale. *Journal of Neurology, Neurosurgery and Psychiatry*, 44, 285–293.

Jennett, S.M. and Lincoln, N.B. (1991). An evaluation of the effectiveness of group therapy for memory problems. *International Disability Studies*, 13, 83–86.

Johnson, D.A. and Gleave, J. (1987). Counting the people disabled by head injury. *Injury*, 18, 7–9.

Johnston, M.V. (1991). Outcomes of community re-entry programs for brain injury survivors. Part 2: Further investigations. *Brain Injury*, 5, 155–168.

Johnston, M.V. and Lewis, F.D. (1991). Outcomes of community re-entry program for brain injury survivors. Part 1: Independent living and productive activities. *Brain Injury*, 5, 141–154.

Johnstone, B., Childers, M.K. and Hoerner, J. (1998). The effects of normal aging on neuropsychological functioning following traumatic brain injury. *Brain Injury*, 12, 569–576.

Jones, M.L. and Evans, R.W. (1992). Outcome validation in post-acute rehabilitation: trends and correlates in treatment and outcome. *Journal of Insurance Medicine*, 24, 186–192.

Jones, R.S. and Eayrs, C.B. (1992). The use of errorless learning procedures in teaching people with learning disability: a critical review. *Mental Handicap Research*, 5, 204–212.

Jordan, B.D., Relkin, N.R., Ravdin, L.D., Jacobs, A.R., Bennett, A. and Gandy, S. (1997). Apolipoprotein E e4 associated with chronic traumatic brain injury in boxing. *Journal of the American Medical Association*, 278, 136–140.

Jorge, R., Robinson, R., Arndt, S., Forrester, A.W., Geisler, F. and Starkstein, S.E. (1993). Comparison between acute and delayed-onset depression following traumatic brain injury. *Journal of Neuropsychiatry and Clinical Neurosciences*, 5, 43–49.

Junqué, C., Bruna, O. and Mataro, M. (1997). Information needs of the traumatic brain injury patient's family members regarding the consequences of the injury and associated perception of physical, cognitive, emotional and quality of life changes. *Brain Injury*, 11, 251–258.

Kant, R., Smith-Seemiller, L., Isaac, G. and Duffy, J. (1997). Tc-HMPAO SPECT in persistent post-concussion syndrome after mild head-injury: Comparison with MRI/CT. *Brain Injury*, 11, 115–125.

Kaplan, E. (1988). A process approach to neuropsychological assessment. In T. Boll and B.K. Bryant (Eds) *Clinical Neuropsychology and Brain Function: Research, Measurement and Practice*. Washington, DC: American Psychological Association.

Katz, J.L. (1982). Three studies in psychosomatic medicine revisited: A tribute to the psychobiological perspective of Herbert Weiner. *Psychosomatic Medicine*, 44, 29–41.

Katzman, S. and Mix, C. (1994). Improving functional independence in a patient with encephalitis through behavior modification shaping techniques. *American Journal of Occupational Therapy*, 48, 259–269.

Kazdin, A. E. (1974). *Behavior Modification in Applied Settings*. Homewood, IL: Dorsey Press.

Kazdin, A.E. (1994). *Behavior Modification in Applied Settings*, 5th Edn. Pacific Grove, CA: Brook/Cole.

Kelly, M.P., Johnson, C.T., Knoller, N., Druback, D.A. and Winslow, M.M. (1997). Substance abuse, traumatic brain injury and neuropsychological outcome. *Brain Injury*, 11, 391–402.

Kertesz, A. (1982). *The Western Aphasia Battery*. New York: Grune and Stratton.

Kewman, D.G., Seigerman, C., Kinter, H., Chu, S. Henson, D. and Reeder, C. (1985). Simulation Training of psychomotor Skills: Teaching the brain-injured to drive. *Rehabilitation Psychology*, 30, 11–26.

Kime, S.K., Lamb, D.G. and Wilson, B.A. (1996). Use of a comprehensive program of external cueing to enhance procedural memory in a patient with dense amnesia. *Brain Injury*, 10, 17–25.

Klauber, M.R., Marshall, L.F., Toole, B.M., Knowlton, S.L. and Bowers, S.A. (1985). Cause of decline in head-injury mortality rate in San Diego County, California. *Journal of Neurosurgery*, 62, 528–531.

Klonoff, P.S., Costa, L.D. and Snow, W.D. (1986). Predictors and indicators of quality of life in patients with closed head injury. *Journal of Clinical and Experimental Neuropsychology*, 8, 469–485.

Kopelman, M.D. (1987). Two types of confabulation. *Journal of Neurology, Neurosurgery and Psychiatry*, 50, 1482–1487.

Kramer, A.F., Strayer, D.L. and Buckley, J. (1991). Task versus component consistency in the development of automatic processing: Psychophysiological assessment. *Psychophysiology*, 28, 425–437.

Kraus, M.F. and Mackie, I.P. (1997). The combined use of amantadine and L-dopa/carbidopa in the treatment of chronic brain-injury. *Brain Injury*, 11, 455–460.

Kreutzer, J. S., Wehman, P., Morton, M.V. and Stonnington, H.H. (1991). Supported employment and compensatory strategies for enhancing vocational outcome following traumatic brain injury. *International Disabilities Studies*, 13, 162–171.

Kreutzer, J.S., Gervasjo, A.H. and Camplair, P.S. (1994). Patient correlates of caregivers; distress and family functioning after traumatic brain injury. *Brain Injury*, 8, 211–230.

Kreutzer, J.S., Marwitz, J.H. and Witol, A.D. (1995). Inter-relationship between crime, substance abuse and aggressive behaviour among persons with traumatic brain injury. *Brain Injury*, 9, 757–768.

LaBerge, D. (1997). Attention, awareness and the triangular circuit. *Consciousness and Cognition*, 6, 149–181.

Lal, S., Merbtiz, C.P. and Grip, J.C. (1988). Modification of function in head-injury patients with sinemet. *Brain Injury*, 2, 225–233.

Lam, C.S., Mchahon, B.T., Priddy, D.A. and Gehred-Schultze, A. (1988). Deficit awareness and treatment performance among traumatic head injury adults. *Brain Injury*, 2, 235–242.

Lancet (1983). Caring for the disabled after head injury (editorial). *Lancet*, ii, 948–849.

Landis, T., Graves, R., Benson, D.F. and Hebben, N. (1982). Visual recognition through kinaesthetic mediation. *Psychological Medicine*, 12, 515–531.

Lashley, B. and Drabman, R. (1974). Facilitation of the acquisition and retention of sight-word vocabulary through token reinforcement. *Journal of Applied Behavioral Analysis*, 7, 307–312.

Lashley, K.S. (1938). Factors limiting recovery after central nervous lesions. *Journal of Nervous and Mental Diseases*, 88, 733–755.

Laurence, S. and Stein, D. G. (1978). Recovery after brain damage and the concept of localization of function. In S. Finger (Ed.) *Recovery from Brain Damage*. New York: Plenum Press.

Lazarus, C. and Logemann, J.A. (1987). Swallowing disorders in closed head trauma patients. *Archives of Physical Medicine and Rehabilitation*, 68, 79–84.

Lazarus, R.S. (1993). From psychological stress to the emotions: a history of a changing outlook. *Annual Review of Psychology*, 44, 1–21.

Leaf, L.E. (1993). Traumatic brain injury: affecting family recovery. *Brain Injury*, 7, 543–546.

Lee, W. (1980). Anticipatory control of postural and task muscles during rapid arm flexion. *Journal of Motor Behavior*, 12, 185–196.

Leri, J.E. (1995). The psychological, political and economic realities of brain injury rehabilitation in the 1990s. *Brain Injury*, 9, 533–542.

Levin, H.S., Grossman, R.G., Rose, J.E. and Teasdale, M.B. (1979a). Long term neuropsychological outcome of closed head injury. *Journal of Neurosurgery*, 50, 412–422.

Levin, H.S., O'Donnell, V.M. and Grossman, R.G. (1979b). The Galveston orientation and amnesia test: A practical scale to assess cognition after head injury. *Journal of Nervous and Mental Diseases*, **167**, 675–684.

Levin, H.S., Lippold, S.C., Goldman, A., Handel, S., High, W.M., Eisenberg, H.M. and Zelitt, D. (1987). Neurobehavioral functioning and magnetic resonance imaging findings in young boxers. *Journal of Neurosurgery*, **67**, 657–667.

Levin, H.S., High, V.M. and Eisenberg, H.M. (1988a). Learning and forgetting during post traumatic amnesia in head injured patients. *Journal of Neurology, Neurosurgery and Psychiatry*, **51**, 14–20.

Levin, H.S., Goldstein, F.C., High, W.M. and Williams, D. (1988b). Automatic and effortful processing after severe closed head injury. *Brain and Cognition*, **7**, 283–297.

Levine, D.N., Calvanio, R. and Rinn., W.E. (1991). The pathogenesis of anosognosia for hemiplegia. *Neurology*, **41**, 1770–1781.

Levine, J., Rudy, T. and Kerns, R. (1994). A two factor model of denial of illness: A confirmatory factor analysis. *Journal of Psychosomatic Research*, **38**, 99–110.

Levy, A.B. and Martin, I. (1975). Classical conditioning of human 'evaluative' responses. *Behavior Research and Therapy*, **13**, 221–226.

Lewin, W., Marshal, T.F. and De Cad Roberts, A.H. (1979). Long term outcome after severe head injury. *British Medical Journal*, **2**, 1533–1538.

Lezak, M.D. (1978). Living with the characterologically altered brain injured patient. *Journal of Clinical Psychiatry*, **39**, 592–598.

Lezak, M.D. (1988). Brain damage is a family affair. *Journal of Clinical and Experimental Neuropsychology*, **10**, 111–123.

Lezak, M. (1993). Newer contributions to neuropsychological assessment of executive functions. *Journal of Head Trauma Rehabilitation*, **8**, 24–31.

Lin, K.-C. (1996). Right-hemispheric activation approaches to neglect rehabilitation post stroke. *American Journal of Occupational Therapy*, **50**, 504–515.

Lincoln, N.B., Whiting, S.E., Cockburn, J. and Bhavnani, G. (1985). An evaluation of perceptual retraining. *International Rehabilitation Medicine*, **7**, 99–101.

Lind, K. (1982). A synthesis of studies on stroke rehabilitation. *Journal of Chronic Diseases*, **35**, 133–149.

Lishman, W.A. (1972). Selective factors in memory. I. Age, sex and personality attributes. *Psychological Medicine*, **2**, 121–138.

Lishman, W.A. (1998). *Organic Psychiatry*, 3rd Edn. Oxford: Blackwell Scientific Publications.

Liu, C.N. and Chambers, W.W. (1958). Intraspinal sprouting of dorsal root axons. *Archives of Neurology and Psychiatry*, **79**, 46–61.

Livingston, M.G. (1986). Assessment of need for coordinated approach in families with victims of head injury. *British Medical Journal*, **293**, 742–744.

Livingston, M.G. (1987). Head injury: the relatives' response. *Brain Injury*, **1**, 8–14.

Livingston, M.G. and Livingston, H.M. (1985). The Glasgow assessment schedual: Clinical and research assessment of head injury outcome. *International Rehabilitation Medicine*, **7**, 145–149.

Lloyd, L.F. and Cuvo, A.J. (1994). Maintenance and generalization of behaviors after treatment of persons with traumatic brain injury. *Brain Injury*, **8**, 529–540.

Logemann, J. (1983). *Evaluation and Treatment of Swallowing Disorders*. San Diego, CA: College-Hill Press.

Logemann, J.A. (1989). Evaluation and treatment planning for the head injured patient with oral intake disorders. *Journal of Head Trauma Rehabilitation*, **4**, 24–33.

Logigan, M.K., Samuels, M.A., Falconer, J. and Zagar, R. (1983). Clinical exercise trials for stroke patients. *Archives of Physical Medicine and Rehabilitation*, **64**, 364–367.

Long, C.J., Gouvier, W.D. and Cole, J.C. (1984). A model of recovery for the total rehabilitation of the individual with head trauma. *Journal of Rehabilitation*, **50**, 39–45.

Lord, J.P. and Hall, K.H. (1986). Neuromuscular reeducation versus traditional programs for stroke rehabilitation. *Archives of Physical Medicine and Rehabilitation*, **67**, 88–91.

Lubinski, R., Steger Moscato, B. and Willer, B.S. (1997). Prevalence of speaking and hearing disabilities among adults with traumatic brain injury for a national household survey. *Brain Injury*, **11**, 103–114.

Lubusko, A.A., Moore, A.D., Stambrook, M. and Gill, D.D. (1994). Cognitive beliefs following severe traumatic brain injury: association with post-injury employment status. *Brain Injury*, **8**, 65–70.

Luerssen, T.G., Klauber, M.R. and Marshall, L.F. (1988). Outcome from head injury related to patient's age. *Journal of Neurosurgery*, **68**, 409–416.

Luzzatti, C. and Verga, R. (1996). Reduplicative paramnesia for places with preserved memory. In P.W. Halligan and J.C. Marshall (Eds) *Methods in Madness*. Hove, East Sussex: Psychology Press.

Mace, F.C., Hock, M.L., Lalli, J.S., West, B.J., Belfiore, P., Pinter, E. and Brown, D.K. (1988). Behavioral momentum in the treatment of non-compliance. *Journal of Applied Behavioral Analysis*, **21**, 123–141.

Mace, F.C., Kratochwill, T.R. and Fiello, R.A. (1983). Positive treatment of aggressive behavior in a mentally retarded adult: A case study. *Behavior Therapy*, **14**, 689–696.

Mackay, L.E., Bernstein, B.A., Chapman, P.E., Morgan, A.S. and Milazzo, L.S. (1992). Early intervention in severe head injury: Long-term benefits of a formalized program. *Archives of Physical Medicine and Rehabilitation*, **73**, 635–641.

Mackworth, N., Mackworth, J. and Cope, D.N. (1982). Towards an interpretation of head injury recovery trends. In *Head Injury Rehabilitation Project: Final Report*, pp. 1–66. San Jose, CA: Santa Clara Valley Medical Center Institute for Medical Research.

Maitz, F.A. (1993). Therapy for families of survivors of head injury: Are we helping, or adding to the burden? Paper presented at the *National Head Injury Foundation USA 12th Annual National Symposium*, 7–10 November 1993, Orlando, FL, 'Research to Reality'.

Manchester, D., Hodgkinson, A. and Casey, T. (1997). Prolonged, severe behavioral disturbance following traumatic brain injury: What can be done? *Brain Injury*, **11**, 605–617.

Manchester, D., Hodgkinson, A., Pfaff, A. and Nguyen, F. (1997). A non-aversive approach to reducing hospital absconding in a head-injured adolescent boy. *Brain Injury*, **11**, 271–277.

Mann, R. (1991). Apathy: a neuropsychiatric syndrome. *Journal of Neuropsychiatry and Clinical Neurosciences*, **3**, 243–254.

Marshall, J.C., Halligan, P.W. and Wade, D.T. (1995). Reduplication of an event after head injury? A cautionary case report. *Cortex*, **31**, 183–190.

Martin, G.L., Koop, S., Turner, G. and Hanel, F. (1981). Backward chaining versus total task presentation to teach assembly tasks to severely retarded persons. *Behavior Research of Severe Developmental Disabilities*, **2**, 117–136.

Martin, I. and Levy, A.B. (1994). The evaluative response: Primitive but necessary. *Behavior Research and Therapy*, **32**, 305–310.

McCracken, H.D. and Stelmach, E.E. (1977). A test of the schema theory of discrete motor learning. *Journal of Motor Behavior*, **9**, 193–201.

McDonnell. J. and Laughlin, B. (1989). A comparison of backward and concurrent chaining strategies in teaching community skills. *Education and Training in Mental Retardation*, **24**, 230–238.

McGlynn, S.M. and Schacter, D.L. (1989). Unawareness of deficits in neuropsychological syndromes. *Journal of Clinical and Experimental Neuropsychology*, **11**, 143–205.

McGregor, K. and Pentland, B. (1997). Head injury rehabilitation in the UK: An economic perspective. *Social Science and Medicine*, **45**, 295–303.

McLaughlin, A.M. and Carey, J.L. (1991). The adversarial alliance: Developing therapeutic relationships between families and the team in brain injury rehabilitation. *Brain Injury*, **7**, 45–57.

McLaughlin, A.M. and Schaffer, V. (1985). Rehabilitate or remold?: Family involvement in head trauma recovery. *Cognitive Rehabilitation*, January/February, 14–17.

McMillan, T.M. (1997). Neuropsychological assessment after extremely severe head injury in a case of life or death. *Brain Injury*, **11**, 483–491.

McMordie, W.R., Rogers, K.F. and Barker, S.L. (1991). Consumer satisfaction with services provided to head injured patients and their families. *Brain Injury*, **5**, 43–57.

McPherson, K.M., Pentland, B., Cudmore, S.F. and Prescott, R.J. (1996). An inter-rater reliability study of the Functional Assessment Measure (FIM+FAM). *Disability and Rehabilitation*, **18**, 341–347.

McShane, R., Keene, J., Gedling, K., Fairburn, C., Jacoby, R. and Hope, A. (1997). Do neuroleptic drugs hasten cognitive decline in dementia? Prospective study with necropsy follow-up. *British Medical Journal*, **314**, 266–270.

Medical Research Council (1976). *Aids to the Examination of the Peripheral Nervous System*. London: Her Majesty's Stationery Office.

Mesulam, M. (1985). *Principles of Behavioral Neurology*. Philadelphia, PA: F.A. Davis.

Milani-Comparetti, A. (1980). Pattern analysis of normal and abnormal development: the fetus, the newborn and the child. In D. Slaton (Ed.) *Development of Movement in Infancy*. Chapel Hill, NC: University of North Carolina Press.

Miller, B.L., Cummings, J.L., McIntyre, H., Ebers, G. and Grode, M. (1986). Hypersexuality or altered sexual preference following brain injury. *Journal of Neurology, Neurosurgery and Psychiatry*, **49**, 867–873.

Miller, E. (1980). The training characteristics of severely head injured patients: A preliminary study. *Journal of Neurology, Neurosurgery and Psychiatry*, **43**, 525–528.

Miller, E. (1984). *Recovery and Management of Neuropsychological Impairments*. Chichester: John Wiley.

Miller, E. (1985). Cognitive retraining of neurological patients. In F.N. Watts (Ed.) *New Developments in Clinical Psychology*. Chichester: John Wiley.

Miller, S. and Hammond, G.R. (1981). Neural control of arm movement in patients following stroke. In M.W. Van Hof and G. Mohnl (Eds) *Functional Recovery from Brain Damage*, pp. 259–274. Amsterdam: Elsevier-New Holland.

Mills, J.M., Nesbeda, T., Katz, D.I. and Alexander, M.P. (1992). Outcomes for traumatically brain injured patients following post-acute rehabilitation programmes. *Brain Injury*, **6**, 219–228.

Monakow, C. Von. (1914). *Die Lokalisation im Grosshirn und der Abbau der Funktion Durch Kortikale Herde*. Weisbaden: Bergmann.

Morgan, A. S. (1994), The trauma center as a continuum of care for persons with severe brain injury. *Journal of Head Trauma Rehabilitation*, 9, 1–10.

Morton, M.V. and Wehman, P. (1995). Psycho Social and emotional sequelae of individuals with traumatic brain injury: a literature review and recommendations. *Brain Injury*, 9, 81–92.

Moscowvitch, M. and Melo, B. (1997). Strategic retrieval and the frontal lobes: Evidence from confabulation and amnesia. *Neuropsychologia*, 35, 1017–1034.

Mozzoni, M.P. and Bailey, J.S. (1996). Improving training methods in brain injury rehabilitation. *Journal of Head Trauma Rehabilitation*, 11, 1–17.

Muir, C.A., Haffey, W.J., Ott, K.J., Karaica, D., Muir, J. and Sutko, M. (1983). Treatment of behavioral deficits. In M. Rosenthal, E. Griffith, M.R. Bond and J.D. Miller (Eds) *Rehabilitation of the Head Injured Adult*, pp. 381–393. Philadelphia, PA: F.A. Davis.

Mulder, T. and Hulstijn, W. (1984). Sensory feedback therapy and theoretical knowledge of motor control and learning. *American Journal of Physical Medicine*, 63, 226–244.

Mulder, T. and Hulstijn, W. (1985). Sensory feedback in the learning of a novel motor task. *Journal of Motor Behavior*, 17, 110–128.

Murray, G., Shea, V. and Conn, D. (1987). Electroconvulsive therapy for poststroke depression. *Journal of Clinical Psychiatry*, 47, 258–260.

Nation, J.R. and Woods, D.J. (1980). Persistence: The role of partial reinforcement in psychotherapy. *Journal of Experimental Psychology: General*, 109, 175–207.

National Head Injury Foundation (1991). *Directory of Head Injury Rehabilitation Services*. Southborough, MA: NHIF.

National Head Injury Foundation (1992). *Directory of Head Injury Rehabilitation Services*. Southborough, MA: NHIF.

National Head Injury Foundation (1993). *Directory of Head Injury Rehabilitation Services*. Southborough, MA: NHIF.

National Head Injury Foundation (1994). *Directory of Head Injury Rehabilitation Services*. Southborough, MA: NHIF.

National Head Injury Foundation (1995). *Directory of Head Injury Rehabilitation Services*. Southborough, MA: NHIF.

Neilsen, J.M. (1938). Disturbances of the body scheme. Their physiologic mechanism. *Bulletin of Los Angeles Neurological Society*, 3, 127–135.

Nelson, T.O. and Narens, L. (1994). Why Investigate Metacognition. In J. Metcalf and P. Shimamura (Eds) *Metacognition: Knowing about Knowing*. Cambridge, MA: MIT Press.

Neubauer, R.A., Gottlieb, S.F. and Kagan, R.L. (1990). Enhancing 'idling' neurons (letter). *Lancet*, 542.

Newell, A. and Rosenbloom, P.S. (1981). Mechanisms of skill acquisition and the law of practice. In J.R. Anderson (Ed.) *Cognitive Skills and their Acquisition*. Hillsdale, NJ: Lawrence Erlbaum Associates.

Newell, K.M. and Walter, C.B. (1981). Kinematic and kinetic parameters and information feedback in motor skill acquisition. *Journal of Human Movement Studies*, 7, 235–254.

Newman, M.F., Croughwell, N.D., Blumenthal, J.A., Lowry, E., White, W.D., Spillane, W., Davis, R.D. Jr., Glower, D.D., Smith, L.R., Mahanna, E.P. *et al.* (1995). Predictors of cognitive decline after cardiac operation. *Annals of Thoracic Surgery*, 59, 1326–1330.

Niemeier, J.P. (1998). The Lighthouse Strategy: use of a visual imagery technique to treat visual inattention in stroke patients. *Brain Injury*, 12, 399–406.

Nihira, K., Leland, H. and Lambert, N. (1993). *Adaptive Behavior Scale – Residential and Community*, 2nd Edn. Austin, TX: Pro-Ed Inc.

Nisbett, R.E. and Wilson, T.D. (1977). Telling more than we can know: Verbal reports on mental processes. *Psychology Review*, **84**, 231–259.

Norman, D.A. and Shallice, T. (1980). Attention to action: Willed and automatic control of behavior. Center for Human Information Processing (Technical Report No. 99). (Reprinted in revised form in R.J. Davidson, G.E. Schwartz and D. Shapiro [Eds.] [1986] *Consciousness and Self Regulation* [Vol. 4]. New York: Plenum Press.)

Novak, T.A., Satterfield, W.T., Lyons, K., Kolski, G., Hackmeyer, L. and Conner, M. (1984). Stroke onset and rehabilitation: time lag as a factor in treatment outcome. *Archives of Physical Medicine and Rehabilitation*, **65**, 316–319.

Novak, T.A., Dillon, M.C. and Jackson, W.T. (1996). Neurochemical mechanisms in brain injury and treatment: A review. *Journal of Clinical and Experimental Neuropsychology*, **18**, 685–706.

Oddy, M., Humphrey, M. and Uttley, D. (1978). Stresses upon the relatives of brain-injured patients. *British Journal of Psychiatry*, **41**, 611–616.

Olver, J.H., Ponsford, J.L. and Curran, C.A. (1996). Outcome following traumatic brain injury: A comparison between 2 and 5 years after injury. *Brain Injury*, **10**, 841–848.

Oostra, K., Everaert, K. and Van Laere, M. (1995). Urinary incontinence in brain injury. *Brain Injury*, **10**, 459–464.

Osberg, J.S., Brooke, M.M., Baryza, M.J., Rowe, K., Lash, M. and Kahn, P. (1997). Impact of childhood brain injury on work and family finances. *Brain Injury*, **11**, 11–24.

Ovsiew, F. (1992). Bedside neuropsychiatry: eliciting the clinical phenomena of neuropsychiatric illness. In *The American Psychiatric Press Textbook of Neuropsychiatry*, 2nd Edn. Washington, DC: American Psychiatric Press.

Pantano, J.C., Baron, J.C., Samson, Y., Bousser, M.G., Derouesne, C. and Comar, D. (1968). Crossed cerebellar diaschisis: further studies. *Brain*, **109**, 677–694.

Panting, A. and Merry, P.H. (1972). The long-term rehabilitation of severe head injuries with particular reference to the need for social and medical support for the patient's family. *Rehabilitation*, **38**, 33–37.

Pattern, B.M. (1972). The ancient art of memory: Usefulness in treatment. *Archives of Neurology*, **26**, 25–31.

Pavlov, I.P. (1927). *Conditioned Reflexes*. London: Oxford University Press.

Petrides, M. (1985). Deficits on conditional associative-learning tasks after frontal and temporal-lobe lesions in man. *Neuropsychologia*, **23**, 601–614.

Piaget, J. and Inhelder, B. (1969). *The Psychology of the Child*. New York: Basic Books.

Pick, A. (1898). Beitrage zur Pathologie und Pathologische Anatomie des Central Nervensystems mit Bermerkungen zur Normalen Anatomie Desslben. Berlin: Karger.

Ponsford, J.L. and Kinsella, G. (1988). Evaluation of a remedial program for attentional deficits following closed-head injury. *Journal of Clinical and Experimental Neuropsychology*, **10**, 693–708.

Ponsford, J.L., Olver, J.H., Curran, C. and Ng, K. (1995). Prediction of employment status 2 years after traumatic brain injury. *Brain Injury*, **9**, 11–20.

Ponte-Allan, M. and Giles, G.M. (in press). Functional outcomes and goal setting in rehabilitation. *American Journal of Occupational Therapy*.

Pope, H., McElroy, S., Satlin, A., Hudson, J.I., Keck, P.E. Jr. and Kalish, R. (1988). Head injury, bipolar disorder and response to valproate. *Comprehensive Psychiatry*, **29**, 34–38.

Posner, M.I. and Peterson, S.E. (1990). The attentional system of the human brain. *Annual Review of Neuroscience*, **13**, 25–42.

Powell, G.E. (1981). *Brain Function Therapy*. Aldershot, Hants: Gower.

Powell, J. and Greenwood, R. (1998). Homerton: the RNRU experience. Paper presented at the *National Traumatic Brain Injury Study (NTBIS) Meeting*. 1 December 1998.

Powell, J.H., Al Adowi, S., Morgan, J. and Greenwood, R.J. (1996). Motivational deficits after brain-injury: Effects of bromocriptine in 11 patients. *Journal of Neurology, Neurosurgery and Psychiatry*, 60, 416–421.

Pribram, K.H. (1968). Towards a neuropsychological theory of person. In K.H. Pribram (Ed.) *The Study of Personality: An Interdisciplinary Approach*. New York: Holt, Rinehart & Winston.

Prigatano, G.P. and Altman, I.M. (1990). Impaired awareness of behavioral limitations after traumatic brain injury. *Archives of Physical Medicine and Rehabilitation*, 71, 1058–1064.

Prigatano, G.P., Fordyce, D.J., Zeiner, H.K., Roueche, J.R., Pepping, M. and Wood, B.C. (1984). Neuropsychological rehabilitation after closed head injury in young adults. *Journal of Neurology, Neurosurgery and Psychiatry*, 47, 505–513.

Prigatano, G.P., Klonoff. P.S. and Bailey, I. (1987). Psychosocial adjustment associated with traumatic brain injury: Statistics BNI neurorehabilitation must beat. *BNI Quarterly*, 3, 10–17.

Pulaski, K.H. and Emmett, L. (1994). Case Report – The combined intervention of therapy and bromocriptine mesylate to improve functional performance after brain injury. *American Journal of Occupational Therapy*, 48, 263–270

Rader, M.A., Alston, J.B. and Ellis, D.W. (1989). Sensory stimulation of severely brain injured patients. *Brain Injury*, 3, 141–147.

Rafferty, F.T., Hawley, L. Cirton, C., Ducker, C. and Berry, V. (1984). Tertiary care of post head trauma patient. *The Psychiatric Hospital*, 15, 193–197.

Ragnarsson, K.T., Thomas, J.P., Zasler, N.D. (1993). Model systems of care for individuals with traumatic brain injury. *Journal of Head Trauma Rehabilitation*, 8, 1–11.

Raichle, M.E. (1997). Brain imaging. In M.S. Gazzaniga (Ed.) *Conversations in the Cognitive Neurosciences*. Cambridge, MA: MIT Press.

Ramachandran, V.S. (1996). The evolutionary biology of self-deception, laughter, dreaming and depression: Some clues from anosognosia. *Medical Hypothesis*, 47, 347–362.

Rappaport, M., Hall, K.M., Hopkins, K., Belleza, T. and Cope, D.N. (1982). Disability rating scale for severe brain trauma; Coma to community. *Archives of Physical Medicine and Rehabilitation*, 63, 118–123.

Read, A., Beaty, P., Corner, J. and Sommerville, C. (1996). Reducing naltrexone-resistant hyperphagia using laser acupuncture to increase endogenous opiates. *Brain Injury*, 10, 911–921.

Reason, J. (1984). Absent-mindedness and cognitive control. In J.E. Harris and P.E. Morris (Eds) *Everyday Memory Actions and Absent-Mindedness*. London: Academic Press.

Reed, E.S. (1982). An outline of a theory of action systems. *Journal of Motor Behavior*, 14, 98–134.

Rescorla, R.A. (1988). Pavlovian Conditioning: It's not what you think it is. *American Psychologist*, 43, 151–160.

Riccio, D.C., Rabinowiitz, V.C. and Axelrod, S. (1994). Memory: when less is more. *American Psychologist*, 49, 917–926.

Richardson, J.C., Chambers, R.A. and Hayward, P.M. (1959). Encephalopathies of anoxia and hypoglycaemia. *Archives of Neurology*, 1, 178–190.

Rimel, R. and Jane, J. (1983). Characteristics of the head-injured patient. In M. Rosenthal, E. Griffith, M.R. Bond and J.D. Miller (Eds) *Rehabilitation of the Head Injured Adult*, pp. 9–21. Philadelphia, PA: F.A. Davis.

Rimel, R., Giordani, M., Barth, J., Boll, T. and Jane, J. (1981). Disability caused by minor head injury. *Neurosurgery*, 9, 221–228.

Rizzo, M. and Tranel, D. (1996). *Head Injury and Post-Concussive Syndrome.* New York: Churchill Livingstone

Roberts, A.H. (1969). *Brain Damage in Boxers.* London: Pitman.

Roberts, A.H. (1979). *Severe Accidental Head Injury: An Assessment of Long-Term Prognosis.* London: Macmillan.

Robertson, I. and North, N. (1992). Spatio-motor cueing in unilateral left neglect: The role of hemispace, hand and motor activation. *Neuropsychologia*, 30, 553–563.

Robertson, I., Gray, J. and McKenzie, S. (1988). Microcomputer based cognitive rehabilitation of visual neglect: 3 multiple baseline single case studies. *Brain Injury*, 2, 151–163.

Robertson, I.H., Ward, T., Ridgeway, V. and Nimmo-Smith, I. (1994). *The Test of Everyday Attention.* Bury St. Edmunds: Thames Valley Test Company.

Robinson, R. and Starkstein, S. (1990). Current research in affective disorders following stroke. *Journal of Neuropsychiatry and Clinical Neurosciences*, 2, 1–14.

Robinson, R.O. (1986). Mechanisms of brain recovery. *Journal of the Royal Society of Medicine*, 79, 430–433.

Rolls, E.T., Hornak, J., Wade, D. and McGrath, J. (1994). Emotion-related learning in patients with social and emotional changes associated with frontal lobe damage. *Journal of Neurology, Neurosurgery and Psychiatry*, 57, 1518–1524

Ross, L. (1977). The intuitive psychologist and his shortcomings: Distortions in the attribution process. *Advances in Experimental Social Psychology*, 10, 173–220.

Ross-Swain, D. (1996). *Ross Information Processing Assessment*, 2nd Edn. Austin, TX: Pro-Ed Inc.

Roth, M. and Myers, D. (1969). The diagnosis of dementia. *British Journal of Hospital Medicine*, 2, 705–717.

Rothi, L.J. and Horner, J. (1983). Restitution and substitution: two theories of recovery with application to neurobehavioral treatment. *Journal of Clinical Neuropsychology*, 5, 73–81

Rothstein, A.L. and Arnold, R.K. (1976). Bridging the gap: Application of research on videotape feedback and bowling. *Motor Skills: Theory into Practice*, 1, 35–62.

Royal College of Physicians (1986). Physical disability in 1986 and beyond. *Journal of The Royal College of Physicians of London*, 20, 177–178.

Russell, W.R. and Smith, A. (1961). Post-traumatic amnesia in closed head injuries. *Archives of Neurology*, 5, 16–29.

Sahgal, V. and Heinemann, A (1989). Recovery of function during inpatient rehabilitation for moderate traumatic brain injury. *Scandinavian Journal of Rehabilitation Medicine*, 21, 71–79.

Sahrmann, S.A. and Norton, B.J. (1977). The relationship of voluntary movement spasticity in the upper motor neuron syndrome. *Annals of Neurology*, 2, 460–465.

Santos, A.B., Wohlreich, M.M. and Pinosky, S.T. (1982). Managing agitation in the critical care setting. *Journal – South Carolina Medical Association*, 88, 386.

Sarno, M.T. (1984). Verbal impairment after closed head injury: Report of a replication study. *Journal of Nervous and Mental Diseases*, 172, 475–479.

Schacter, D.L. (1992). Consciousness and awareness in memory and amnesia: Critical issues. In A.D. Milner and M.D. Rugg (Eds) *Neuropsychology of Consciousness*, pp. 179–200. London: Academic Press.

Schacter, D.L., McAndrew, M.P. and Moscowvitch, M. (1988). Access to consciousness: dissociations between implicit and explicit knowledge in neuropsychological syndromes. In L. Weiskrantz (Ed.) *Thought without Language*, pp. 242–278. Oxford: Oxford University Press.

Schalen, W., Nordstrom, G. and Nordstrom, C. H. (1994). Economic aspects of capacity for work after severe traumatic brain lesions. *Brain Injury*, **8**, 37–47.

Schmidt, N.D. (1997). Outcome-oriented rehabilitation: a response to managed care. *Journal of Head Trauma Rehabilitation*, **12**, 44–50.

Schmidt, R.A. (1988). *Motor Control and Learning: A Behavioral Emphasis*, 2nd Edn. Champaign, IL: Human Kinetics Press.

Schmidt, R.A. and Young, D.E. (1987). Transfer of movement control in motor skill learning. In S.M. Cormier and J.D. Hagman (Eds) *Transfer of Learning: Contemporary Research and Application*. Orlando, FL: Academic Press.

Schmidt, R.A., Young, D.E., Swinnen, S. and Shapiro, D.C. (1989). Summary knowledge of results for skill acquisition: support for the guidance hypothesis. *Journal of Experimental Psychology: Learning, Memory, Cognition*, **15**, 352–359.

Schmitter-Edgecombe, M. and Rogers, W.A. (1997). Automatic process development following severe closed head injury. *Neuropsychology*, **11**, 296–308.

Schoenbaum, M. (1997). Do smokers understand the mortality effects of smoking? Evidence from the health and retirement survey. *American Journal of Public Health*, **87**, 755–759.

Schoenfeld, T.A. and Hamilton, L.W. (1977). Secondary brain changes following lesions: A new paradigm for lesion experimentation. *Physiology and Behavior*, **18**, 951–967.

Schuell, H. (1963). *The Minnesota Test for the Differential Diagnosis of Aphasia*. Minneapolis, MN: University of Minnesota Press.

Schulz, C.H. (1994). Helping Factors in a peer developed support group for brain injured individuals. Part II. survivor interview perspective. *American Journal of Occupational Therapy*, **48**, 305–309

Schwartz, M.F., Mayer, N.H., Fitzpatrick DeSalme, E.J. and Montgomery, M.W. (1993). Cognitive theory and the study of everyday action disorders after brain damage. *Journal of Head Trauma Rehabilitation*, **8**, 59–72.

Schwartzberg, S.L. (1994). Helping factors in a peer developed support group for brain injured individuals. *American Journal of Occupational Therapy*, **48**, 297–304.

Scranton, J., Fogel, M.L. and Erdman, W.J. (1970). Evaluation of functional levels of patients during and following rehabilitation. *Archives of Physical Medicine and Rehabilitation*, **51**, 1–21.

Seelig, J.M., Becker, D.P., Miller, J.D., Greenberg, R.P., Ward, J.D. and Choi, S.C. (1981). Traumatic acute subdural hematoma major mortality reductions in comatose patients treated within four hours. *New England Journal of Medicine*, **304**, 1245–1249.

Seligman, M. (1975). *Helplessness: On Depression, Development and Death*. San Fransisco, CA: W.H. Freeman.

Shallice, T. and Evans, M.E. (1978). The involvement of the frontal lobes in cognitive estimation. *Cortex*, **14**, 294–303.

Shaw, L., Brodsky, L. and McMahon, B.T. (1985). Neuropsychiatric intervention in the rehabilitation of head injured patients. *Psychiatric Journal of the University of Ottawa*, **10**, 237–240.

Shea, J. B. and Morgan, R.L. (1979). Contextual interference effects on the acquisition, retention and transfer of a motor skill. *Journal of Experimental Psychology: Human Learning and Memory*, **5**, 179–187.

Shiffrin, R.M. and Schneider, W. (1977). Controlled and automatic information processing: II. Perceptual learning, automatic attending and a general theory. *Psychological Review*, **84**, 127–190.

Shumway-Cook, A. and McCollum, G. (1991). Assessment and treatment of balance deficits. In P. Montgomery and B. Connolly (Eds) *Motor Control and Physical Therapy: Theoretical Framework and Practical Application*, pp. 123–140. Hixon, TN: Chattanooga Group Inc.

Shumway-Cook, A. and Olmscheid, R. (1990). A systems analysis of postural dyscontrol in traumatically brain-injured patients. *Journal of Head Trauma Rehabilitation*, 5, 51–62.

Silvestri, S. and Aronson, S. (1997). Severe head injury: Prehospital and emergency department management. *The Mount Sinai Journal of Medicine*, 64, 329–338.

Sirigu, A., Zalla, T., Pillon, B., Grafman, J., Agid, Y. and Dubois, B. (1995). Selective impairments in managerial knowledge following pre-frontal cortex damage. *Cortex*, 31, 301–316.

Skinner, B.F. (1938). *The Behavior of Organisms: An Experimental Analysis*. New York: Appleton-Century-Crofts.

Skinner, B.F. (1948). 'Superstition' in the pigeon. *Journal of Experimental Psychology*, 38, 168–172.

Skinner, B.F. (1976), *About Behaviorism*. New York: Vintage.

Skord, KG. and Miranti, S.V. (1994). Towards a more integrated approach to job placement and retention for persons with traumatic brain injury and premorbid disadvantages. *Brain Injury*, 8, 383–392.

Slifer, K.J., Tucker, C.L., Gerson, C.A., Sevier, R.C., Kane, A.C., Amari, A. and Clawson, B.P. (1997). Antecedent management and compliance training improve adolescent's participation in early brain injury rehabilitation. *Brain Injury*, 11, 877–889.

Small, M. and Ellis, S. (1996). Denial of hemiplegia: An investigation into the theories of causation. *European Neurology*, 36, 353–363.

Smith, E. (1997). Infusing cognitive neuroscience into cognitive psychology. In R.L. Solso (Ed.) *Mind and Brain Sciences in the 21st Century*. Cambridge, MA: MIT Press.

Smith, H.W. (1975). *Strategies of Social Research*. Englewood Cliffs, NJ: Prentice-Hall

Social Services Inspectorate (1996). *A Hidden Disability. Traumatic Brain Injury Rehabilitation Project Report*. London: Department of Health, UK.

Soderback, I. and Normell, L.A. (1986a). Intellectual function training in adults with acquired brain damage: An occupational therapy method. *Scandinavian Journal of Rehabilitation Medicine*, 18, 139–146.

Soderback, I. and Normell, L.A. (1986b). Intellectual function training in adults with acquired brain damage: Evaluation. *Scandinavian Journal of Rehabilitation Medicine*, 18, 147–153.

Sohlberg, M.M. and Mateer, C.A. (1986). *APT: Attention Process Training Manual*. Puyallup, WA: Association for Neuropsychological Research and Development.

Sohlberg, M.M. and Mateer, C.A. (1987). Effectiveness of an attention training program. *Journal of Clinical and Experimental Neuropsychology*, 9, 117–130.

Spencer, J., Young, M.E., Rintala, D. and Bates, S. (1995). Socialization to the culture of a rehabilitation hospital: an ethnographic study. *American Journal of Occupational Therapy*, 49, 53–62.

Spettel, C.M., Ellis, D.W., Ross, S.E., Sandel, M.E., O'Malley, K.F., Stein, S.C., Spivak, G. and Hurley, K.E. (1991). Time or rehabilitation admission and severity of trauma: effect on brain injury outcome. *Archives of Physical Medicine and Rehabilitation*, 72, 320–325.

Spooner, F. (1981). An operant analysis of the effects of backward chaining and total task presentation. *Dissertation Abstracts International*, 41(3), 992A.

Spooner, F. (1984). Comparison of backward chaining and total task presentation in training severely handicapped persons. *Education and Training of the Mentally Retarded*, **19**, 15–22.

Starkstein, S., Federoff, P., Price, T., Leiguarda, R. and Robinson, R. (1992). Anosognosia in patients with cerebrovascular lesions: A study of causative factors. *Stroke*, **23**, 1446–1453.

Stern, J.M., Melamed, S., Silberg, S., Rahmani, L. and Groswasser, L. (1985). Behavioral disturbance as an expression of severity of cerebral damage. *Scandinavian Journal of Rehabilitation Medicine: Supplement*, **12**, 36–41.

Stern, P.H., McDowell, F., Miller, J.M. and Robinson, M. (1970). Effects of facilitation exercise techniques in stroke rehabilitation. *Archives of Physical Medicine and Rehabilitation*, **51**, 526- 531.

Stilwell, J., Hawley, C., Stilwell, P., Davies, C. and Fletcher, J. (1998). *National Traumatic Brain Injury Study: Summary of Report*. Coventry: Centre for Health Services Studies, University of Warwick.

Strauss, D.H., Spitzer, R.L. and Mushkin, P.R. (1990). Maladaptive denial of physical illness: A proposal for DSM-IV. *American Journal of Psychiatry*, **147**, 1168–1172.

Strick, S.J. (1956). Diffuse degeneration of the cerebral white matter in severe dementia following head-injury. *Journal of Neurology, Neurosurgery and Psychiatry*, **19**, 163–195.

Strick, S.J. (1969). The pathology of brain-damage due to blunt head-injuries. In A.E. Walker, W.F. Caveness and M. Critchley (Eds) *The Late Effects of Head Injury*, Vol. 51. Springfield, IL: Charles C. Thomas.

Sunderland, A., Harris, J.E. and Badderley, A.D. (1983). Do laboratory tests predict everyday memory? A neuropsychological study. *Journal of Verbal Learning and Verbal Behavior*, **22**, 341–357.

Svartdal, F. (1991). Operant modulation of low level attributes of rule governed behavior by non verbal contingencies. *Learning and Motivation*, **22**, 406–420.

Tangeman, P.T., Banaitis, D.A. and Williams, A.K. (1990). Rehabilitation of chronic stroke patients: changes in functional performance. *Archives of Physical Medicine and Rehabilitation*, **71**, 876–880.

Tate, R.L., Lulham, J.M., Broe, G.A., Strettles, B. and Pfaff, A. (1989). Psychosocial outcome for the survivors of severe blunt head injury: the results from a consecutive series of 100 patients. *Journal of Neurology, Neurosurgery and Psychiatry*, **52**, 1128–1134.

Tatemichi, T.K., Desmond, D.W., Stern, Y., Sano, M. and Bagiella, E. (1994). Cognitive impairment after stroke: frequency, patterns and relationship to functional abilities. *Journal of Neurology, Neurosurgery and Psychiatry*, **57**, 202–207.

Taub, E. (1976). Motor behavior following deafferentation in the developing and motorically mature monkey. *Advances in Behavioral Biology*, **18**, 675–705.

Teasdale, G.M. (1995). Head injury. *Journal of Neurology, Neurosurgery and Psychiatry*, **58**, 526–539.

Teasdale, G. and Jennett, B. (1974). Assessment of coma and impaired consciousness: A practical scale. *Lancet*, ii, 81–84.

Teasdale, G. and Mendelow, D. (1984). Pathophysiology of head injuries. In D.N. Brooks (Ed.) *Closed Head Injury: Psychological Social and Family Consequences*. London: Oxford University Press

Teasdale, G.M., Nicoll, J.A.R., Murray, G. and Fiddes, M. (1997). Association of apolipoprotein E polymorphism with outcome after head injury. *Lancet*, **350**, 1069–1071.

Teasdale, T., Skovdahl Hansen, H., Gade, A. and Christensen, A.-L, (1997). Neuropsychological test scores before and after brain injury rehabilitation in relation to return to employment. *Neuropsychological Rehabilitation*, 7, 23–42.

Teuber, H.-L. (1975). Recovery of function after brain injury in man. In CIBA Foundation Symposium 34. New Series. *Outcome of Severe Damage to the Central Nervous System*. Amsterdam: Elsevier.

Thomsen, I.V. (1974). The patient with severe brain injury and his family: a follow-up of 50 patients. *Scandinavian Journal of Rehabilitation Medicine*, 6, 180–183.

Thomsen, I.V. (1981). Neuropsychological treatment and long term follow-up of an aphasic patient with very severe head trauma. *Journal of Clinical Neuropsychology*, 3, 43–51.

Thomsen, I.V. (1984). Late outcome of severe blunt head trauma: a 10–15 year second follow-up. *Journal of Neurology, Neurosurgery and Psychiatry*, 47, 260–268.

Thomsen, I.V. (1989). Do young patients have worse outcomes after severe head trauma? *Brain Injury*, 3, 157-162.

Thomsen, I.V. (1992). Late psychological outcome in severe traumatic brain injury. Preliminary results of a third follow up study after 20 years. *Scandinavian Journal of Rehabilitation Medicine: Supplement*, 26, 42–52.

Thorndike, E.L. (1911). *Animal Intelligence*. New York: Macmillan.

Tizard, B. (1959). Theories of brain localization from Flourens to Lashley. *Medical History*, 3, 132–145.

Toglia, J.P. (1993). *Contextual Memory Test; Manual*. Tucson, AZ: Therapy Skill Builders,

Toglia, J.P. (1998). A dynamic interactional model to cognitive rehabilitation. In N. Katz (Ed.) *Cognition and Occupation in Rehabilitation. Cognitive Models for Intervention in Occupational Therapy*. Bethesda, MD: American Occupational Therapy Association.

Treadwell, K. and Page, T.J. (1996). Functional analysis: Identifying the environmental determinants of severe behavior disorder. *Journal of Head Trauma Rehabilitation*, 11, 62–74.

Trower P., Bryant, B.M. and Argyle, M. (1978). *Social Skills and Mental Health*. London: Methuen.

Tyerman, A. (1997).Working out: vocational rehabilitation project. Paper presented at *Social Reintegration after Brain Injury Conference*, Birmingham.

Tyerman, A. (1999).*Working out; A Joint DOH/ES Traumatic Brain Injury Vocational Rehabilitation Project: Short Report.*

Tyerman, A.D. and Humphrey, M.E. (1986). Self concept change following severe head injury. Paper presented at *Models of Brain Injury Rehabilitation Conference*, London.

Tzidkiahu, T., Sazbon, L. and Solzi, P. (1994).Characteristic reactions of relatives of post coma unawareness patients in the process of adjusting to loss. *Brain Injury*, 8, 159–165.

Ullman, P. and Krasner, L. (1969). *A Psychological Approach to Abnormal Behavior*. Englewood Cliffs, NJ: Prentice-Hall.

Ullman, U., Ashenhurst, E.M., Hurwitz, L.J. and Gruen, A. (1960) Motivational and structural factors in the denial of hemiplegia. *Archives of Neurology*, 3, 306–318.

Uniform Data System for Medical Rehabilitation (1993). *Guide for the Uniform Data Set for Medical Rehabilitation (Adult FIM), Version 4.0 effective 1 January 1994*. Buffalo, NY: UB Foundation Activities, Inc.

Vallar, G., Sterzi, G., Bottini, G., Cappa, S. and Rusconi, M.L. (1990). Temporary remission of left hemiaesthesis after vestibular stimulation: and sensory neglect phenomenon. *Cortex*, 26,123–131.

Van Zomeren, A.H. and Deelman, B.G. (1978). Long-term recovery of visual reaction time after closed head injury. *Journal of Neurology, Neurosurgery and Psychiatry*, 41, 452–457.

Van Zomeren, A.H., Brouner, W.H., Rothengatter, J.A. and Snoek, J.W. (1988). Fitness to drive a car after recovery from severe head injury. *Archives of Physical Medicine and Rehabilitation*, 69, 90–96.

Vargha-Khadem, F., Gadian, D.G., Watkins, K.E., Connelly, A., Van Paesschen, W. and Mishkin, M. (1997). Differential effects of early hippocampal pathology on episodic and semantic memory. *Science*, 277, 376–380.

Varnee, N.R. and Menefee, L. (1993). Psychosocial and executive deficits following closed head injury: Implications for orbital frontal cortex. *Journal of Head Trauma Rehabilitation*, 8, 32–44.

Verfaellie, M. and Heilman, K.M. (1987). Response preparation and response inhibition after lesions of the medial frontal lonbe. *Archives of Neurology*, 44, 1265–1271.

Vogenthaler, D. R., Smith, K.R. and Goldfader, P. (1989). Head injury, an empirical study: describing long-term productivity and independent living outcome. *Brain Injury*, 3, 355–368.

Vollmer, D.G., Torner, J.C., Jane, J.A., Sadovnic, B., Charlebois, D., Eisenberg, H.M., Foulkes, M.A., Marmarou, A. and Marshal, L.F. (1991). Age and outcome following traumatic coma: Why do older patients fare worse? *Journal of Neurosurgery*, 75, s37–s49.

Wade, D.T., Skillbeck, C.E., Hewer, R.L. and Wood, V.A. (1984). Therapy after stroke: amount, determinants and effects. *International Rehabilitation Medicine*, 6, 105–110.

Wade, D.T., Crawford, S., Wenden, F.J., King, N.S. and Moss, N.E.G. (1997). Does routine follow-up after head injury help? A randomized controlled trial. *Journal of Neurology, Neurosurgery and Psychiatry*, 62, 478–484.

Wade, D.T., King, N.S., Wenden, F.J., Crawford, S. and Caldwell, F.E. (1998). Routine follow up after head injury: a second randomized controlled trial. *Journal of Neurology, Neurosurgery and Psychiatry*, 65, 177–183.

Wanatanabe, T.K., Black, K.L., Zafonte, R.D., Millis, S.R. and Mann, N.R. (1998). Do calendars enhance posttraumatic temporal orientation?: a pilot study. *Brain Injury*, 12, 81–85.

Watson, J. (1924), *Behaviorism*. Chicago, IL: Phoenix Books.

Webb, C., Rose, F.D., Johnson, D.A. and Attree, E.A. (1996). Age and recovery from brain injury: clinical opinions and experimental evidence. *Brain Injury*, 10, 303–310.

Weddell, R., Oddy, M. and Jenkins, D. (1980). Social adjustment after rehabilitation: two year follow up of patients with severe head injury. *Psychological Medicine*, 10, 257–263.

Wehman, P., Kregel, J., West, M. and Cifu, D. (1994). Return to work for patients with traumatic brain injury. Analysis of costs. *American Journal of Physical Medicine and Rehabilitation*, 73, 280–282.

Wehman, P., Sherron, P., Kregel, J., Kreutzer, J., Tran, S. and Cifu, D. (1993). Return to work for persons following severe traumatic brain injury. Supported employment outcomes after five years. *American Journal of Physical and Medical Rehabilitation*, 72, 355–363.

Weingartner, H., Gold, P., Ballenge, J.C., Smallberg, S., Summers, R., Rubinow, D.R., Post, R.M. and Goodwin, F.K. (1981). Effects of vasopressin on human memory function. *Science*, 211, 601-603.

Weinstein, E.A. and Cole, M. (1963). Concepts of anosognosia. In L. Halpern (Ed.) *Problems in Dynamic Neurology: Functions of the Human Nervous System*, pp. 254–273. Jerusalem: Jerusalem Post Press.

Weinstein, E.A. and Kahn, R.L. (1950) The syndrome of Anosognosia. *Archives of Neurology and Psychiatry*, **64**, 772–791.

Weinstein, E.A. and Kahn, R.L. (1955). *Denial of Illness: Symbolic and Physiological Aspects.* Springfield, IL: Charles C. Thomas.

Weiskrantz, L. (1997). *Consciousness Lost and Found.* Oxford: Oxford University Press.

Weitz, R. (1989). Uncertainty and the lives of persons with AIDS. *Journal of Health and Social Behavior*, **30**, 270–281.

West, M.D. (1995). Aspects of the workplace and return to work for persons with brain injury in supported employment. *Brain Injury*, **9**, 301–313.

Whitlock, J.A. (1992). Functional outcome of low-level traumatically brain-injured admitted to an acute rehabilitation programme. *Brain Injury*, **6**, 447–559.

Willer, B., Rosenthal, M., Kreutzer, J., Gordon, W.A and Rempel, R. (1993). Assessment of community integration following rehabilitation for traumatic brain injury. *Journal of Head Trauma Rehabilitation*, **8**, 75–85

Willer, B.S., Allen, K.M., Liss, M. and Zicht, M.S. (1991). Problems and coping strategies of individuals with traumatic brain injury and their spouses. *Archives of Physical Medicine and Rehabilitation*, **72**, 460–464.

Williams, D.H., Levin, H.S. and Eisenberg, H.E. (1990). Mild head injury classification. *Neurosurgery*, **27**, 422–428.

Wilms, W. (1984). Vocational education and job success: The employer's view. *Phi Delta Kappa*, **65**, 347–350.

Wilson, B.A. (1991). Long term prognosis of patients with severe memory disorders. *Neuropsycholgical Rehabilitation*, **1**, 117–134.

Wilson, B.A. (1996). Cognitive functioning of adult survivors of cerebral hypoxia. *Brain Injury*, **10**, 863–875.

Wilson, B.A. and Evans, J.J. (1996). Error-free learning in the rehabilitation of people with memory impairment. *Journal of Head Trauma Rehabilitation*, **11**, 54–64.

Wilson, B.A. and Moffat, N. (1984). *Clinical Management of Memory Problems.* London: Croom Helm.

Wilson, B.A., Cockburn, J. and Baddeley, A. (1991). *The Rivermead Behavioral Memory Test*, 2nd Edn. Bury St. Edmunds: Thames Valley Test Company.

Wilson, B.A., Badderley, A.D., Evans, J. and Shiel, A. (1994). Errorless learning in the rehabilitation of memory impaired people. *Neuropsychological Rehabilitation*, **4**, 307–326.

Wilson, S.L. and McMillan, T.M. (1993). A review of the evidence for the effectiveness of sensory stimulation treatment for coma and vegetative states. *Neuropsychological Rehabilitation*, **3**, 149–160.

Wilson, S.L., Powell, G.E., Elliott, K. and Thwaites, H. (1991). Sensory stimulation in prolonged coma: four single case studies. *Brain Injury*, **5**, 393–400.

Wilson, S.L., Cranny, S. and Andrews, K. (1992). The efficacy of music for stimulation in prolonged coma-four single case experiments. *Clinical Rehabilitation*, **6**, 181–187.

Wilson, S.L., Brock, D., Powell, G.E. and Thwaites, H. (1996). Vegetative state and responses to sensory stimulation: An analysis of 24 cases. *Brain Injury*, **10**, 807–818.

Winchel, R. and Stanley, M. (1991). Self-injurious behavior: a review of the behavior and biology of self-mutilation. *American Journal of Psychiatry*, **148**, 306–317.

Winstein, C.J. (1987). Motor learning considerations in stroke. In P.W. Duncan and M.B. Badke (Eds) *Stroke Rehabilitation: The Recovery of Motor Control*, pp. 109–134. Chicago, IL: Yearbook Medical Publisher.

Winstein, C.J. (1991). Designing practice for motor learning: clinical implications. In M. Lister (Ed.) *11 STEP Contemporary Management of Motor Control Problems*, pp. 65–76. Virginia: Foundation for Physical Therapy, Inc.

Winstein, C.J. and Schmidt, R.A. (1990). Reduced frequency of knowledge of results enhances motor skill learning. *Journal of Experimental Psychology: Learning, Memory, Cognition*, 16, 677–691.

Winstein, C.J., Gardner, E.R., McNeal, D.R., Barto, S. and Nicholson, D.E. (1989). Standing balance training: effect on balance and locomotion in hemiparetic adults. *Archives of Physical Medicine and Rehabilitation*, 70, 755–762.

Wolery, M., Griffen, A.K., Ault, M.J., Gast, D.L. and Doyle, P.M. (1990). Comparison of constant time delay and the system of least prompts in teaching chained tasks. *Education and Training in Mental Retardation*, 25, 243–257.

Wood, R. and Burgess, P. (1988). Management of Behaviour disorders following brain injury. In I. Fussey and G.M. Giles (Eds) *Rehabilitation of the Severely Brain Injured Adult: A Practical Approach*, pp. 43–68. London: Croom Helm.

Wood R.L. (1987). *Brain Injury Rehabilitation: A Neurobehavioural Approach*. London: Croom Helm.

Wood, R.L. and Eames, P. (1981). Application of behaviour modification in the treatment of the traumatically brain-injured adults. In G. Davey (Ed.) *Applications of Conditioning Theory*. London: Methuen.

Wood, R.L. and Fussey, I. (1987). Computer based cognitive retraining: a controlled study. *International Disability Studies*, 9, 149–153.

Wood, R.L. and Yurdakul, L.K. (1997). Change in relationship status following traumatic brain-injury. *Brain Injury*, 11, 491–502.

World Health Organization (1980). *International Classification of Impairment Disabilities and Handicaps*. Geneva: World Health Organization.

World Health Organization (1997). *ICIDH-2: International Classification of Impairments, Activities and Participation. A Manual of Dimensions of Disablement and Functioning. Beta-1 Draft for Field Trials*. Geneva: World Health Organization.

Yarnell, P.R. and Rossie, G.V. (1988). Minor whiplash head injury with major debilitation. *Brain Injury*, 2, 255–258.

Ylvisaker, M. and Urbancyk, B. (1994). Assessment and treatment of speech, swallowing and communication disorders following traumatic brain injury. In M.A. Finlayson and S.H. Garner (Eds) *Brain Injury Rehabilitation: Clinical Considerations*. Baltimore, MD: Williams and Wilkins.

Yorkston, K.M., Honsinger, M.J., Mitsuda, P.M. and Hammen, V. (1989). The relationship between speech and swallowing disorders in head-injured patients. *Journal of Head Trauma Rehabilitation*, 4, 1–16.

Young, A. W. and Leafhead, K.M. (1996). Betwixt life and death: Case studies of the Cotard delusion. In P.W. Halligan and J.C. Marshall (Eds) *Methods in Madness*. Hove, East Sussex: Psychology Press.

Youngjohn, J.R. and Altman, I.M. (1989). A performance-based group approach to the treatment of anosognosia and denial. *Rehabilitation Psychology*, 34, 217–222.

Yu, J. (1983). Animal models of recovery with training after central nervous system lesions. *International Rehabilitation Medicine*, 4, 190–194.

Yudofsky, S.C., Silver, J.M., Jackson, W., Endicott, J. and Williams, D. (1986). The overt aggression scale for the objective rating of verbal and physical aggression. *American Journal of Psychiatry*, 143, 35–39.

Yuen, H.K. (1994). Neurofunctional approach to improve self-care skills in adults with brain damage. *Occupational Therapy in Mental Health*, **12**, 31–45.

Yuen, H.K. and Benzing, P. (1996). Guiding behavior through redirection in brain injury rehabilitation. *Brain Injury*, **10**, 229–238.

Zencius, A.H., Wesolowski, M.D., Burke, W.H. and McQuade, P. (1989). Antecedent control in the treatment of brain injured clients. *Brain Injury*, **3**, 199–205.

Zencius, A.H., Wesolowski, M.D. and Rodriguez, I.M. (1998). Improving orientation in head injured adults by repeated practice, multi-sensory input and peer participation. *Brain Injury*, **12**, 53–61.

Zervas, I.M., Augustine, A. and Fricchione, G.L. (1993). Patient delay in cancer. *General Hospital Psychiatry*, **15**, 9–13.

Index

A

A–B–C record **232**
activities of daily living 4, 16, 20, 59, 78, 105, 121, 123
   see also functional skills
acute rehabilitation 1, 4, 14, 16, 25, 54–7, 58, 59, 65, 76, 77, 78, 79, 97, 105, 174, 175, 208, 263, 267, 277
ADL, *see* activities of daily living
affective disorders 23, 37, 42–3, 44, 45, 51, 52, 83
age
   incidence of traumatic brain injury 3, 205, 212, 228, 272
   outcome 3, 31, 212, 228, 254
agitation 31, 38, 40, 47, 48, 51, 56, 62, 72, 73, 82, 165, 215, 218
   assessment of 62, 68, 81, 95
   see also confusion
aggression 43–5, 50–2, 61, 62, 63, 64
agitated behaviour scale 88
alcohol 6, 21, 37, 48, 123
   and outcome from traumatic brain injury 3, 75, 221
amnesia 196
   anteriograde 114
   memory 114, 196
   retraining 119, 128, 275
   retrograde 114, 117
   see also memory, post-traumatic amnesia
amotivation 41–2
   see also motivation
antecedent control 21, 64, 86, 92, 95, 101–2, 234
   and confusion 275
   behaviour disorder 21, 87, 88, 93, 101, 234
   functional skills 87
   recording 21, 92, 99, 130, 232
anticonvulsants 42, 19, 51
apathy 41–2, 47, 50, 64
apolipoprotein E4: 4
apraxia 173–4
   see also speech

assessment
   baselining 87, 99
   early 55, 167, 168–9
   ecological 100, 276
   functional/behaviour 99
   neuropsychological 5, 6, 30, 60
   observation 66
   standardized 87–8, 100, 177, 178
   see also Overt Aggression Scale, recordings
attention 6, 18, 36, 67, 71, 98, 104, 108, 110–4, 115, 121, 122, 123, 124, 126, 132, 146, 147, 198, 199–201, 202, 203, 204, 205, 208, 213, 216, 219, 273
   assessment 110–11
   automatic processing 108, 110
   control processing 104, 107, 108, 122
   models of 204
   needs for 69, 71, 86, 88, 92, 93, 235–6
   retraining 113–14
   treatment 111–13
attentional
   deficit 23, 69, 111–14, 115, 127, 170, 207, 208, 216
   processing 60
   see also attention

B

Barry Rehabilitation Inpatient Screening of Cognition (BRISC) 60, 61, 62
behaviour
   assessment 21
   compensation 11–12
   cognition and 22, 24, 38, 273
   disorders 21, 23, 24, 62–4, 65, 66, 67, 81–4, 85, 86, 87, 88, 91, 95, 96, 102, 103, 153, 154, 155, 183, 233, 274
   see also negative behaviour disorder, positive behaviour disorder
   management 57–8, 66–7, 68, 69, 85–8, 232–9
   vs modification 66–7

timing of intervention and 57, 58, 66
   treatment of 54–79, 102–6
behavioural
   momentum 94–5, 103
   syndromes 41–6
biasing cognitive set 102
brain injury
   assessing 2
   causes of 29–30
   educational attainment, effect on 212
   imaging 11
   see also magnetic resonance imaging
   mechanisms 1, 8, 9, 29–30
   medical considerations
   mild 5–6, 28
      see also post-concussion syndrome
   prevalence of 262
   repeated, effects of 6, 32
   risk factors
   severity of 2, 15, 28, 212
   social consequences of 7–8
   theories of recovery 18–20
   types of 29–30, 59–61

C

case management 227, 248, 256, 259, 263, 278
chaining 63, 78, 119, 236
   backward 106
   forward 106
   whole task method 106
checklists 99, 119, 121, 263
cognitive behaviour therapy 209, 275, 276
   deficits 146–7, 213
cognitive retraining 16–18, 175, 180, 276
collateral sprouting 10
coma 47, 48, 49, 50, 51, 52, 55, 58, 61, 165, 166, 246
   assessment 4, 34, 68, 70, 72, 73, 77, 167–9, 170, 171, 172, 173, 174, 175, 176, 177, 178
   duration and recovery 29, 165, 166–7, 170
      see also recovery
   stimulation 54, 97, 134
   treatment 178

Community Integration
  Questionnaire (CIQ) 5
community
  intervention 263
  reintegration 264–69
  skills 5, 97, 126–30, 134
compensatory strategies 98,
  136, 138
computerized tomography
  (CT) 6, 33, 35
computers, use in
  rehabilitation 17
conditioning 21, 22, 78
  classical 66, 84, 187
  operant 81, 84, 92, 106
  see also learning theory
confabulation 45, 195–7, 205
confusion 31, 35, 43, 62, 70,
  101, 102, 119, 168, 192,
  199, 201, 205, 230, 264,
  275
  see also agitation
continence 123–4, 134
cooking skills, retraining in
  128, 129, 227
coping strategies 192–3
cost management 80
  see also funding
counselling 248–50
cues 12, 21, 46, 94, 99, 106,
  107, 109, 110, 123, 125,
  126, 127, 130, 131, 144,
  145, 146, 147, 150, 151,
  179, 183, 196, 236

D

data collection 65–6
  see also recording
debriefing 110
delusions 197–8
dementia 32
denervation supersensitivity
  9–10
denial 184–5, 186, 187, 188,
  190–1, 193–8, 199,
  206–8, 210, 246–7, 248
  see also lack of insight
depression 13, 37, 42–43,
  49–50, 83, 190–1
diaries 119, 120–121
diaschisis 9
differential reinforcement
  procedures 89, 106
disability rating scale 4, 5, 88,
  168
discharge planning 76, 243,
  256

dissociative disorder 83
distraction 104, 105
distrubance of mood 42–3
dressing retraining 20, 78, 105,
  106, 109, 125–6, 278
driving 104, 116, 127–8, 272
  see also mobility
dysarthria 173–4
  see also speech
dysphagia management 173
  see also speech
dysphonia 173–4
  see also speech

E

eating 41, 105, 125, 172, 173,
  202, 227, 236, 240
employment 6, 8
  supported 223
  see also work
encephalitis 29, 45, 50, 124,
  125
environment 2, 20, 38, 39, 51,
  56–7, 64–8, 79, 86, 89,
  90–3, 96, 101, 105, 109,
  121, 122, 127, 130, 139,
  140, 145, 149, 151, 165,
  169, 170, 171, 172,
  178–179, 181, 183, 190,
  191–2, 193, 204, 234,
  240, 263, 275–6, 277, 279
epilepsy 23, 31, 32, 33, 35,
  36
episodic dyscontrol 23, 82, 85
equipotentiality 10
errorless learning 95, 149
  and compliance 95, 103
  behaviour training 95, 123,
  275
  skills training 95, 123, 275
extinction 24, 78, 85, 87, 89,
  91–2, 95

F

fading 107
family 7, 8, 27, 55, 88,
  239–40, 241–50
  economic effects on 245
  effect of brain injury on
  relationships 7, 8, 21,
  114, 170, 184, 218, 261,
  263, 264
  involvement 77
  long-term care and 259–61
  needs at acute stage 241–6,
  251, 252, 253, 258, 259
  profiles 251–7

relationships with staff 8,
  38, 41, 69, 74, 75, 76, 77,
  165, 173, 175, 187, 206,
  231, 233, 239–40, 257–8,
  270, 271
  stress levels 7, 26, 76, 81,
  273, 274
  types of response 25, 32,
  39, 40, 47, 48, 63, 77, 78,
  167, 173, 187, 239–40,
  268
feedback 17, 108, 110, 111,
  112, 148, 150–2, 179,
  199, 207, 208, 224,
  278–9
feeding 125
functional analysis 234
Functional Assessment
  Measure (FAM) 5
functional behavioural-
  learning approach 21–5
Functional Independence
  Measure (FIM) 4, 5, 278
functional skills 121–4
  see also activities of daily
  living
funding 262

G

Galveston Orientation and
  Amnesia Test (GOAT) 60,
  61, 117
gastrosomy feeding 34
generalization 16, 20, 55, 76,
  77, 78, 79, 99, 103, 113,
  114, 151, 159, 188
genetic factors and role in
  brain injury 4
Glasgow Assessment Schedule
  (GAS) 4
Glasgow Coma Scale (GCS) 2,
  3, 4, 5, 15, 28, 48, 50,
  52, 53, 166, 167, 168,
  201, 212, 216
Glasgow Outcome Scale
  (GOS) 4, 15
goal
  achievement 103
  setting 109, 152, 279
grief 32
group treatment 180

H

hearing 174–5
heterotopic ossification 56,
  57, 138, 142, 155
  and behaviour 19, 57

highlighting 108
hospital, length of stay 15
hyperbaric oxygen 34

I

incontinence 35, 36, 123–4, 161, 186, 194
inconvenience training 275
initiation 20, 39, 48, 51, 52, 62, 63, 69, 92, 139–40, 166, 172
implicit guidance 102
insight 37, 59, 76, 99, 128, 169, 180, 181, 183, 213–4, 244, 246, 261, 263, 272, 277
  psychological model *204*
  see also lack of insight
intervention, timing of 57, *58*

J

job coaches 223–4

K

kitchen skills, *see* cooking
knowledge
  category specific 116
  explicit 116
  implicit 116, 187
  of performance 148, 149
  of results 17, 110, 113, 148, 149, 150, 152

L

lack of insight 7, 37, 109, 134, 184–210, 276
  factors associated with **205**
  forms of **202**
  schematic presentation of theory *199*
language 12, 38, 55, 59–60, 61, 131, 158, 164–5, 166, 170, 171–83, 188, 272, 273
  assessment 31, 35, 219
  expressive 78, 171, 166, 176, 182
  receptive 166, 167, 171, 176, 182
  see also speech
learner illusion 273
learning 11–12, 18, 20, 21–5, 39, 60, 64, 67–9, 71, 78, 81–5, 88–96, 100, 106, 107–9, 112, 116, 163, 181, 187, 192, 199, 234, 237–8, 239, 273–6

deficit 60
discriminant 237
learning theory 2, 21, 81, 84, 96, 112
  methods of 22, 91
  motor learning 114, 135–152
leisure time 227–8
life expectancy 32
long-term care 15, 76, 120, 247
  future needs 259–62

M

magnetic resonance imaging (MRI) 33, 35
mania 42, 43, 49, 51, 83
medication 32, 33, 37, 38, 40
  functional skills and
memory 37, 66, 75, 101, 146, 153, 187, 195–201, 203, 245
  assessment of 28, 60, 61, 114, 116–18, 196
  impairment 49, 52, 55, 60, 185, 202, 205, 210, 275
  memory books 99, 100, 119–21, 181, 183
  retraining of 19, 20, 23, 98, 118–21, 153
  types of 114–16
  see also amnesia, orientation
metacognition 17, 108–9, 181, 191
migraine 32–3
milieu 105, 276
minimally responsive patient, evaluation of 141–4, 165
mobility 36–8, 126–8, 139
modelling 237
models of therapy 18–21
motivation 23, 63, 69, 82, 146, 152, 192, 193
motor control
  assessment 141–5
  impairment 136–40
  model 135–40
motor learning 114, 135–52
  assessment 114, 141–4
  factors affecting 146–52
  principles of 145–6
  regulation strength tone 142–3

N

negative behaviour disorder 23–4, 61, 62, 83

neglect 16, 56, 77, 110, 112, 113, 126, 127, 140, 142, 195, 200, 201, 205
network theory 10–11
neural Darwinism 11–12
neural networks 11
neurobehavioural rating scale 277
neurological substitution 11
neuropsychiatric disorders 22, 27, 28, 30–1, 41, 185, 278
neuropsychological disorder 3, 5–6, 22, 23, 27–8, 30–1, 60
  assessment of 60–2
non-participation 64

O

observations, *see* recordings
obsessive–compulsive disorder 23, 37
occupational activities, *see* work
operant conditioning 81, 92, 106
  see also conditioning
oral motor 171–4
organization of patient care 54, 80, 170
orientation 61, 70, 87, 112, 116–7, 119, 120, 127, 170, 171, 172, 204, 221, 231
outcome of patients 2–8, 12–8, 20, 25–6, 28, 32, 38–9, 60, 97, 212, 220, 241–2, 259–60, 274, 276–9
  studies 134
overlearning 20, 94, 98, 100, 107, 237, 275
overstimulation 104
Overt Aggression Scale 88
  neurobehavioural revision 88

P

parallel distributed processing 10
paraphasias 176
patient
  assessment 46–7, 55–6
  see also assessment
  involvement 68–9
perseveration 47, 166, 176

persistent vegetative state 2, 3
personality, risk factor for traumatic brain injury 46, 53, 55, 74–5, 77, 82, 184, 194
change of 7, 24, 77, 193, 244, 245, 246, 251, 252, 255, 261
pharmacological intervention 8, 22, 39, 46, 47, 48, 49, 50, 51, 52, 53, 63, 82, 83, 240, 274
planning 44, 53, 60, 64, 76, 79, 80, 87, 120, 123, 125, 128, 164, 177, 198, 200, 201, 202, 205, 213, 222, 227, 243, 255, 256, 257, 259–60, 265, 267, 269, 271, 278, 279
community reintegration 267–8, 271
skills 199–202, 205, 213, 222, 227
treatment 53, 60, 64, 79, 80, 87, 164, 243, 278–9
plasticity 9, 11, 12, 272
positive behaviour disorder 23, 24, 61, 62
see also behaviour, negative behaviour disorder
post-acute evaluation 175, **176**
post-concussion syndrome 6
post-traumatic amnesia 3–4, 9, 13, 28, 31, 61, 115, 119, 212, 214, 216, 218, 222, 225, 246
see also memory, amnesia
practice 24, 107–108, 114, 118, 128, 139, 149–50, 154, 183
pre-morbid personality 74–5
priming 122–3, 275
prompts 76, 107–8, 129, 131, 153, 157, 158, 161, 236
see also cues
psychosis 33, 37, 45–6, 52, 75

R
Rancho Los Amigos scales of cognitive functioning 15, 57, 68, **169**, 172
recording information 21, 41, 65, 68, 70, 87, 90, 99, 100, 117, 130, 167, 177, 194, 232

by patient 70, 120–1
forms for 65, 117
memories 114, 120–1
staff response 88
see also assessment
recovery 5–6, 15, 18–19, 25–6, 27–8, 30, 34, 35, 55, 68, 81–2, 97, 108, 115, 117, 119, 120, 125, 139, 146–7, 181, 207, 208, 217, 221, 234, 247, 262, 269, 274, 275, 277
measurement of 4–5, 6, 14, 68
mechanisms of 1, 33
natural history of 31–3, 189, 197, 210, 277
post-acute 97–8, 103, 165–74, 179
rate of 77, 167
stages of 27
theories of 8–12
redundancy of function 10, 12, 33
see also equipotentiality
reduplicative paramnesia 185, 199
rehabilitation
developments in 274–9
effectiveness of 12–16, 28–9
models 16–18
teams 229–30
see also community rehabilitation, recovery, work
reinforcement 22, 23, 24–5, 55, 57, 60, 63, 64, 69, 70, 71, 84–5, 88–96, 106, 108, 124, 132, 154, 155, 156, 160, 161, 162, 190, 199, 234, 235, 237, 238, 278
reserve capacity 6
response cost 72, 73, 74, 92
retraining methods 101
reward 23, 89, 163, 183
see also reinforcement
Rivermead Behavioural Memory Test (RBMT) 118
road safety 126
see also street crossing

S
safety 56–7
self-injurious behaviour 46, 53
self-awareness 188–90, 191–2, 201, 203

sensory loss 59–60
sessional practice 100, 125, 179–80
severity of injury 2, 15, 28, 115, 205, 212, 228
sexual problems 209, 250
dysfunction/dysinhibition 7, 37, 41, 44, 50, 52, 93, 134
family reactions 7, 170, 250, 256, 270
shaping 63, 69, 77, 78, 124, 162, 237
shopping 20, 118, 128, 133, 147, 159, 177, 227
social
isolation 8, 130
retraining 182
skills 108, 130–1, **132**, **133**, 134, 226
assessment 5, 221
deficits 99, 100, 134, 225
training 25, 130, 131–4, 180, 182, 212, 225
worker, role of 219, 246–8, 249, 255–61
speech 15, 34, 35, 43, 47, 48, 60, 111, 125, 130–3, 155, 161, 164, 165, 168, 170–83, 219, 229, 233, 247, 259, 278
staff
characteristics 8, 28, 34, 46, 54, 56, 57, 64, 67, 68, 79, 85, 103, 104, 120, 124, 165, 178, 179, 209, 223, 224, 230–1, 242, 271
stress 26, 96, 104, 105
training 77, 78, 79, 86–7, 88, 89, 96, 100, 173, 178, 179, 229, 231, 235, 278
use of specific 103
see also family
stimulus control training 93–4, 181, 236, 239, 275
strategies 19, 54, 57, 69, 77, 100, 109, 119, 121, 175, 250, 256, 258, 275
behavioural 77, 174
compensatory 136, 180, 181, 183
cognitive 19
coping 8, 217
external 119, 121, 181
internal 118
intervention 2, 18, 46–7, 111–13, 135, 210
learning 136

strategies (*continued*)
  movement 136–7, 138–9
  problem solving 213
  reinforcement 69
  stress 193
  substitute 11
  see also behaviour
    management,
    reinforcement
street crossing 99, 107, 122,
    236
  see also road safety
stress 192–3
  see also family, staff
structure 64, 105
support groups 8
swallowing disorder 34, 69,
    125, 153, 155, *156*, 157,
    160, 171–2, 173, 239,
    240

T
target
  behaviours 65, 69–70, 87,
    90, 99, 100–1, 232, 238
  setting 234
task analysis 106, 126, 223,
    234, 236, 278
task-specific training 98

teams 27, 29, 79, 178,
    229–31, 242, 246, 258,
    262
test of everyday attention 111
therapeutic environment 64, 96
  activities 102–3
  intervention 5, 13, 19, 23,
    109, 135, 151, 164, 165,
    178, 276
  see also milieu
three-part training approach
    21, 197
time out 25, 63, 71, 72, 73,
    91–2, 94, 157, 235, 258
  see also time-out-on-the-spot
time-out-on-the-spot
    (TOOTS) 24, 71, 92
token systems 24, 58, 68,
    70, 72–3, 88, 90–1,
    92, 183
training programmes
    100–1
transfers 125, 134, 139,
    144–5, 147, *162*, 163
treatment
  environment 178–9, 181
  goals 164–5
  group 180
  history 75–7

individual 179–80
  planning 87, 164
  programme 153–63, 180
therapeutic intervention 5,
    13, 19, 23, 109, 135,
    151, 164, 165, 178, 276
  see also strategies, treatment
triggers 30, 104

V
visual neglect 127, 140

W
walking 105, *161*
  see also mobility
washing 20, 99, 106, 109,
    121, 125–6
work
  assessment 219–220, 228
  factors affecting 211–16
  placements 221–15
  rehabilitation 220–1
  skills 121, 212, 215, 217,
    225
  training of 216, 220–221,
    222, 224

Z
z-deficit scores 3